Essential Paediatrics

Essential
Paediatrics

David Hull
BSc, MB, FRCP, DObst RCOG, DCH
Professor of Child Health, University of Nottingham

Derek I. Johnston
MA, MD, FRCP, DCH
Consultant Paediatrician, University Hospital, Nottingham

ILLUSTRATED BY GEOFFREY LYTH BA

SECOND EDITION

CHURCHILL LIVINGSTONE
EDINBURGH LONDON MELBOURNE AND NEW YORK 1987

CHURCHILL LIVINGSTONE
Medical Division of Longman Group UK Limited

Distributed in the United States of America by
Churchill Livingstone Inc., 1560 Broadway, New York,
N.Y. 10036, and by associated companies, branches and
representatives throughout the world.

First published 1981
    Reprinted 1981
    Reprinted 1982
    Reprinted 1984
    Reprinted 1986
Second edition 1987
    Reprinted 1988
    Reprinted 1990

ISBN 0-443-03295-5

British Library Cataloguing in Publication Data

Hull, David
    Essential paediatrics, —2nd ed.
    1. Children—Diseases
    I. Title   II. Johnston, Derek I.
    618.92   RJ45

Library of Congress Cataloging in Publication Data

Hull, David.
    Essential paediatrics.

    Includes bibliographies and index.
    1. Pediatrics. 2. Children—Diseases. I. Johnston,
Derek I.   II. Title.   [DNLM: 1. Pediatrics.   WS 200 H913e]
RJ45.H873   1987   618.92   86-17580

Produced by Longman Singapore Publishers (Pte) Ltd.
Printed in Singapore

Preface

This book is intended primarily for medical students, to help them master the essentials of paediatrics in the brief time provided for this purpose in their clinical course. It may also serve as a useful introduction to paediatrics for other health professionals.

Attention is mainly directed toward the common conditions. Genetics and heart disorders are considered in more detail than other areas because we believe it is important that they be understood thoroughly from the beginning. Many of the rare disorders are mentioned by name only just to note their existence. Occasionally they are discussed at more length because they are life-threatening or have genetic consequences or simply because they are of interest.

Many people, both known and unknown to us, have written pointing out areas needing adjustment and errors needing correction in the first edition. Reviewers too have highlighted the book's limitations. We are grateful to them all and for this second edition we have altered some sections, introduced others and updated the whole as best we are able, while staying within the original brief that we set ourselves.

No book is an alternative to clinical experience acquired by talking to and examining children and discussing their problems with their parents. It is our hope that, by providing a text which covers most aspects of paediatic practice, readers may feel more able to approach a sick child with confidence and that time spent in paediatric wards and clinics will be remembered with pleasure.

Again the authors are indebted to the contributors, listed on page vii, who offered expert advice regarding the accuracy, relevance and balance of the sections dealing with their respective specialties. We also acknowledge our debt to medical artist Mr Geoffrey Lyth, whose contribution to the text is invaluable, and to Mrs Janet Joy for her advice on the Formulary. Finally, we should like to thank Miss Kath Reed who typed tape recordings and handwritten drafts with unbelievable speed and accuracy.

Nottingham, 1987
D. H.
D. I. J.

Contributors

B. Roger Allen
MB, ChB, FRCP
Consultant Dermatologist, University Hospital, Nottingham.

Peter R. H. Barbor
JP, MB, FRCP
Consultant Paediatrician, University Hospital, Nottingham.

Christopher L. Colton
MB FRCS
Consultant Orthopaedic Surgeon, University Hospital, Nottingham.

David A. Curnock
MA, MB, BCh, MRCP, DCH, DObst, RCOG
Consultant Paediatrician, City Hospital, Nottingham.

John S. Fitzsimmons
MB, FRCP(E), DCH
Consultant in charge of the Clinical Genetic Service, City Hospital, Nottingham.

E. Joan Hiller
BSc, MB BS, FRCP, DObst RCOG
Consultant Paediatrician, City Hospital, Nottingham.

Leela Kapila
MB, BS, FRCS
Consultant Paediatric Surgeon, City and University Hospitals, Nottingham.

Margaret J. Mayell
MB, ChB, FRCS(Ed)
Consultant Paediatric Surgeon, City Hospital, Nottingham.

David H. Mellor
MD, FRCP, DCH
Consultant Paediatric Neurologist,
City and University Hospitals, Nottingham.

Anthony D. Milner
MD, FRCP, DCH
Professor of Paediatric Respiratory Medicine and Honorary Consultant
Paediatrician, University of Nottingham.

Nicholas Rutter
BA, MD, FRCP
Senior Lecturer in Child Health and Honorary Consultant Paediatrician,
University of Nottingham.

Alan R. Watson
BSc, MB, ChB, MRCP
Consultant Paediatric Nephrologist, City Hospital, Nottingham.

Contents

1
The Ill Child and his Doctor

In paediatric practice it is not possible to make a full diagnosis or draw up an appropriate care programme without some knowledge of the child, his age, size, abilities and personality. Furthermore, a child is part of a family; to understand him one must know something of his family, particularly his parents, their life styles, their family life, their capacity to look after their children and in particular their relationships to our patient and attitudes towards his illness. Families live in communities and as the child grows older and becomes more independent he relates more directly to the community, in particular to his school and his peers. Thus, it is helpful to know the main features of that community and the child's and family's relationship to it. The mode of presentation, the symptoms and even the signs of disease may be influenced by the nature of the child, his family and their surroundings and experiences. Likewise, treatment will depend on the reserves and resources of the family and community.

THE INTERVIEW

First impressions are important. Even very young children are quick to sense an atmosphere and the reactions of their parents to it. As they grow older they become expert at masking their feelings. In uncertain situations they are more likely to demonstrate what they think by actions rather than words. They will look to and reach for those they trust. Children, not unlike adults, warm to those who like and admire them, and they are less suspicious than adults of ulterior motives. A relaxed, friendly beginning to the interview not only eases its passage, but is essential for its success.

It is a matter of sensitivity and judgement to know how to make the first introductions. In the U.K. shaking hands is probably right for most parents but not for most children. It is impolite not to know the child's name and what he would like to be called. All Susans do not like to be called 'Suzie'. The sex of the child is not always evident from appearances. Sometimes the dress and hair style may be very misleading and you may wonder why. Even under such circumstances, to call a boy 'she' is a mistake. His mother will not like it and

1

neither will he if he is old enough to understand. Never refer to the baby as 'it'. Next ascertain the names and the relationship to the child of the adults who accompany him. Children belong to their parents, parents are responsible for their children so it is the parents' point of view that, in the first instance, you want to know. Not infrequently parents differ in their interpretation of their child's symptoms and signs. Neither parent has a monopoly on objectivity. Sometimes unaccompanied mothers will say, referring to her husband, that 'he disagrees with me and says I fuss too much', or alternatively that 'he told me to bring the child along because he is not right'. Some grandparents are a tremendous support to their children when they start their own families but others tend to be interfering busybodies. The latter, if they are present at the interview, should be encouraged not to interrupt or enlarge upon the history given by the parents, though their attempts to do so may help in understanding the total situation.

The ability and willingness of children to describe their own symptoms varies widely. If in doubt always ask. It is instructive, for example, to find out why the child thinks he has been brought to see you. The answers are often revealing if not too helpful with the diagnosis. Another very important question, possibly best asked at the end of the interview, is what does the child and what do the parents think is the cause of the child's illness? In particular, what do they fear it might be?

In the main, children are not interested in adult talk so as the interview gets underway the majority of the younger ones will become restless and seek ways of entertaining themselves; but never make the mistake of thinking that they are not listening to what is being said. Toys for every age group should be scattered on the desk, shelves and floor. Play will not only occupy the youngster, it will also give valuable clues to his motor skills, mental abilities, interests and personality. So whilst taking the history watch the child. In particular, watch the way he moves, how he uses his eyes and ears and hands and feet. Does he follow up a challenge? Is he constructive? Is he relaxed? Watch the interplay between the child and his parents, and the child and yourself. It will not only help interpret the history but also give some indication of how best to examine the child later to get the most information. For example, if a four-year-old stays on his mother's knee and demands that the toys be brought to him, he is obviously feeling very

The interview

Suggested types of toys which should be at hand for children of varying ages

threatened or is limited either by his illness or in his abilities. In these circumstances it is probably wisest to make the preliminary examination at least, whilst the child is on his mother's knee. Know something about the toys in the room; for example, at what stage can a child be expected to put a square block in a square hole, or to lift it out to find pictures underneath, or to name what he sees. If he does not do it you have not learnt much — it might be simply because of the situation — but if he does you may have learnt a great deal.

History

Every doctor develops his or her own way of collecting information. It is best to start by noting the main complaint or complaints. If there are a number, then a simple opening problem list helps. Then enlarge and define each problem and enquire about associated problems. An obsessional enquiry about all the bodily functions is not usually necessary, it wastes time and may interrupt the flow of the interview. However for most medical problems, and always for any child admitted to hospital, certain background information is essential.

Firstly, it is important to collect information about the child's own life. Was the pregnancy, labour and birth normal? What was the birth weight? How was he in the first days of life? It may be important to note whether he was breast or bottle fed and when he was weaned. Has he had the common childhood infections? Has he been immunised? Has he been treated in hospital and, if so, when and where and for what?

Secondly, an assessment should be made as to how the child is progressing. Full assessment of motor and language achievement and mental and social responses demands considerable skill and experience. However, for most purposes a simple enquiry about the principal stages of development is all that is required and should be within the competence of anyone presuming to advise parents about the care of their children. Plot on the charts of normal development, what his parents say he can do — and they are usually right — and what he is observed to do in clinic. For the older child, ask about progress at school. It is not acceptable to make a note that the child is slow or retarded without indicating the basis for that conclusion. Indeed, labels of that nature are best avoided altogether. If a child is not speaking at three years of age, write that he has delayed speech, but do not guess at the likely cause, even if, for instance,

Steps in development

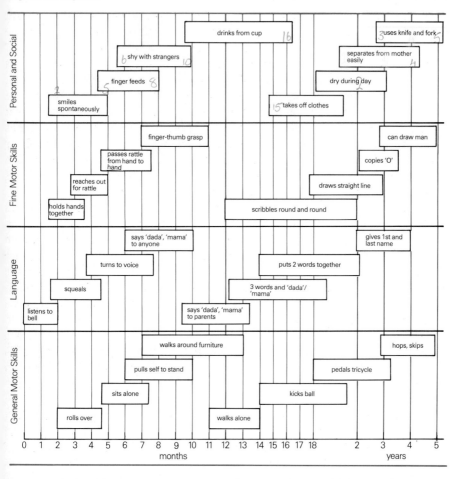

his mother appears not to understand even your simplest questions.

Always ask about the health of the rest of the family. This is important for a variety of reasons. The first, and perhaps the most obvious, is that the child might have an inherited disorder. Collect the information carefully and record it using accepted symbols and notation (see Ch. 2). Secondly, if environmental factors are important, then other members of the family may also be affected. This might include anything from respiratory infections to the inhalation of lead. Thirdly, the presence of chronic illness in other members of the family may be the reason why the parents are concerned about the child before you. It may be that the family's stress has helped precipitate the child's problems. The fourth, though not the most important, is probably the most interesting reason. There are often family complaints, headaches, stomach aches, weariness, which determine the family language of disease and colour the way the child and his parents interpret his symptoms and signs. This will be particularly so if there is a strong behavioural component to his problem.

Examination

Examining children can be fun, but it may involve games when you do not want to play, and occasionally it can be singularly frustrating. Children, even the smallest infants, will try and work out your intentions by looking into your eyes. People with kind eyes do not mean to hurt! The parents may be more nervous about what you might do than the child himself, so they need reassurance as well. Some parents attempt to comfort their child by telling him not to worry 'the doctor won't hurt you'. Up until that time it may not have entered his head that you might, so be prepared for the protests. Some mothers may say such things in an attempt to put you off any examination which might be uncomfortable or embarrassing. Always encourage the parents to help you with the examination by holding or distracting the child, unless, of course, the youngster is approaching puberty when his independence is to be respected.

Clinicians have different practices about clothes. Undressing disturbs babies and they do not like it. Older infants hold onto their clothes as a protection, so they may object to their removal. From three years onwards there is usually no problem until puberty. Then the youngster must be handled with all the care and sensitivity you would extend to royalty! So it can be very useful to make observations whilst the child is clothed and undisturbed. Palpation and auscultation can easily be performed through vest and pants. On the other hand, some babies and children will remain undisturbed and, indeed, may expect you to undress them, and you can learn a great deal by the handling involved. It is a form of palpation which the children understand and further palpation afterwards is usually acceptable. But if the child shows uncertainty ask the parents to undress him. Even the most defensive child is usually happy for you to observe him naked from a distance.

Although the collection of the information may be disorderly, its recording in the notes must not be. In most situations it is important to record aspects of the child's size. Weight and length or height must be measured accurately. In certain situations, skull circumference and very occasionally skin fold thicknesses may also be measured. The data is recorded in the notes and on the appropriate charts.

Note the child's general behaviour and awareness. You may wish to make your own evaluation of the child's capabilities and record them with the parents' reports of his achievements.

Next, observe the child. Much of the information you seek may be obtained by careful observation. In general terms, is his appearance at all unusual? If so, try to define why, is it the shape of his head, the mould of his ears, the position of his eyes, his bodily proportions or the posture? Does he look like his parents? Has he got any of the recognised major or minor anomalies?

Then specifically assess his general size, proportions and nutritional state. Note the nature and distribution of any skin lesions or rashes. Then examine the system or systems that are the source of the complaint.

Respiratory disorders are often most easily observed. Avoid percussion or auscultation until you have noted the respiratory rate and the movement of the diaphragm and chest wall with quiet breathing and the effect of a stronger respiratory effort performed on request in an older child, or with a cry in a baby.

listen to the heart

percuss the lower
and upper border
of liver

Determine whether or not the lung is over-inflated by percussion of the upper edge of the liver.

Interpretation of breath sounds and additional noises can be difficult in the very young. Fine crackling noises on inspiration (crepitations) may be heard on careful auscultation in apparently normal babies. If they are persistent and bilateral in a distressed toddler they usually indicate bronchiolitis or, very rarely, left heart failure. Coarse intermittent noises during both inspiration and expiration (rales) usually signify liquid debris in the larger airways. They may be transmitted from the back of the throat. Harsh and more persistent noises superadded on the breath sounds (rhonchi), indicating a more persistent obstruction, are less frequently heard in children. Continuous noises, hardening and extending the breath sounds (bronchial breathing) may be heard in babies over most of the upper back, and usually are transmitted sounds from the main airway. When the airway is partially obstructed the noise becomes harsher and more vibrant and is called a stridor. This term covers a wide range of sounds, some fine and high pitched, some low and coarse. The character depends on the site, the nature of the obstruction and the narrowness of the aperture. Wheezing is heard when the mid airways are narrowed; always check if it is bilateral.

Examination of the cardiovascular system begins by recording the rate, rhythm, strength and character of the peripheral pulses. Palpate and percuss the anterior chest wall to determine the heart size, the site and nature of the apex beat and to detect the presence, if any, of a thrill. Then listen to the first heart sound, then the second, then the sounds in between and then the murmurs between the heart sounds. For each murmur you will wish to know its timing, character, loudness, site and distribution. Check if it is transmitted into the neck.

Always observe the abdomen before you palpate. Look for swellings and movements. Ask if anywhere is tender, and if you can, watch the child's face and not his abdomen whilst you palpate. After general palpation in the four quadrants, systematically determine the position and size of the liver, spleen, kidneys and bladder. If an organ is enlarged, note its position, size, surface and texture, the character of the edge if it has one, and whether or not it is tender. When examining the back of the chest, look at the spine, particularly the lower end.

Again, examination of the locomotor and nervous systems is more by observation than manipulation. In babies and infants always palpate the anterior fontanelle or head 'soft spot'. It usually closes in the middle of the second year.

Examination

palpate the
anterior fontanelle

examine the ear

Note if it is pulsating: it usually does. You can record the heart rate from it. The fontanelle may be full or flat. Ask yourself the following questions: Can the child see? Can he hear? Does he move his eyes and head well and in all directions? Does he move all limbs, is the movement normal and full? Is the contour and position of each limb normal? Is the power good? When you handle the infant, note the tone on passive movement of the limb. Is there any limitation in the movement at any joint? Are the joints unduly lax and hyperextendable? Again, watch the child's face whilst you move his limbs. Eliciting the reflex responses rarely adds useful information in children but it is as well to keep up the habit for the odd occasion when it does. In the infant the percussing finger can be used as the hammer.

Finally, examine with the light. If necessary, check the eyes and then the ear drums and finally the throat. Never force yourself upon the child. Never force his mouth open against his will: be patient. Ask yourself, is the information you wish to gather as important as all that? Why use a nasty dry stick to depress the tongue when a smooth tea-spoon handle will do just as well, and spoons are meant to go into mouths anyway.

Before you finish, should you bother to record the blood pressure? If disease of the kidney or heart is suspected, the answer is yes.

This completes the general examination. During it you may have included specific observations or examinations, for example, to see if the testes are in the scrotum, femoral pulses are present, the hips in joint, the characteristic of unusual lumps, the presence of the signs of puberty, etcetera.

Once the clinical enquiry is complete the next step is to re-examine the initial list of problems, some may be easily dealt with by appropriate advice, on the other hand new problems may have arisen. Draw up a new list and indicate what steps by way of further enquiry, investigation or treatment you propose to follow, and discuss these with the parents and to the extent that he may understand it, with your patient.

THE PROBLEMS

Every week a practising pediatrician sees a condition, anomaly, or a sign that he has never seen before and in such a situation his actions depend on his basic scientific knowledge. Every month he will treat a condition which is known but rare, then he relies on colleagues who have reported their observations in the medical literature. However, the substance of a doctor's practice is with diseases he has seen before, and his management of these problems will be influenced as much by his own previous experience and by his knowledge of his own patients and their community, as it is by therapies recommended in text books. What are these common problems? Obviously, this will vary from place to place and from community to community, and on whether the doctor works in family practice, child health clinic, or district hospital.

Family practice

If we assume that each family doctor has about 2500 people in his practice — in the U.K. the average is a little less — then with a birth rate running at 12.0 births per 1000 population, there will be 30 births in the practice each year and 450 child patients spread between 0 and 15 years of age. Between 15 and 20 per cent of the family doctor's work is with children. Disorders of the respiratory system are by far the commonest, followed by skin conditions, infectious diseases, gastrointestinal disorders, problems with eyes, ears and teeth. Social and administrative problems form the bulk of the remainder. Only 10 per cent of children's disorders are judged to be serious and in need of specific therapy, though it is likely that medicine will be prescribed in over half the cases.

Only occasionally will an individual family doctor have to care for a child with some of the conditions which are often seen in hospital. Thus, on average, a family doctor will see a child presenting with mental retardation, diabetes or spina bifida every five years or so, a child with Down syndrome every 20 years, cystic fibrosis every 40 years and muscular dystrophy every 480 years!

Hospital service

Children who fall ill suddenly are usually brought directly to the hospital emergency and accident department. Over half of the children admitted to hospital are brought by their parents directly to hospital. Here the conditions commonly seen are home and road accidents, accidental poisoning, acute respiratory illness, fevers, convulsions and acute bowel upsets.

Patients referred to the Paediatric consultancy service usually have less acute conditions. The commoner problems include recurrent respiratory infections,

Paediatric experience in general practice and in hospital

Paediatric services (Sickness service)

Population · Family Practice · Hospital Practice

asthma, failure to thrive, small size, suspected developmental delay, convulsions or suspected convulsions, nocturnal enuresis and constipation. There are usually special clinics for children with chronic illnesses, for example for children with diabetes, leukaemia, neurology, short stature, cystic fibrosis and renal disorders. Children with physical and mental handicaps are assessed in a special developmental assessment unit by a team which includes physiotherapists, occupational therapists, psychologists, teachers, audiometricians as well as doctors from various disciplines.

Child health and school medical service
Many family doctors work in group practices in health centres. Working with them in the primary care team are health visitors. In some centres one doctor in the group, with the health visitors, holds regular child health clinics in order to examine routinely every child and provides a preventive health service. In

Child health services (Health service); a = assessment, s = support, c = care

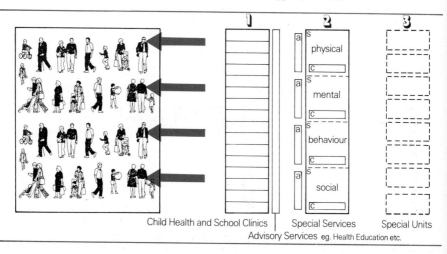

Child Health and School Clinics · Special Services · Special Units
Advisory Services eg. Health Education etc.

others a special clinical medical officer attends the clinic. Healthy babies are examined routinely at six weeks of age and then at regular intervals afterwards. The predominant problems in the early months are related to feeding, nutrition, bowels and general growth and development. Hearing is assessed at 6 to 9 months of age. The infants are examined for vision abnormalities and the development of squints. The clinics also have responsibilities for the immunisation programme and health education. After the age of five years surveillance is continued by the school health services.

The preventive role of the child health clinic

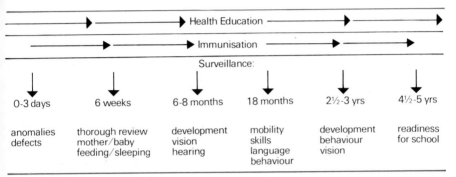

The distribution of health problems differs across the town. Certain inner city areas, deprived by most material and social standards, have a higher incidence of most medical problems and the children who live there are, in general, less physically, mentally and socially able. At a disadvantage from birth, these children 'born to fail', are less able to form secure relationships and thus are themselves less likely to establish a strong family environment for their own children. Breaking this circle of events is one of the major tasks of community paediatric care. It is a challenge that the health service staff share with social workers and teachers.

Problems of people living in the inner city areas in Nottingham, from Social Services Survey, 1983

	Average (%)	Inner City (%)
Single parent family	14	36
Low birth weight < 2500 g	6	11
Children in care or on child abuse register	0.6	2.4
Youth 10–16 years in trouble with police	4	8
Youth 16–19 years unemployed	16	37
Adult 20 years+ unemployed	8	21

MORTALITY

Happily, infant and child mortality rates continue to fall. The rates are highest for the very young. In over 40 per cent of neonatal deaths, the infant has a congenital abnormality incompatible with independent life, and over 40 per cent

Mortality rates

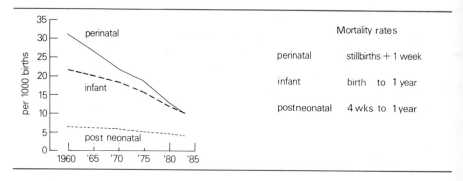

are very immature and even with artificial respiratory and nutritional support do not survive the first few days after birth. Improvements in general health, antenatal care, and appropriate genetic counselling may accelerate the fall in the perinatal mortality rate.

Older infants rarely die in hospital. The majority of children dying between four weeks and one year, post-neonatal infant deaths, die suddenly at home. The 'sudden infant death syndrome' or 'cot death' has received considerable attention recently. There is undoubtedly a small group of infants who die suddenly and nothing abnormal is found at post mortem. Some consider that death might be due to a confusion in respiratory control precipitated by a respiratory infection or unexpected regurgitation. However, many of the infants who die unexpectedly do have evidence of known disease, or non-specific signs of illness at autopsy. The incidence is higher in families living in poor housing, when the parents are inexperienced or of limited ability, or when there is domestic stress. Early infant death occurs more often in babies born prematurely or experiencing problems in the newborn period. These characteristics can be identified at birth and if the families are given extra advice and support during the early months the number of post-neonatal infant deaths can be reduced.

An unexpected death of a child over the age of one year is rare. Many are due

Postneonatal infant deaths

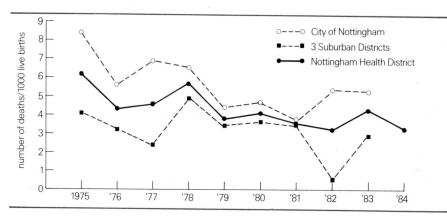

Major causes of death in childhood

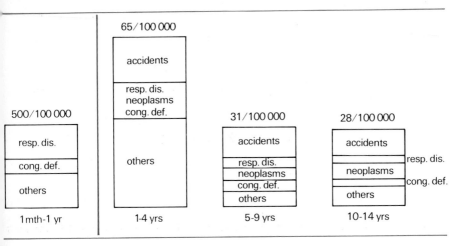

to accidents; others are due to previously diagnosed malignancies. The remainder include children with inherited diseases, for example, cystic fibrosis, muscular dystrophies, and progressive encephalopathies. Acute infections, which used to be a major cause of death, are usually controllable; but occasionally the onset can be so sudden and death follows so quickly that therapeutic measure cannot be introduced in time, for example in meningitis with septicaemia or an intravascular coagulopathy, severe gastroenteritis, acute epiglottitis and fulminating respiratory infections.

BIBLIOGRAPHY

Fit for the future. the report of the Committee on Child Health Services. Chairman Court S D M. 1876 H.M.S.O. London. Cmnd. 6684
Hicks D 1976 Primary health care — a review. H.M.S.O., London
Polnay L, Hull D Eds 1985 Community Paediatrics. Churchill Livingstone
The country deprived area study 1983 Nottinghamshire County Council

2

Genes

i generation

ii generation

iii generation

Pedigree: congenital cataracts

The differences between people result from the interaction between their genetic inheritance, or genotype, and the environment in which they develop and live. Most of us are fortunate and the eventual product of this interaction, our phenotype, is normal. Others, as a result of faulty gene action with or without a hostile environment, may be subject to various types of disease. This effect may be obvious at birth as a congenital abnormality or it may become evident only later in life as a consequence of growth or environmental factors. Since about 1 in 40 pregnancies results in the birth of a child with a serious congenital abnormality and about 30% of children admitted to paediatric wards have a significant inherited disease, some knowledge of genetics is essential for those working with children. In many patients, it may be difficult to decide the importance of genetic or environmental factors and it is <u>important, therefore, in all patients, to take a detailed family history</u>. In those patients suffering from a disorder thought to be the result of abnormal gene action a comprehensive <u>family pedigree</u> is essential. The pedigree may be of considerable help with the diagnosis and without them affected families cannot be offered sensible advice for the future.

Diseases in man thought to be genetic in origin may be divided into those

Pedigree notation

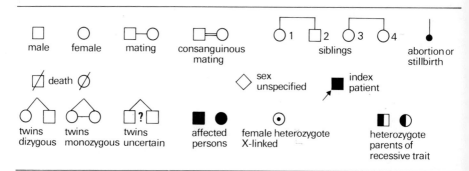

resulting from the action of single major genes, those due to chromosomal abnormalities and those in which there is evidence of a genetic component acting in conjunction with environmental factors.

SINGLE GENE INHERITANCE

The mode of single gene inheritance may be autosomal or sex-linked, dominant or recessive.

Autosomal dominant inheritance

Over 1000 diseases are known to result from this mode of inheritance. Although individually rare and responsible for less than 1 per cent of total human illness, they may nevertheless present very striking clinical features.

In this form of inheritance the abnormal gene responsible for the disease is carried on one of a pair of autosomes, and the heterozygote manifests the condition. In most instances the specific chromosome involved is not known but both sexes are affected. As each parent contributes only one of the two genes to the gamete, each offspring has a 1 in 2 chance of inheriting the abnormal gene and hence manifesting the disease. The risk remains the same for each successive pregnancy, irrespective of the outcome of the preceding one. This all sounds very obvious, but when parents have had two affected children they do feel that the next should be normal or at least the risk should be better than 50:50. Unfortunately, it is not.

As in many other forms of disease, irrespective of the cause, the severity of the condition may vary considerably from one individual to another. This variation is referred to as expressivity and points to the importance of examining patients thoroughly before declaring them free of the disease. Some of those affected may have only minor manifestations but, by passing on the responsible gene, may have a child with much more serious problems. This is very well illustrated by a family with tuberous sclerosis. The features of this disease are mental retardation, a characteristic facial rash and epilepsy. In the family illustrated below, the mother has epilepsy and the facial rash but she was able to attend a secondary modern school where she managed, albeit with some difficulty. Early in life her daughter developed a particular form of epilepsy called infantile spasms, and she was left severely mentally retarded. She has not yet,

Dominant inheritance

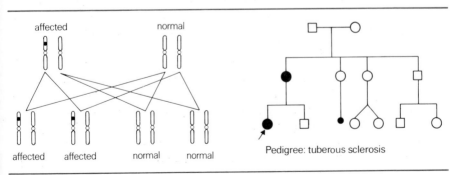

affected   normal

affected   affected   normal   normal

Pedigree: tuberous sclerosis

Dominantly inherited conditions

achondroplasia	Marfan syndrome	retinoblastoma
Apert syndrome	myotonic dystrophy	Treacher-Collins syndrome
brachydactyly	neurofibromatosis	tuberous sclerosis
ectodermal dysplasia	Noonan syndrome	Ullrich-Noonan syndrome
Ehlers-Danlos syndrome	peroneal muscular atrophy	von Willebrand syndrome
Holt-Oram syndrome	polycystic kidneys (Adult)	Waardenburg syndrome

but may later, develop the characteristic facial rash. When these parents were informed of the genetic implications of the condition, they decided not to have further children.

This particular form of mental retardation, as with other types of dominantly inherited disease, may occur in the offspring of normal parents. When this happens the abnormal gene is not found in either parent but arises as a mutation in the gametes, either in the ova or sperm. The risk of another mutation in future pregnancies is very low but the affected child will have the same risk of passing on the abnormal gene as any other affected person. In achondroplasia, a skeletal abnormality producing dwarfism, as many as 80% have normal parents, and are the result of a new mutation. Paternal age at the time of conception appears to be a significant factor in the mutation rate in achondroplasia as in many other inherited disorders and the older the father the greater the risk. It occasionally happens that a gene disorder present in one generation fails to appear in the next but reappears in subsequent generations. In these circumstances the gene is said to lack penetrance. Such a skip-generation is not a common occurrence and apparent cases of it may well only illustrate our inability to detect minor expressions of the abnormal gene.

The concept of dominance and recessiveness is useful but it is as well to remember that genes cannot work in isolation and their actions may be modified by many factors, including other genes.

Autosomal recessive inheritance
There are approximately 700 diseases known to be transmitted by the autosomal recessive mode. Whereas autosomal dominant diseases tend to produce gross structural defects and clinically obvious abnormalities, recessively inherited disorders commonly result in biochemical disturbances. Although in some the defect may be of a single enzyme, the clinical effects may be widespread and very serious. In phenylketonuria, for example, the end result of such a deficiency may be severe mental retardation, whilst in congenital adrenal hyperplasia it may cause a life-threatening electrolyte disturbance.

In recessive inheritance neither parent shows any signs of the disease but the risk of their offspring being affected is 1 in 4. There is a 1 in 2 chance of a child being a carrier like the parent and only a 1 in 4 chance that their offspring will be normal both phenotypically and genotypically. Those with the disease do not usually have affected children and the asymptomatic carriers will only have become aware of their carrier status with the birth of an affected child.

Many of us carry abnormal genes but fortunately our spouse, although also

Recessive inheritance

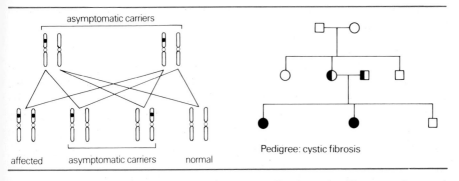

asymptomatic carriers

affected   asymptomatic carriers   normal

Pedigree: cystic fibrosis

carrying some abnormal genes, usually carries different ones. However the possibility of the spouse carrying the same abnormal gene is considerably increased in first cousin marriages. First cousins share one eighth of their total genetic complement, their genome, with each other and thus the opportunity for similar recessive genes to come together and hence produce disease is increased. As the resulting biochemical deficiency may well cause mental retardation it is not surprising that there is concern about first cousin marriages.

As with dominantly inherited disease, the action of the gene is not an all or none phenomenon and in recessive disease the heterozygote may well manifest some biochemical evidence of the condition. This is illustrated by Tay-Sach's disease. This disorder is seen most fequently in the Ashkenazi Jewish population on the North-Eastern American seaboard. It causes mental retardation, blindness and a variety of neurological abnormalities, all the result of the deficiency of the enzyme hexosaminidase-A. Minor deficiencies of this enzyme can be detected in heterozygotes, but they remain clinically unaffected. As individual carriers can be detected it is possible to screen large populations at special risk. Such a screening programme has had considerable success in American Ashkenazi Jews in selected areas.

The gene loci responsible for most recessive disease have not been assigned to specific chromosomes. One exception however is the gene responsible for a particular type of congenital adrenal hyperplasia, the variety associated with 21-hydroxylase deficiency. It has recently been demonstrated that this gene lies close to the gene loci for the important histocompatibility antigens comprising the HLA system. These gene loci are known to be on chromosome No. 6 and

Recessively inherited conditions

congenital adrenal hyperplasia	galactosaemia	porphyria
agammaglobulinaemia	glycogen storage disease	retinitis pigmentosa
albinism	homocystinuria	sickle cell disease
cystic fibrosis	Laurence-Moon-Biedl syndrome	Tay-Sach disease
deafness (some types)	lipodoses	thalassaemia
epidermolysis bullosa	mucopolysaccharidoses	Werdnig-Hoffman disease

although this association does not help in the management of the disease, it may offer an opportunity for prenatal diagnosis when techniques for identification of specific genes become available.

Sex-linked disorders

There are 100 or so sex-linked diseases described to date. They include several common and serious childhood problems. So far, no serious disability has been reported due to genes carried on the Y chromosome and sex-linked normally means X-linked. In addition, although dominantly inherited sex-linked disorders do occur, for example a variety of vitamin D resistant rickets is transmitted in this fashion, they are rare and the common sex-linked diseases are recessively inherited. Because the gene for colour blindness is carried on the X chromosome, mapping of the gene loci on this chromosome is further advanced than on most others.

In these disorders the abnormal gene is carried on the X chromosome. In the female, the presence of the normal allele on her other X chromosome protects from the disease but she is a carrier. In the male, however, the abnormal gene on his X chromosome is not balanced by a normal allele and he manifests the disease. Any son born to a carrier female will have a 1 in 2 chance of having the condition. Equally any daughter has a 1 in 2 chance of being a carrier, like mother. Because it is the X chromosome which carries the abnormal gene an affected male can never transfer the disease to his sons but all his daughters will be carriers.

Sex-linked recessive inheritance

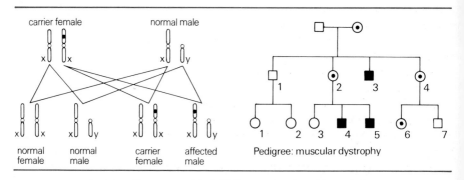

Pedigree: muscular dystrophy

The illustrated pedigree is of a family in which several children are affected by Duchenne muscular dystrophy. In generation II, a male child (II.3) developed evidence of the disease by the age of four years and subsequently died from the condition at the age of 16 years. Unfortunately, unaware of the genetic implications of her brother's disease, his sister already having one daughter, had another child, a boy, and before his disease became obvious she had a second affected son. Both developed clinical evidence of the disease before starting school and both will probably die before the age of 20. Her sister was more fortunate and despite the fact that she was subsequently shown to be a carrier, she already had a son who was unaffected and a daughter who in turn was shown to be a carrier.

Sex-linked inherited conditions

albinism	glucose-6-phosphate dehydrogenase deficiency
Becker muscular dystrophy	haemophilia
Christmas disease	kinky hair syndrome
diabetes insipidus	pseudohypertrophic muscular dystrophy
ectodermal dysplasia	red-green colour blindness
fragile X mental retardation	X-linked agammaglobulinaemia

Duchenne muscular Dystrophy

X-linked recessive mental retardation

Some males and females with mental retardation have an abnormality of the X chromosome referred to as a fragile site and localised to the distal part of the long arm of the X chromosome. It produces the appearance of a constriction and it is most easily demonstrated when the chromosomes are cultured in a medium deficient in folic acid. Many males with this abnormality have an associated enlargement of the testes but the cause of this is unknown. This type of mental retardation is second only in frequency to Down syndrome and occurs in 1 in 2000 males. It is possible to demonstrate the fragile X chromosome in either fetal blood or fetal fibroblasts and the condition can be diagnosed prenatally.

CHROMOSOMAL ABNORMALITIES

Whereas genes, a specific sequence of nucleotide bases, cannot be visualised, it is possible to detect alterations in both the number and the structure of chromosomes by direct examination of cells during cell division. Peripheral blood lymphocytes are the cells usually studied. Mitotic division is stimulated by agents such as phytohaemaglutinin and then the chromosomes are fixed, stained, identified and arranged in matching pairs, the karyotype.

Normal male karyotype; female XX in box

Chromosomes consist of two halves, the chromatids, joined at a point called the centromere. With special stains the chromosomes can be shown to have heterochromic bands alternating with lighter non-staining areas. For very accurate identification these light and dark areas are assigned special numbers so that it is possible to detect loss or deletion of even a small portion of a chromosome.

Chromosomes contain many hundreds of genes and loss of any of these may have serious consequences. For reasons which are less clear, additional genetic material in the form of an extra chromosome may have just as serious an effect.

There are 46 chromosomes in the nucleus of each body cell, of these 22 are matching pairs with matching genes and are called autosomes. The remaining pair, the sex chromosomes, are alike in the female and labelled XX but in the male there is only one X and a smaller chromosome, Y. In the gamete, ovum or sperm, there are only 23 chromosomes, half the somatic cell number, and this ensures that at fertilisation the normal human chromosomal complement is reconstituted.

Somatic cells grow by the process of mitosis, each daughter cell having the same chromosomal complement as the parent cell. This is made possible by each chromosome splitting longitudinally into two. Gametes are the result of a different process called meiosis in which, as a result of two nuclear divisions, the total number of chromosomes is halved. By this means the germ cells contain only one of each pair of chromosomes and hence only one of each equivalent pairs of genes. This reduction division is an essential factor in the inheritance of diseases resulting from abnormalities of genes. Meiosis also affords the opportunity for exchange of genetic material between homozygous chromosomes and hence forms the basis of the wide variation of human characteristics.

Diseases associated with chromosomal abnormalities may result from changes in the number of either the autosomes or sex chromosomes, aneuploidy; or from alterations in chromosomal structure, for example loss or deletion of a portion of a chromosome; or interchange of chromosomal material from one chromosome to another, translocation.

Down syndrome, trisomy 21

The illustrated karyotype is from a female infant with Down syndrome, one of the common causes of mental retardation. There is an extra chromosome in the No 21 group or Group G. This is referred to as trisomy 21. Theoretically it is possible to have trisomy of any of the autosomes but for some, as yet unknown reason, trisomy 21 is by far the commonest. In normal circumstances, during meiosis there is equal distribution of single chromosomes to each daughter cell. In trisomies where there is an extra chromosome, normal separation fails to occur, one pair of chromosomes remain together and the result is one gamete with two homologous chromosomes and another gamete devoid of these chromosomes. At fertilisation the union of a normal gamete carrying one chromosome and the abnormal gamete containing two of the same chromosome produces trisomy for that particular chromosome. This unequal distribution of chromosomes is referred to as non-disjunction.

The incidence of Down syndrome as with some other trisomic anomalies increases with maternal age. It is possible that as the female ages, her ovaries are increasingly subject to environmental hazards. However, mothers of any age can have infants with Down syndrome and, as few women over the age of 40 years have babies, the majority of affected infants are born to younger women and non-disjunction is the usual cause. However, not all infants with trisomy 21 are a consequence of non-disjunction. About 6 per cent are associated with chromosomal re-arrangements, so-called translocations, and approximately 2 per cent with mosaicism.

Non-disjunction 92%.
Translocations . 6%.
Mosaicism 2%.

Incidence of trisomy 21 according to maternal age

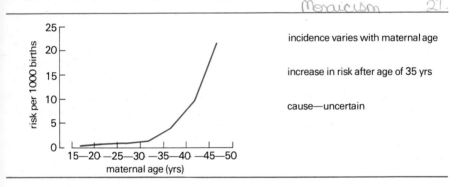

In mosaicism some of the body cells have a normal complement of chromosomes, 46, others have 47 chromosomes, the extra one being an additional No. 21. This abnormality may be a result of mitotic non-disjunction after formation of the zygote. Babies with Down syndrome due to mosaicism usually do not differ from those with the full trisomy 21 abnormality, but some may be less obviously unusual either in their physical appearance or intellectual ability. It might be expected that the higher the proportion of trisomic cells the greater the degree of abnormality. However, such an obvious linear relationship is not always apparent either in the mosaicism of Down syndrome or other conditions. It may be that the proportion of abnormal cells gradually alters during the child's growth.

Clinical features. The diagnosis of Down syndrome is usually suspected soon after birth. In the majority a confident diagnosis can be made on clinical criteria alone but occasionally the diagnosis may not be suspected for weeks, or in some cases, months after birth. Chromosome studies are important to help in the diagnosis when there is doubt, and to identify the rarer chromosomal anomalies even when the diagnosis is certain. As in other chromosomal anomalies, abnormalities of the dermal ridge patterns may occur and in association with other

Trisomy 21. Clinical features

How did it Happen?
Will it happen again? ?
Will it be as bad.
Are there Any Tests

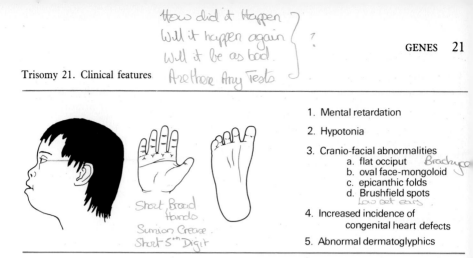

Short Broad Hands
Simian Crease.
Short 5ᵗʰ Digit

1. Mental retardation
2. Hypotonia
3. Cranio-facial abnormalities
   a. flat occiput *Brachy...*
   b. oval face-mongoloid
   c. epicanthic folds
   d. Brushfield spots
   Low set ears
4. Increased incidence of congenital heart defects
5. Abnormal dermatoglyphics

features may suggest the need for chromosomal analysis in some dysmorphic infants. Once the diagnosis is firm it is important to discuss the implications thoroughly with both parents. Medical opinion varies as to whether this is best done in the first few days after birth or sometime later when parental attachment is stronger. Making the diagnosis is usually the easiest aspect of the problem; helping the parents to accept the child and make the most of his disabilities may be more difficult.

A number of societies are very helpful. They provide a forum for parents to discuss their problem with others who have had similar experience. The parents will ask many questions, in particular why did it happen to their child, and will it happen again? If mother is under 36 the risk of a further child being affected is not high and certainly not greater than 1/100. However, despite this low risk, many couples are sufficiently concerned to request diagnostic amniocentesis in future pregnancies. This is usually performed between the 14th and 16th week of pregnancy and involves taking a sample of amniotic fluid containing fetal cells, which are cultured in vitro and the chromosomal complement analysed. The procedure is technically easy; but the delay between the performance of the amniocentesis and the completion of the cytology examination is very upsetting for some parents. In some situations chorionic villus biopsy at 8–10 weeks of pregnancy may be offered. Happily in the majority the findings are normal and the parents can be reassured. In those families where the child has a translocation however, the risks of recurrence are very much greater.

Trisomy 18. Edward syndrome

1. Mental retardation

2. Cranio-facial anomalies
   a. micrognathia
   b. prominent occiput
   c. low-set, faun-like ears

3. Abnormalities of limbs

4. Cardiac and other abnormalities

5. Abnormal dermatoglyphics

The other trisomies

Trisomy of some of the other chromosmes have been described but they are rare. In most cases the patients suffer from a combination of physical abnormalities and mental retardation. Despite their rarity, new syndromes resulting from chromosomal abnormalities are regularly described, and it is important to examine the karyotype of any baby with an unexplained cluster of congenital abnormalities, particularly any infant who has an odd facial appearance and developmental delay.

Sex chromosome anomalies

Survival without one of a matching pair of autosomes does not appear to occur. However it is possible to lose one X chromosome and survive. This is referred to as monosomy and is usually written XO.

Turner syndrome (XO). The diagnosis can be confirmed by chromosomal analysis but additional information may be obtained by examining the buccal mucosal cells for the presence of the Barr body. This chromatin mass, almost certainly an inactivated X chromosome, is seen in a higher percentage of cells in the female than in the male, females are normally reported as chromatin positive and males as chromatin negative. In Turner syndrome, with only one X chromosome, girls are chromatin negative. When there is an extra X chromosome, for example in an XXX female, there are two Barr bodies to be seen in the buccal cells. The XO constitution is common in abortuses but due to a high fetal loss rate the incidence of Turner syndrome is only about 1 in 2500 live births.

Turner syndrome (XO), Clinical features

Short stature

Cranio-facial abnormalities
  a. webbing of neck
  b. down-turned mouth
  c. micrognathia
  d. downward slanting palprebral fissures

Abnormalities of limbs and trunk
  a. lymphoedema
  b. cubitus valgus
  c. widely-separated nipples   *Shield Chest.*

Ovarian dysgenesis with infertility *(Streak ovaries)*

Increased incidence of heart defects
  — Coarctation of Ao.

Klinefelter syndrome (XXY). Although the Y chromosome is small, it does carry the coded information for maleness and even though there is an extra X chromosome in this syndrome the patients are male in appearance. It occurs in 1 in every 1000 males births and often passes undetected. The men are usually tall and thin, and have infertility and hypogonadism.

They contrast with those males with an XYY chromosomal constitution. Individuals with an extra Y chromosome are thought to be more common in prison communities and to have an increased tendency to psychiatric illness. *False!*

Klinefelter syndrome (XXY). Clinical features

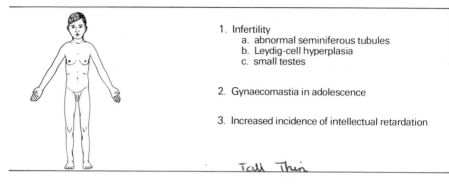

1. Infertility
   a. abnormal seminiferous tubules
   b. Leydig-cell hyperplasia
   c. small testes

2. Gynaecomastia in adolescence

3. Increased incidence of intellectual retardation

Tall Thin

Structural changes in chromosomes

Sometimes a portion of one chromosome is transposed or translocated onto another chromosome. If during this process of translocation no important genetic information is lost, then there may be no obvious clinical effects of the rearrangement and the translocation is said to be balanced. However, the possessor of this abnormality, particularly if it is the mother, is very prone to produce offspring with an unbalanced translocation with resultant serious congenital abnormalities. This type of structural rearrangement between chromosomes is responsible for about 6% of all children with Down syndrome and commonly involves chromosomes in Groups D and G. It is possible for it to arise *de novo* in the infant but more commonly it results from a parental balanced translocation. If the latter is the case the risk of Down syndrome in further children is high, around 1 in 8 if the mother carries the translocation and 1 in 20 if the father is the carrier. It is important to study all the siblings and the chromosomal make-up of the relatives of the carrier parent, if the risk of their producing abnormal infants is to be recognised and reduced.

⊙ balanced carrier 13/21

⊕ unbalanced
translocation 13/21
(Down syndrome)

Translocations may be found in other conditions, for example in about 10 per cent of women who have frequent miscarriages or failed pregnancies. Should such a person have a successful pregnancy there is a real risk that her child will have an unbalanced translocation and be abnormal.

Down syndrome 13/21 translocation karyotype

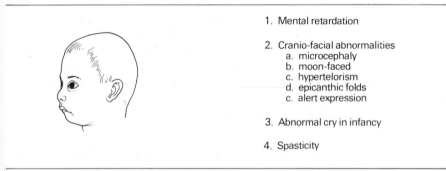

13/21

21

It has been suggested that chromosomal abnormalities occur in 0.5% of all newborn. This figure may be an under-estimate. In a recent report 7% of infants dead at birth or dying in the first year of life were found to have a chromosomal anomaly. A chromosomal anomaly is found in about 25 to 30% of early abortions.

Deletions

Loss of a portion of a chromosome may result in a clinical syndrome often characterised by mental retardation in association with multiple physical abnormalities. The deletion may involve the terminal portion of a chromosome or, more frequently, may be interstitial when the chromosome reunites following two breaks. The Cri-du-chat syndrome due to deletion of part of the short arm of Chromosome 5 is the most common of the deletion syndromes seen in man.

Cri-du-chat (deletion short arm, chromosome 5)

1. Mental retardation

2. Cranio-facial abnormalities
   a. microcephaly
   b. moon-faced
   c. hypertelorism
   d. epicanthic folds
   c. alert expression

3. Abnormal cry in infancy

4. Spasticity

POLYGENIC OR MULTIFACTORIAL INHERITANCE

The inherited diseases discussed so far have resulted from either a fault in a single gene or an alteration in chromosomal structure or number. There are, however, many commoner disorders in which there is a genetic component but the inheritance pattern cannot be explained simply in terms of dominant or recessive traits or chromosomal rearrangement. In these it appears that it is the cumulative action of a number of genes, a polygenic effect, which is important and it is this

Polygenic inheritance

liability (sum of genetic and environmental influences)

factor which is responsible for the familial tendency or predisposition to various diseases. However, as the expression of the disease depends on environmental factors as well as genetic ones, the aetiology of this group of conditions is more correctly described as multifactorial. Many human traits, for example height and intelligence, are inherited in this way and these characteristics in a given population follow a Gaussian or normal distribution. The liability of any individual to develop a disease of multifactorial aetiology also has a normal distribution, and the condition occurs when a certain threshold level is exceeded.

When one member of a family is affected then relatives sharing some of the responsible genes are at an increased risk and as expected this risk is higher for a first degree relative, that is sons and daughters, than for second degree relatives, cousins and nephews.

The neural tube defects are the most common serious congenital abnormalities in the U.K. and their distribution within the community fits a multifactorial aetiology. Thus in communities with an incidence of 5 per 1000 births the risk of any mother having a baby with this condition is 1 in 200. Following the birth of an affected child the risk for subsequent infants will be 1 in 20. Should she be unlucky enough to have a second affected child then the risk for subsequent pregnancies rises to approximately 1 in 8. With three affected children the risk rises even higher, probably 1 in 4. Families with such tragic histories were encountered before it was possible to diagnose the condition early in pregnancy. The chances of both identical twins being affected is less than 10%.

Conditions with polygenic inheritance, example: spina bifida

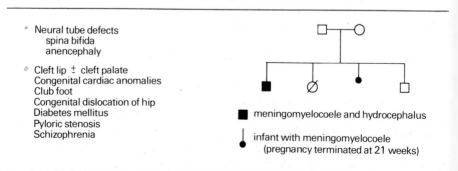

- Neural tube defects
     spina bifida
     anencephaly

- Cleft lip ± cleft palate
     Congenital cardiac anomalies
     Club foot
     Congenital dislocation of hip
     Diabetes mellitus
     Pyloric stenosis
     Schizophrenia

■ meningomyelocoele and hydrocephalus

infant with meningomyelocoele
(pregnancy terminated at 21 weeks)

The geographical distribution of this abnormality emphasises its multifactorial origin. In Belfast the incidence is 7:1000 and in South Wales even higher, whereas in East Anglia and South East England the incidence is only about 2:1000. The increased tendency of those of celtic stock to have affected children persists even in those celts who move to live in other parts of the world. This suggests a genetic contribution. The births of children with neural tube abnormalities have a definite seasonal incidence; they are more commonly in lower social classes; and they are more likely to affect the first and fourth children in a family. These various elements could be considered to reflect environmental factors.

Epidemiological studies in the future should identify further environmental factors in multifactorial conditions. Recently, it has been reported that deficiency of some vitamins, particularly of the B group may play a part in the aetiology of neural tube defects. Supplements of folic acid given early in pregnancy to mother may reduce the number of recurrences of this anomaly.

Pre-natal diagnosis of the condition has been possible for some time. In anencephaly or open meningomyelocele a normal fetal blood constituent, alpha-fetoprotein, is increased in the amniotic fluid. This increase can be detected sufficiently early for termination of the pregnancy to be offered to the parents. Initially, amniocentesis and estimation of the alpha-fetoprotein was only considered in those couples who already had an affected child. However, when it was confirmed that a rise in the maternal serum alpha-fetoprotein was also present in many cases of neural tube detect it became possible to offer a routine screening procedure for all mothers irrespective of their previous history. Despite the problems inherent in such a widescale population screening procedure it is already producing a significant decrease in the number of children born with this abnormality in our community.

GENETIC COUNSELLING

When genetic disease occurs in a family or an individual it is important that the relevant members of the family receive genetic counselling. The counsellor's main task is to establish or confirm the diagnosis; assess the genetic implications of this and compute the risk of the disorder to offsprings or siblings. The individuals concerned must be made aware of the options for dealing with the risk and

Genetic counselling

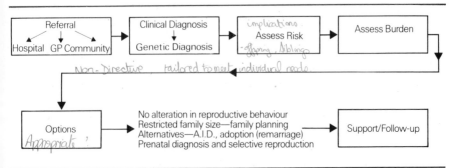

should be helped to choose a course of action which seems appropriate to them. To be really successful the counsellor must also be very sensitive to the difficulties in imparting medical information in a non-directive way and must be aware of the psychological consequences of genetic disease. Effective communication between the counsellor and those counselled is obviously essential and it is important that the problem is dealt with in a sympathetic and unhurried manner. When prenatal diagnosis is under consideration the genetic risk may become secondary to the concern about the interruption of a pregnancy and the emotional, religious or ethical price to be paid for this. The counsellor must try and help families come to terms with this uncertainty and the conselling, although remaining non-directive must be tailored to meet individual needs.

PRENATAL DIAGNOSIS

This has become increasingly available for a variety of conditions and although primary prevention is always preferred, this approach is increasingly requested by couples at high risk of a serious disorder in their children. At present, it is indicated in about 10% of all pregnancies and in most cases (over 90%) prenatal testing provides reassurance that the fetus is not affected.

Techniques available for prenatal diagnosis

amniocentesis
chorionic villous biopsy
fetoscopy ± fetal blood sampling
fetal imaging
  ultrasound
  X-ray

chorion

amniocentesis

chorionic villous biopsy

DNA DIAGNOSIS AND GENE PROBING

It is now possible to diagnose a small number of genetic diseases by direct identification of the abnormal gene or indirectly as a consequence of its known associations with minor variations in the DNA molecule. This has been made possible by the discovery of a group of enzymes referred to as restriction endonucleases which are present in various bacteral species and are capable of cleaving the large DNA molecules into smaller pieces containing the specific genes of interest. There are now several hundred such enzymes and they are named according to the organism from which they are derived, eg Eco R1 from *E. coli*. All have the ability to recognise and cleave DNA at specific sites. The fragments obtained after such cleavage are double stranded but a variety of techniques are available to render them single stranded. If these are then exposed to a radio-active copy of a specific gene the fragments that contain the complimentory DNA sequence will bind with this gene. These can then be examined and their size estimated. Sufficient DNA for analysis can be obtained from blood or from tissue such as chorionic villus materal obtained early in pregnancy. Although only a few diseases can be presently diagnosed by this new technique it will undoubtedly become increasingly used in the diagnosis and prevention of other genetic disorders.

BIBLIOGRAPHY

Emery A E H 1983 Elements of medical genetics, 6th edn. Churchill Livingstone, Edinburgh
Connor J M, Ferguson-Smith M A 1984 Essential medical genetics, Blackwell Scientific
    Publications
Harper P S 1984 Practical Genetic Counselling, 2nd edn, Wright Publications
McKusick V A 1983 Mendelian inheritance in man, 6th edn. The Johns Hopkins University
    Press, Baltimore
Salmon M A, Lenderbaum R H 1978 Developmental defects and syndrome. H. M. & M.
    Publishers

3
Fetus

Since the fetus lies hidden, unobserved within the uterus, he can fall ill, lose parts, even die, without the mother being aware of what is happening. In the main, he is protected against diseases which attack the mother, and his favoured status allows him to thrive and grow even though the mother's reserves are under pressure. Paradoxically there are some situations, fortunately rare, when the fetus is seriously harmed by agents which either have little effect on the mother, for example the virus of german measles, or which might even benefit her, for example various drugs. Towards the end of pregnancy fetal demands for oxygen and nutrients reach a point where they may challenge the capacity of the utero-placental unit to supply them. At this stage, any disturbance of that supply line might interfere with fetal growth or damage sometimes permanently the delicate rapidly growing tissues, particularly in the brain.

EXAMINATION OF THE FETUS

In the past, the assessment of fetal growth depended on a knowledge of the date of the last menstrual period and the estimation of fetal size by palpation; now ultrasound techniques provide more accurate means of measuring growth.

Measurement of fetal head growth and two indices of placento-fetal well being. The examples are serial measurements in individual situations where the fetus was in difficulties

29

However, evaluation of fetal health is more difficult. Some indication of fetal well-being is gained by measuring maternal blood levels of placental lactogen, a protein synthesised by the placenta, or the maternal 24-hour urinary output of oestrogens which reflect the rate of steroid synthesis by the feto-placental unit. Normal values of these biochemical measurements are available for the different stages of gestation. Repeated measurements which show falling levels indicate that the fetus is under increasing difficulty.

If it is suspected that the fetus is structurally or biochemically abnormal, then more invasive procedures which involve entering the uterus might be justified. With chorion biopsy there is a risk of abortion, with amniocentesis there is a slight risk of fetal injury or premature birth. They do, however, allow analysis of fetal cells for a wide range of inherited biochemical disorders and chromosomal abnormalities. In later pregnancy an index of the maturity of the fetal lungs, and thus the capacity of the infant to survive if delivered prematurely, can be gained from measuring the ratio of lecithin to sphingomyelin in the amniotic fluid. In rhesus incompatibility, when the infant is suspected of being severely affected, the concentration of bilirubin in amniotic fluid can be a guide to management.

Fetoscopy requires the introduction of an instrument with a larger bore, but it does permit the fetus to be viewed, in part at least, so that it is possible to identify a placental vessel and collect some fetal blood samples. The latter procedure enables conditions to be diagnosed which would escape detection. This technique has allowed programmes for the antenatal detection of thalassaemia to be successfully established.

Once labour starts some indication of the ability of the fetus to tolerate it can be gained by analysis of the fetal heart rate, particularly in relation to the uterine contractions, and pH measured on capillary blood samples from the presenting part may indicate the degree of asphyxia that the fetus is experiencing.

FETAL INFECTIONS

The list of organisms that have been proven to cross the placenta and affect the fetus is relatively short. It is possible that a much larger number might on rare occasions cause fetal disease or death, but gathering evidence for this relationship is difficult.

Fetal infections

Transplacental:

Treponema pallidum
(syphilis)

Rubella virus
Cytomegalovirus
Plasmodia (malaria)
Toxoplasma gondii
HIV (AIDS agent)

TORCH

Birth canal:

Neisseria gonorrhoea
Listeria monocytogenes
Herpes virus hominis
Hepatitis B

Candida albicans
enteropathogenic
—Escherichia coli
Streptococcus Group B

Rubella

A small percentage of women have their first attack of german measles during early pregnancy, and they may or may not have a suggestive rash. The risks to the fetus are considerable, particularly if a viraemia occurs in the first trimester; a large percentage of pregnancies abort or the surviving fetus is seriously damaged. The viraemia may persist throughout pregnancy and the infant may continue to excrete virus for many years afterwards. During this time the disease process continues. It is because of these terrible consequences of this otherwise trivial infection, that rubella immunisation is offered to all teenage girls. Older women may be immunised but should not become pregnant for at least three months.

Rubella. Clinical features in mothers; the antibodies in the affected and non-affected infants after birth; and the percentage of children at different age groups with antibody

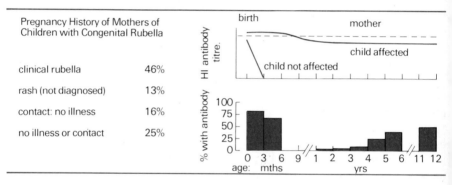

Pregnancy History of Mothers of Children with Congenital Rubella	
clinical rubella	46%
rash (not diagnosed)	13%
contact: no illness	16%
no illness or contact	25%

Clinical features. A surviving fetus may be left with congenital heart defects, defects of the ears with deafness, the eye disorders, particularly cataracts. A small percentage present at birth with purpura, thrombocytopenia, hepatosplenomegaly and have X-ray evidence of bony lesions. Many have an associated encephalopathy and are subsequently mentally retarded.

If a pregnant woman has contact with suspected rubella it is essential to determine whether she is vulnerable to primary infection or whether she has protection from previous exposure. If the diagnosis is suspected, blood is taken and tested for serum haemagglutinin inhibition antibodies (HI) for rubella. If

Congenital rubella. Clinical features

antibodies are high within the incubation period, the patient can be considered to be protected by a previous infection. If they are low, a further sample should be taken 7 to 10 days and if possible 17 to 21 days after first exposure. A rise in titre confirms primary infection and the risk of fetal damage and many consider this grounds for a therapeutic abortion. Diagnosis in the newborn is confirmed by the presence of a specific rubella IgM antibody.

Infections which affect the fetus (from Hanshaw et al 1985)

Agent	Abortion	Stillbirth	Low birth weight	Main congenital defects
Rubella	+	+	+	cataract, deafness, congenital heart defect
Cytomegalovirus	?	+	+	microcephaly, deafness
Herpes virus hominis	–	–	+	microcephaly
Varicella-zoster	?	?	+	hypoplasia of limbs cutaneous scars
Syphilis	+	+	+	rashes, bloody snuffles, widespread organ disease

Cytomegalovirus disease (CMV)

In common with rubella virus, CMV produces a mild disease in adults. It is also widespread in the community; 50 per cent of pregnant English women have antibodies to CMV. It has been estimated that between 1 and 6 per cent of pregnant women contract CMV infections and that the fetus is affected in around 50 per cent. Infection in early pregnancy may cause abortion or a spectrum of malformations including growth failure, microcephaly, mental retardation and deafness. CMV may be a significant cause of mental handicap, epilepsy and nerve deafness, problems which become manifest in later life when the relationship with intrauterine infection is less likely to be appreciated. CMV infection in late pregnancy may produce a systemic illness comprising purpura, hepatospleno-megaly, pneumonia and encephalitis.

Due to the absence of clinical illness in the adult, the infection in the mother often passes undetected. Even routine screening of the newborn for raised CMV specific IgM levels can be misleading. However, the presence of virus in the urine of the newborn with raised cytomegalovirus specific IgM antibody confirms the diagnosis. At present there is no reliable vaccine available for the protection against CMV infections.

Toxoplasmosis

Toxoplasma gondii, a protozoon parasite, is found around the world and affects animals as well as man. Again, the maternal infection may not produce any clinical symptoms. Only a small percentage of women contract the infection in the first part of pregnancy but when they do so the organism may invade the placenta and spread to the fetus.

Toxoplasmosis has widespread effects on the developing brain, causing hydro-cephalus or microcephaly with cerebral calcification and a chorioretinitis. There is usually resultant mental handicap with other neurological abnormalities.

A diagnosis is made on the basis of rising antibody titres. In the newborn, the toxoplasma specific IgM fluorescent antibody test will be positive in those infants who have been infected, but the absence of antibodies does not rule out the possibility of a congenital infection. Infants thought to have the disease should be followed up both clinically and serologically.

Others
Syphilis used to be the most commonly recognised organism that attacked the fetus but happily it is now very rare in the U.K. The same is true for congenital tuberculosis. Malaria commonly affects the placenta and may interfere with the fetal growth. Mothers with malaria have babies of relatively low birth weight. Occasionally the parasites cross to the fetus and cause fetal disease.

INFECTIONS ACQUIRED DURING PASSAGE THROUGH THE BIRTH CANAL

A sterile infant passing through the birth canal is at risk of contracting a wide range of infections, particularly from pathogenic organisms in the maternal bowel. If the membranes have ruptured prematurely, the infant may be infected two or three days prior to birth by organisms entering the uterus via the birth canal. There has been some concern that, even without rupture of the membranes, infection can pass up the birth canal to produce an infection of the placenta and the fetus.

Gonococcal ophthalmia
Infection due to *Neisseria gonorrhoea* acquired during the birth can lead to a purulent conjunctivitis, which if not treated promptly, results in corneal ulceration and perforation. Frequent irrigation with antibiotic eye drops is recommended together with a course of systemic penicillin or, if the organism is insensitive to penicillin, a broad spectrum antibiotic.

Pneumonia and meningitis
So-called congenital pneumonia is in most instances not due to a bacterial infection. However, occasionally listeria or group B streptococcal organisms in the birth canal can be drawn into the respiratory tract and produce a bacterial pneumonia in the first few days of life. The possibility needs to be recognised and vigorous antibiotic therapy given for septicaemia and meningitis may quickly follow.

Herpes virus infections
Herpes virus Type 2 infection is a sexually transmitted disease. The cervicitis is frequently asymptomatic but it creates a major risk for the fetus. Ascending infection may result in abortion or, in later pregnancy, premature birth. There is a high (40 per cent) risk of direct infection during the infant's passage through the birth canal. Neonatal herpes infection is frequently fatal and some obstetricians regard herpetic cervicitis an indication for elective Caesarean section.

Hepatitis B virus

Hepatitis B (incubation 50–180 days) is a major health problem in developing countries. It contributes to a high mortality from cirrhosis and hepatocellular carcinoma. The pool of chronic carriers is perpetuated by maternal–child transfer at birth. Active and passive immunisation programmes are being established in an attempt to protect subsequent generations.

DRUGS ACROSS THE PLACENTA

There is no doubt that some drugs cause embryopathy. There is some suspicion that many others may under some circumstances have harmful effects, but it is very difficult to establish beyond doubt that they made a contribution to the production of an abnormality in one particular child. Difficulty establishing the association is due in part to the fact that the drug may only occasionally have this harmful effect, and in part to the fact that the end pathology may not be specific.

Drugs affecting the embryo and fetus

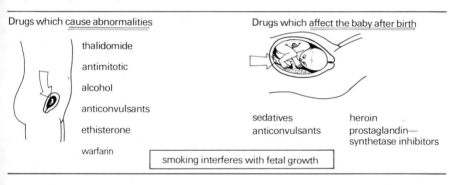

Drugs which cause abnormalities	Drugs which affect the baby after birth	
thalidomide		
antimitotic		
alcohol		
anticonvulsants	sedatives	heroin
ethisterone	anticonvulsants	prostaglandin— synthetase inhibitors
warfarin		

smoking interferes with fetal growth

Thalidomide

It was the damaging effect of this drug which highlighted the need for caution when introducing new agents for treating women during pregnancy. The drug damaged a large percentage of the fetuses of women who received it in early pregnancy. Characteristically it affected the skeletal system, causing unusual defects of the arms and legs, phocomelia. The limbs may be absent, shortened, or hypoplastic. Less frequently there may be abnormalities of the intestinal tract, of the heart or kidneys, or there may be a harelip and eye defects.

Other drugs causing embryopathies

Cytotoxic agents may kill the fetus, indeed aminopterin was used to terminate pregnancies, but if the pregnancy continues the fetus may survive with many deformities. Progesterone preparations will masculinise the female fetus. Alcohol can cause facial abnormalities, growth retardation and mental handicap. Such abnormalities are not unusual in babies of women who are chronic alcoholics. Anti-convulsant drugs e.g. hydantoin, primidone and the anticoagulant, warfarin, have been associated with dysmorphic features and a variety of abnormalities. Certainly there is sufficient evidence to recommend that they are not given during pregnancy unless there are sound clinical indications.

Drugs given to fetus which affect neonatal behaviour

Drugs administered to the mother during the time prior to delivery may affect the baby's behaviour immediately after birth. Obviously sedatives and anaesthetics which cross the placenta will make the baby sleepy and inactive. This is the reason why many babies after Caesarean section used to require resuscitation. Mothers who are on long-term anticonvulsant therapy may have babies with withdrawal symptoms. The babies on the second and third day become hyperactive and difficult to feed and some have 'jittery' episodes. It is important to reassure mother of the nature of these episodes as she may fear that her baby is going to have fits like herself. Mothers who are drug addicts have babies who are undersized but their maturation may be advanced so that they have a lower incidence of respiratory distress syndrome. However, the babies may show severe withdrawal symptoms and require careful management over the first few weeks of life. Any drugs that the obstetrician uses to accelerate labour, may interfere with the fetus and the development of the baby after birth. For example, it has been suspected that the prostaglandin and antiprostaglandin agents may interfere with the balance between patency and closure of the ductus arteriosus. Oxytocin administered to control labour causes a small increase in bilirubin levels in the infants after birth.

MATERNAL IMMUNOGLOBULINS

The immune defence mechanisms develop early in fetal life, but in the absence of stimulation, specific antibodies are not produced. The human fetus gains some specific protection by the transfer of maternal IgG across the placenta. In general the maternal immunoglobulins confer benefit but they can produce disease. The commonest example is the transfer of maternal antibodies against the fetal blood cells as in rhesus and ABO incompatibility. Less commonly, mothers suffering from the so-called autoimmune diseases may transfer damaging antibodies to the fetus. Thus, mothers with platelet antibodies, who may or may not themselves have clinical features of idiopathic thrombocytopenia, may have babies who

Transient disorders in the newborn caused by maternal immunoglobulin

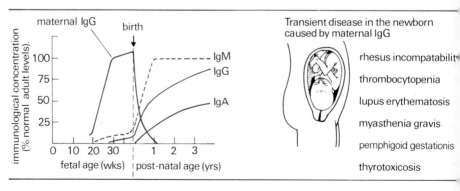

develop purpura in the first 2–3 days of life due to the transfer of antiplatelet antibodies across the placenta. Similarly, mothers with systemic lupus erythematosis may have infants who have either systemic disease, which is usually lethal, or transient lupus rashes on the face. Likewise, babies of mothers with myasthenia gravis may have transient but severe hypotonia, and infants of mothers with ulcerative colitis may have transient melaena. Finally, mothers with circulating thyroid antibodies, irrespective of whether they are themselves thyrotoxic or even in a hypothyroid state during pregnancy, may have infants who develop all the signs of thyrotoxicosis after birth including exophthalmos. There may be little indication that the baby is affected until they develop heart failure in the second week or so of life. It is as well to keep an eye on all infants at risk.

BIBLIOGRAPHY

Boyd R, Battaglia F C 1983 Perinatal medicine. Butterworths International Medical Reviews, London
Chiswick M 1983 Recent advances in perinatal medicine I. Churchill Livingstone, Edinburgh
Hanshaw J B, Dudgeon J A, Marshall W 1985 Virus diseases of the fetus and newborn. Saunders, Philadelphia
de Swiet M 1985 Maternal autoimmune disease and the fetus. Archives of Disease in Childhood 60: 794–797

4
Newborn

In our concern to provide every mother and her child with a safe birth we may overlook the importance of their first meeting face to face. They have a deep basic need to 'recognise' and respond to each other. Fascinating research in recent years has demonstrated how very aware and responsive the human newborn is to his new environment. If the mother is ill or the delivery is difficult or the newborn infant is sick or weak it is even more important for the caring staff to encourage the establishment and the strengthening of the bond between mother and child. Failure to do so may lead subsequently to poor feeding patterns, failure to thrive, and the longer term consequences of maternal neglect. When mother and infant have failed to establish a mutually satisfying relationship there is an increased risk of child abuse and post-neonatal infant death.

ROUTINE EXAMINATION OF THE NEWBORN

'Is my baby all right?' is often the first question that mothers ask after delivery and it is so difficult to answer if he is not! As soon as the baby is born a quick but careful scrutiny of the face, eyes, mouth, chest, abdomen, spine and limbs should exclude major abnormalities; a lusty cry and the development of a suffuse pink blush over the face and body denotes satisfactory immediate adjustment to independent existence. Together they are sufficient to answer the mother's pressing question. If you are not sure of the sex of the infant do not make a guess. Explain to the parents that occasionally it can be difficult to tell immediately and that tests may be necessary. If there is difficulty establishing adequate breathing, then the appropriate steps in resuscitation should be taken. If the baby is small, immature or injured, he must be given extra support and protection. If the mother has had hydramnios then a firm tube must be passed into the stomach to exclude oesophageal atresia, a congenital abnormality which is usually associated with a tracheo-oesophageal fistula.

Over the next 48 hours all infants should be examined thoroughly and at leisure, preferably in the mother's presence, ideally with both parents, and only

Incidence of the commoner malformations in Great Britain (these figures are only approximate; see Carter 1976)

Malformation	per 1000 live births
Anencephaly	2.0
Spina bifida	2.5
Cleft lip ± cleft palate	1.0
Club foot	1.2
Congenital hip dislocation	1.5
Congenital heart malformations	6.0
Down syndrome	1.7
Pyloric stenosis	3.0

after the details of the medical history of the family, the pregnancy and labour are known. This first medical examination is a screening procedure, and its aim is to discover disorders which are open to early management. The baby should be naked in a warm room, and the mother should be able to see clearly what you are doing. The examination should be thorough and in a logical sequence; first assess overall size, proportions and maturity, then look for structural abnormalities, starting with the head and eyes and then the ears, mouth, chest, abdomen and limbs, hands and feet. Note any accessory tags, digits and dimples. Many abnormalities follow failure of complete union in the midline, and so a quick check along the midline is worthwhile, and this should include a close look at the palate and anus. Respiratory disorders are more easily seen than heard. Palpating the peripheral pulses may suggest, if full, a ductus arteriosus, or, if weak, a major defect causing poor systemic cardiac output. The presence or absence of femoral pulsations must always be noted. Abnormal heart sounds and murmurs are more difficult to interpret; if there is doubt, it is better to find an opportunity to re-examine the baby later. If the murmur persists but the baby is otherwise well, then the parents are told of the finding and a follow-up examination is arranged. Two other conditions are specifically sought; congenital dislocation of the hips, and in boys, the presence of testes in the scrotum.

The third stage of this examination is to assess the baby's behaviour and responsiveness. The mother and the midwife will usually be quick to tell you about the baby's feeding, behaviour, crying and sleeping patterns. An unduly floppy or sleepy baby, an irritable or restless baby, or a poor 'suckler' all call for more careful evaluation, particularly in relation to the establishment or otherwise of satisfactory breast feeding. Finally give the mother an opportunity to ask any other questions.

Minor anomalies

Parents should be reassured about the following minor anomalies:

Capillary or macular haemangioma (stork bites, salmon patch) around the eyes and at the nape of the neck are seen in 30 to 50 per cent of babies. Those around the eyes usually disappear in the first year. Those at the nape may persist.

Blue-black pigmented areas (Mongolian blue spots) at the base of the back and on the buttocks are unimportant and are common in infants of dark skinned parents but can also occur in Caucasian infants. They usually fade over the first year or so.

Urticaria of the newborn is a fluctuating, widespread, erythematous rash with a raised white dot at the centre of the red flare. It is usually most marked on the trunk and is most evident on the second day. It disappears spontaneously, requiring no treatment.

Heat rash (miliaria) is seen in mature infants nursed in warm humid atmospheres. Both red, macular patches and superficial, clear vesicles may be seen, most evident on the forehead and around the neck. The lesions clear in a cool environment.

Breast enlargement Both girl and boy infants may develop breast enlargement and even secrete small amounts of milk (witches milk). Girls may discharge a mucous plug from the vagina and there may be a little vaginal bleeding on about the fourth day. "Newborn Period"

White pimples (milia) on the nose and cheeks are very common and are found in about 40 per cent of infants. They are blocked sebaceous glands and clear spontaneously.

Cysts in the mouth occur on the palate near the midline (Epstein's pearls) and larger ones of the gums (epulis) and on the floor of the mouth. Epstein's pearls and most of the others resolve spontaneously. Teeth may be present at birth: some are loose and have to be removed.

Accessory skin tags on the face, anterior to the ears (accessory auricles) or loosely attached, vestigial, extra digits can usually be dealt with easily but this should preferably be done by the surgical team.

Sacral dimples should be explored gently to exclude underlying sinuses.

Minor anomalies

accessory auricle
white pimples
capillary naevi
third fontanelle
Wormian bone
urticaria
Mongolian spots
breast enlargement
accessory digit
single palmar crease
two cord vessels
fused labia
sacral dimples

Some anomalies, although relatively unimportant in themselves, may be associated with more important abnormalities. The fontanelles (head 'soft spots') are occasionally very wide and not infrequently extra bones float in the space,

Wormian bones. If skin defects overlie the posterior fontanelle the possibility of chromosomal abnormalities should be considered. A third fontanelle is occasionally found between the anterior and posterior fontanelles and is common in trisomy 21. Oddly shaped ears and two cord vessels may be associated with renal abnormalities. A single palmar crease, instead of the usual two, may sometimes be associated with other abnormalities, including Down syndrome.

Congenital postural deformities

The posture of the infant after birth often reflects his position *in utero*. However, with more freedom, the infant soon chooses to curl into a compact shape with arms and legs flexed. If there is less than an average amount of amniotic fluid to cushion the fetus, then towards the end of gestation the infant may be so tightly packed within the uterus that deformations of the musculoskeletal system develop. These congenital postural deformities may mould the head into odd shapes (dolichocephaly, plagiocephaly) suppress or distort the chin, resulting in its being unduly small (micrognathia), or cause mandibular asymmetry or neck muscle contractures and torticollis. The shoulders may be dislocated, the chest wall compressed, the hands and feet distorted (club hand, club foot). These effects are usually multiple and are seen in their extreme form when the kidneys are absent in renal agenesis, and very little amniotic fluid is present (oligohydramnios). The presenting part is often the most deformed. One special example of postural deformity associated with intrauterine position is dislocation of the hip, which is more common in breech presentation.

Intrauterine postures

Biochemical screening

The number of inherited biochemical disorders or variations which can be recognised by relatively simple and cheap biochemical tests increases yearly. It is the simplicity and cheapness of the test which makes it feasible to test the blood of every newborn infant. The tests are primarily intended to screen for phenylketonuria (the Guthrie test) and hypothyroidism, but other conditions including galactosaemia, maple syrup urine disease and homocystinuria may be identified. The blood test is performed when milk feeding has been established, usually on the fourth or fifth day of life.

BIRTH INJURIES

The short journey down the birth canal is not without hazards for the infant but fortunately the risks are becoming less as the technique for recognising fetal distress improve. Infants who are judged to be too big for the birth canal or who fail to advance during labour and become distressed are now delivered by Caesarean section, making heroic obstetric manipulations to achieve vaginal birth rarely necessary. The risk of birth trauma is greater in breech deliveries, in premature births, in precipitate deliveries and when the baby is unexpectedly large.

Some of the damage caused by the birth is unsightly but quickly resolves. Inevitably, the presenting part becomes oedematous and bruised. This caput succedaneum is commonly found on the back of the head and happily it clears spontaneously in a few days. However, the swelling looks uncomfortable when it involves the breech and scrotum and very unpleasant in a face presentation. The face also looks bloated, blue and bruised when the cord is pulled tightly around the neck (an appearance called 'traumatic cyanosis'), and there may also be retinal and conjunctival haemorrhages. As the fetal head is pushed down the birth canal it rotates and the apex of the parietal bones may catch the ischial spines and be dented like a ping pong ball or the outer shelf may be cracked and crepitus may be felt, or the periosteum may separate and a cephalhaematoma form beneath the periosteum producing a lump the size of a small hen's egg. Again, these injuries are of little import although the cephalhaematoma may take many months before it finally disappears. Rarely a bleed may occur under the aponeurosis (sub-aponeurotic haemorrhage) when the bleeding is not confined to a single cranial bone like a cephalhaematoma but spreads rapidly over the head and down towards the eyes. A significant fraction of the blood volume may be lost into this haematoma.

Severe compression with extreme moulding of the skull can tear the tentorium cerebelli and its accompanying vein. The resulting haemorrhage is likely to cause permanent damage or death. The baby may be born in a state of shock and may

Birth injuries

Fractures:
  clavicle
humerus
ribs

Nervous tissue damage:
  brain bleed (tentorial tear)
  spinal cord
  upper brachial plexus
    →Erbs Palsy.

Dislocations
  shoulder
  hip

caput succedaneum
common

subaponeurotic haemorrhage
very rare

cephalhaematoma
rare

not respond to resuscitative procedures.

Manipulation of the spine and arms, which is most likely to be required for breech deliveries, may damage the cervical spinal cord with residual palsies in arms and legs, or lead to stretching and damage of the upper part of the brachial plexus causing weakness or paralysis of abduction at the shoulder, flexion at the elbow and extension and supination of the wrist (Erb's palsy). The arm is dropped into the position a waiter adopts in the expectation of a tip. The weakness usually resolves spontaneously in a few weeks.

Rough handling may lead not only to fracture of the skull but also of the clavicle, humerus or ribs. These injuries may pass undetected immediately after birth, but can be recognised when a lump appears due to callus formation around the fracture.

Forceps blades may compress the facial nerve as it leaves the parotid gland. Usually the resultant facial palsy is transient, but occasionally the pressure causes overlying fat necrosis with permanent scarring and a residual palsy.

BIRTH ASPHYXIA

The fetus, floating in the amniotic fluid, 'breathes', 'feeds' and 'excretes' through the placenta. The fetal lungs are filled with fluid secreted by the alveolar cells to a volume close to the functional residual capacity found after birth. Following delivery, the placenta is discarded and 'dies' whilst the independent infant activates his own system for obtaining oxygen and nutrients and discarding waste.

The most urgent requirement is to breathe. To do this the lung liquid must be displaced by air. During a vaginal birth the thorax is squeezed in the birth canal and the lung liquid can sometimes be seen pouring out of the baby's nose when his head is just emerging from the birth canal. Once the infant gasps, air is drawn into the lung and lung liquid disappears to the periphery of the respiratory tree. From there it is cleared by the pulmonary circulation and lymphatics. Failure to complete this process satisfactorily is one important factor leading to transient tachypnoea.

As the infant passes down the birth canal his head is squeezed and then released and exposed to the cooling air. His limbs are pushed, pulled and finally allowed to drop into positions they have never occupied before. His umbilical cord is intermittently obstructed, stretched and finally clamped. His arterial concentration of oxygen falls and that of carbon dioxide rises. Many of these stimuli are known to provoke a gasp.

On average, newborn infants gasp after six seconds and the majority have done so by twenty seconds. With these efforts the lungs rapidly fill with air and a residual lung volume is formed. Once this is achieved, tidal breathing begins. It occurs on average after thirty seconds and the majority of infants are breathing regularly by ninety seconds.

As the lungs expand and fill with gas, the pulmonary vascular resistance falls, the pulmonary blood flow increases and the pressure in the left atrium rises closing the foramen ovale. As a consequence of these changes, oxygenated blood passes through the ductus arteriosus; oxygen has a direct effect on the muscle of the ductus causing contraction and physiological closure, anatomical closure

The onset of breathing and circulatory adjustments after birth

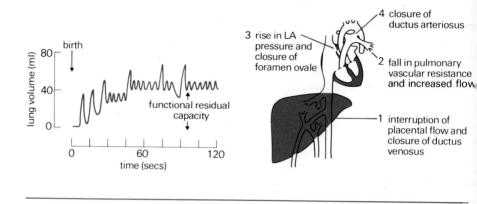

proceeds more slowly over the following weeks. Occasionally, in cyanosed infants, the ductus may remain open or the physiologically closed ductus may reopen, and so add to the infant's problems sometimes to the point of precipitating heart failure.

Infants may be asphyxiated *in utero* for a variety of reasons. If the disorder is not reversed they will be asphyxiated at birth and they must be resuscitated immediately. Many of the babies who appear all but dead at birth but who respond promptly to active resuscitation may make a full recovery. More commonly, infants are reasonably oxygenated at birth but due to previous asphyxia or sedative drugs given to the mother they fail to begin adequate ventilation, and then become asphyxiated and require resuscitation. Many factors are associated with birth asphyxia including the general well being of the mother and the maturity and nutrition of the infant.

Causes of intrauterine asphyxia

maternal asphyxia; lung, heart disease

poor uterine perfusion, shock, posture, vascular disease

disease and separation of placenta

interruption of cord; prolapse

fetal anaemia and heart failure

With increasing asphyxia the infant becomes blue and then white, hypotonic, unresponding, and the heart rate begins to fall. These features, colour, tone, response to stimulation, respiration and heart rate were arranged into a scoring

Assessment of neonatal asphyxia

			Apgar Score		
			0	1	2
1. response to stimulation	—		none	facial grimace	cry
2 respiration	—		absent	gasping	regular
3 heart rate	—		0	<100	>100
4. colour of trunk	—		white	blue	pink
5. muscle tone	—		flaccid	some flexion	normal with movement

system by an American anaesthetist, Dr Virginia Apgar. The main features to watch are the infant's attempts to breathe and the rate and strength of the pulse. Those who fail to breathe and become asphyxiated should be actively resuscitated when the heart rate begins to fall.

Resuscitation

The newly born baby is gently dried and wrapped in a warm towel. The time of birth is noted. The upper airway is cleared by gentle suction of excess fluid →<5 cm and any inhaled vernix, blood or meconium. If during this procedure the infant fails to make any respiratory effort then a gasp may be provoked by blowing cold H₂O oxygen on the nose. If this is not effective then the other bizzare methods used in the past, for example pinching, slapping, injecting respiratory stimulants, or putting champagne or pepper on the nasal mucosa, are not likely to work.

The next step is to expand and ventilate the lungs. Often inflation of the lungs itself will initiate a gasp with spontaneous breathing. If it does not, the lung should be ventilated at a rate between 20 and 30 inflations per minute with pressures limited to 30 cm H_2O. The majority of infants will quickly become pink and begin breathing within two or five minutes.   if Hypoplastic lungs - May need →60 cm H

The most effective method of inflating the lungs is via an endotracheal tube. To insert the tube, the infant's head must be carefully positioned in slight extension, the small finger of the hand holding the endoscope pushes the larynx into view. If either the skill or the equipment is not available for intubation then the

Steps in resuscitation

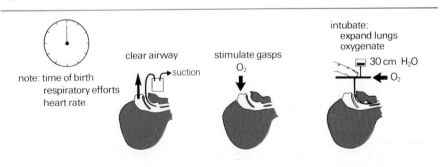

note: time of birth
respiratory efforts
heart rate

clear airway
→suction

stimulate gasps
O_2

intubate:
expand lungs
oxygenate
30 cm H_2O
← O_2

infant can be resuscitated nearly as well with a face mask which fits snugly over his mouth and nose, and a bag which delivers small volumes of gas. It is essential to hold the lower jaw forward to ensure a clear airway; over-inflation of the stomach should be avoided by passing a nasogastric tube and putting gentle hand pressure on the upper abdomen.

If the infant fails to become pink with good expansion of the lung then he is probably in a state of shock. If the apex rate is less than 60 and falling, start cardiac massage using two finger pressure on the lower half of the sternum at 100–120 beats per minute. Metabolic acidosis can be corrected by giving 4.2% sodium bicarbonate 4 ml/kg into the umbilical vein. It is important to flush it through.

If the lungs do not expand then either there is a rare abnormality of the airways or lungs, or the endotracheal tube is not in the trachea. Clumsy insertion of the tube can damage the upper airways; energetic and faulty inflation may damage the lungs. Occasionally, the difficult decision of whether to resuscitate or not has to be made. If the baby is physically normal and can be resuscitated then recent reports suggest that he will probably survive intact, although he may have a stormy few days rather like an older child after a head injury. If the baby is physically abnormal then one must ask oneself firstly, could this child survive even if resuscitation is successful, and secondly, has the infant's brain developed adequately? If the answer to either is no, then resuscitation is not justifiable. If there is uncertainty, call a colleague, remembering that in general parents would wish us to respond to their offspring as we would wish others to respond to our own.

Reasons for failure to resuscitate and the immediate effects of severe birth asphyxia

Reasons for failure to resuscitate	Immediate effects of severe birth asphyxia

1. Brain damage:
    haemorrhage: ischaemia
	Brain:
	    fits, irritability
	    abnormal tone
	    hypo and hyperventilation
	    hypoglycaemia

2. Upper airway obstruction:
    laryngeal spasm
    laryngeal stenosis	

3. Lung pathology:
    pneumothorax
    hypoplasia
    effusion
    diaphragmatic hernia
	Lungs:
	    aspiration, RDS
	    haemorrhage
	
	Kidneys:
	    vein thrombosis
	    tubular necrosis

4. Small chest cage	
5. Shock due to ruptured viscera	Bowels: ileus, perforation

Effects of asphyxia

Birth asphyxia may have both immediate and long term effects. Acute total asphyxia seen, for example with cord prolapse, may by haemorrhage and oedema, damage and interfere with brain function, causing profound hypotonia followed by irritability and fitting; there may be an abnormal cry and poor sucking patterns. The breathing pattern may be so disturbed as to suggest a primary respiratory problem. Loss of homeostatic control may lead to hypoglycaemia, hypocalcaemia and hypothermia. But asphyxia may damage many other organs as well: in the lungs it causes oedema; in the myocardium changes resembling an infarct; in the bowel it causes an ileus or ischaemic perforations; in the kidneys it may result in renal vein thrombosis or tubular necrosis; and in the liver disorders of metabolism and haemostasis may result. In premature infants, birth asphyxia increases the risk of idiopathic respiratory distress syndrome and lethal intraventricular haemorrhages.

The immediate post natal effects of chronic intermittent prenatal asphyxia are more difficult to assess for invariably asphyxia is not the only noxious factor affecting the infant.

Cerebral oedema, haemorrhage or ischaemia may lead to permanent brain damage and resultant cerebral palsy and mental handicap. That less severe degrees of asphyxia can lead to less severe evidence of brain damage, for example, fits, hyperactivity and learning problems is generally accepted but the extent to which it is responsible for these disorders in the community is difficult to assess.

We are still left with the problem of trying to determine which infants asphyxiated before or during the birth are likely to be permanently affected. Some infants make remarkable recoveries so that parents should be encouraged to be reasonably optimistic. It has been estimated that only 1 in 10 of infants showing evidence of brain asphyxia in the week or so after birth are subsequently found to have evidence of brain damage.

SIZE AT BIRTH

The birth weight plotted on growth charts of body weight against gestational age help us to define groups of babies. Those whose birth weights are between the 10th and 90th centile lines are 'normal weight for dates'. Those babies with birth weights over the 90th centile are called 'large for dates', and those with weights under the 10th centile are 'small for dates'. Small for dates babies are also

Weight at birth and fetal weight curves

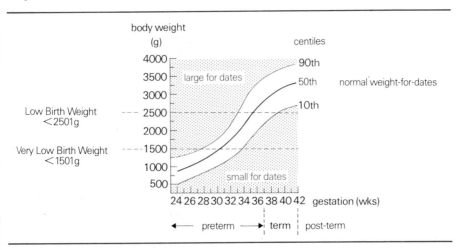

described as 'small for gestation age', 'light for dates', and dysmature. It is important to determine whether a baby is 'large for dates' or 'small for dates' or premature or postmature for each has special problems which can be anticipated and treated.

Large-for-dates infants
The infant of a diabetic mother is large and obese. Not many years ago many of them were stillborn. Now with improved antenatal care the majority survive but they are still at a slightly greater risk of having a congenital abnormality; their broad shoulders may give problems during the birth (shoulder dystocia) and after birth they are more likely to develop hypoglycaemia, respiratory distress and to become jaundiced. Their hyperexcitability, jitteriness and immaturity may initially cause feeding difficulties. With meticulous control of the diabetic state during the whole of pregnancy, many if not all these problems can be avoided. The exciting question is whether or not good control in early pregnancy will reduce the incidence of congenital abnormalities.

Low birth weight
About 7 per cent of UK births are low birth weight, defined as all those weighing 2500 g or less, at birth. The incidence is lower in Scandinavian countries and higher in Third World countries. The low birth weight group include a disproportionate number of the babies with problems. In the U.K. about 8 per cent of stillbirths and 80 per cent of first week deaths are of low birth weight.

Low birth weight is associated amongst other things with poor socio-economic conditions, congenital abnormalities, intrauterine infections, multiple pregnancies, poor placental function, and maternal starvation, illness, smoking, drug and alcohol abuse. Low birth weight may be due to premature birth, before 37 weeks (preterm infant), or poor fetal growth ('small for dates,' infant). Although they may be of the same weight, preterm and 'small for dates' infants look different and have different problems. Some babies are both preterm and small for dates and are at risk of the problems of both groups.

Comparison between the features of the preterm and small-for-dates infant

Preterm (but normal weight-for-dates)	Small-for-dates (but born at term)
small but plump	wasted
red or very pink	white or pale pink
length <50cm	length >50cm
head circumference <c.35cm	head circumference >c.35cm
lanugo hair	thick, dark hair
skin: shiny transparent, thin, oedematous	skin: dry, loose, thick
ears, breast tissue, genitalia —all immature	ears, breast tissue, genitalia —all mature
hypotonic (floppy)	good muscle tone

Small-for-dates infants

It is important to recognise these infants preferably before birth for they are more likely to be in trouble during delivery and be in need of prompt and skilful resuscitation. They are particularly susceptible to damaging hypoglycaemia in the first days of life. Four hourly estimations of blood glucose concentration should be made and early generous feeding commenced. Should the blood glucose concentration fall below 1.1 mmol/l, intravenous glucose therapy is necessary.

Small-for-dates babies have a lower perinatal mortality rate than babies of similar birth weight born preterm, but their eventual outlook may not be so good. Those who are small but perfectly proportioned, suggesting intrauterine growth retardation early in the pregnancy, may remain small, and their abilities are more likely to fall below the average. The situation is complex because of the association with poor socio-economic status.

Some clinical problems of preterm and small-for-dates infants

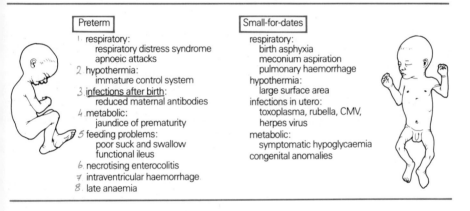

Preterm	Small-for-dates

1. respiratory:
   respiratory distress syndrome
   apnoeic attacks
 2. hypothermia:
   immature control system
 3. infections after birth:
   reduced maternal antibodies
 4. metabolic:
   jaundice of prematurity
 5. feeding problems:
   poor suck and swallow
   functional ileus
 6. necrotising enterocolitis
 7. intraventricular haemorrhage
 8. late anaemia
	respiratory:
	   birth asphyxia
	   meconium aspiration
	   pulmonary haemorrhage
	 hypothermia:
	   large surface area
	 infections in utero:
	   toxoplasma, rubella, CMV,
	   herpes virus
	 metabolic:
	   symptomatic hypoglycaemia
	   congenital anomalies

Preterm infants

The survival rates of preterm babies have improved over the years. Much of this progress is due to the better management. Neonatal care is provided at two levels. Special care is for well preterm infants who need to be carefully watched and monitored in a relatively stable environment and where special expertise is available to help them establish and maintain adequate nutrition. Intensive care is for sick and very immature infants who require a strictly controlled environment, respiratory support and parenteral nutrition.

Structurally normal babies of 32 weeks or more with good birth weights (over 1.5 kg) and without major birth damage now survive and survive intact. The same is true of the majority of babies between 28 and 32 weeks (1.0–1.5 kg). Below 28 weeks (under 1.0 kg) an increasing number of babies are surviving but 15–25 per cent are left with a serious handicap.

Premature birth brings with it a number of problems.

Nutrition As the ability of the weak preterm infant to suckle is limited they often require to be fed for some weeks after birth using a nasogastric tube. Breast milk and various artificial milks have been given with success but recent work

Survival rates in prematurely-born infants

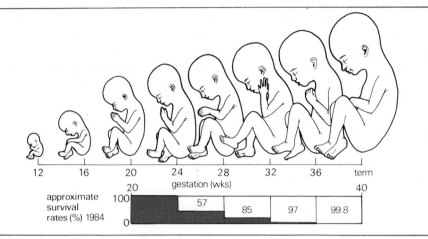

suggests that milks formulated specially for low birth weight infants result in better growth and development. The immature bowel adjusts surprisingly well, although there may be a functional ileus for the first few days of life. ⚓·

Thermal stability. Premature babies have high surface area to body weight ratio and little subcutaneous fat, and over the first few days they lose water rapidly through their skin (transepidermal water loss). These physical character- istics make it difficult for them to maintain thermal stability. As cold exposure jeopardises their survival, great attention must be paid to keeping them warm. To provide a controlled ambient temperature it is current practice to nurse premature infants in incubators or under radiant warmers but it is also important to reduce heat losses by insulating the infant with clothing and a thermal blanket.

Respiratory difficulties. Because of their immaturity many preterm babies have difficulty expanding their lungs and the work of breathing is greatly increased due to the idiopathic respiratory distress syndrome (p. 52). Also their respiratory drive varies, and this is apparent in their periodic breathing pattern which becomes troublesome when it leads to long apnoeic spells (p. 54).

Liver immaturity. Physiological jaundice is often more marked and more prolonged in immature infants but with careful nursing and early establishment of feeding and the use of phototherapy, exchange transfusions should rarely be necessary. It is thought that the preterm brain is more at risk from damage due to high bilirubin levels.

Infections. Because of their delicate surfaces and limited immunological competence, premature babies are more susceptible to infections. Because of their weak defence systems, they do not show the symptoms and signs that are seen in older infants. Their clinical state changes rapidly from bacteraemia, to septi- caemia, to death. Associated meningitis can easily pass undetected. Therefore in any infant suspected of having an infection, it is necessary to perform a 'septic screen' including culture of urine, blood and cerebrospinal fluid and to commence therapy with broad spectrum antibiotics before the results come back.

Intraventricular haemorrhage (IVH). Small haemorrhages into the germinal layer lining the lateral ventricles in the brain are commonly seen on ultrasound scanning of preterm babies, especially those who have experienced asphyxia or severe respiratory problems. These may extend into the ventricular system and a few infants subsequently develop hydrocephalus. However, the majority have small haemorrhages and seem to recover without serious long-term effects. A much poorer outlook in terms of handicap follows ischaemia of the brain parenchyma leading to periventricular leucomalacia.

Necrotizing enterocolitis (NEC). This is a serious condition affecting the bowel during the first three weeks. It is much commoner in the smallest preterm infants. The cause is not known but hypoxic damage to the bowel wall possibly associated with umbilical catheterisation, apnoeic spells, and septicaemia, and the colonization of the bowel with certain organisms are probably precipitating events. Isolated cases occur but so do worrying outbreaks within neonatal units. The baby vomits bile-stained fluid, the abdomen distends and blood and mucus appear in the stools. The diagnosis is confirmed by abdominal x-ray which shows thickened bowel wall containing intra-mural gas. Perforation may occur. Oral feeding is stopped for at least a week and feeds and broad spectrum antibiotics are given intravenously and metronidazole orally. Surgical resection of perforated and necrotic bowel may be needed.

Retrolental fibroplasia (RLF). In the 1960s it was found that preterm infants who inhaled gas mixtures with high oxygen concentrations were at risk of developing abnormal vascularisation at the back of the eye (retrolental fibroplasia or retinopathy of prematurity). Some of these babies became blind. Whilst it was clear, even from these early studies that oxygen excess was not the only cause of RLF, nevertheless it seems wise not to give extra oxygen to preterm infants when they do not need it. However many do, and then it is important to measure the percentage of oxygen in the inspired gas (FiO_2) and the partial pressure of oxygen in arterial blood (PaO_2), if it is at all possible, so that oxygen is not given in excess.

However even with strictly controlled oxygen levels many very immature infants develop retrolental fibroplasia and some go on to partial or complete blindness. Associated disorders include intraventricular haemorrhage, apnoeic attacks, patent ductus arteriosus, septicaemia and metabolic acidosis and any or all may play a part in its causation. Oxygen, it seems, is neither the only nor a necessary aetiological factor.

Nutritional deficiencies. Once they have adjusted to extra-uterine life and feeding has been established, preterm babies can grow at a rate similar to that which they would have achieved *in utero*. This high growth rate can lead to vitamin deficiency, so vitamin supplements are given. The bulk of iron transfer across the placenta occurs during the third trimester of pregnancy. Preterm infants are commonly given iron supplements from the fourth week. Calcium, phosphorus and vitamin D supplementation all appear to be necessary to avoid oesteopathy of prematurity, a condition that develops in some preterm infants in the first months of life and is characterised by pathological fractures and rickets.

Other hazards. Premature babies are often born unexpectedly and are therefore more likely to experience asphyxia during birth and their delicate tissues are more likely to be damaged. They are susceptible to hypoglycaemia, metabolic acidosis, peripheral oedema, and irritability and fits due to birth injury and asphyxia.

The delicate preterm infant is also more easily damaged by nursing and medical procedures. For example, if hypertonic solutions like 10% glucose, calcium or amino acid preparations leak out of a peripheral vein they quickly cause necrosis which can result in a permanent scar.

Prognosis

The outlook of prematurely born infants, particularly those with only moderate problems adjusting to extrauterine life, is good. The majority reach their expected size and ability level. Until recently infants born before 28 weeks' gestation were thought not to be viable. It was exceedingly rare for infants weighing less than 1 kg to survive. Now, with intensive care, including if necessary artificial ventilation and intravenous nutrition, more and more are surviving. It is important to follow them all carefully, 5–10 per cent of babies with birth weights below 1500 g are found to have a major handicap such as cerebral palsy, developmental delay, blindness or deafness.

Inevitably intensive neonatal care interferes with the normal establishment of the parent–child relationship and this, with adverse social factors, is probably responsible for the fact the immature babies are at increased risk of cot death and child abuse.

RESPIRATORY PROBLEMS IN THE NEWBORN

Respiratory distress in newborn babies is recognized by tachypnoea (a respiratory rate of more than 60 per minute); recession of the intercostal spaces, sternum and subcostal areas; expiratory grunting, and cyanosis or the need for oxygen to remain pink. Respiratory failure may be due to a wide variety of both pulmonary and extrapulmonary causes.

Lung disorders due to aspiration

An infant may aspirate foreign material before, during and after birth.

Intrauterine pneumonia. Occasionally babies are born with lung consolidation due to material aspirated from the amniotic fluid. This 'congenital pneumonia' is associated with prolonged rupture of the fetal membranes, amnionitis and fetal asphyxia. If organisms are present they are usually *E. coli, Staphylococcus aureus* and *epidermidis*, and the beta-haemolytic streptococcus group B. The latter can produce a particularly vicious infection leading to septicaemia and meningitis. The babies develop respiratory distress in the first 2–3 days after birth. A chest x-ray shows patchy shadowing. Broad spectrum antibiotics should be given on suspicion. Group B streptococcus can also cause a fulminating septicaemia and meningitis in the 2–6 week postnatal period. Less common but important lung infections are caused by *Listeria monocytogenes* and by Chlamydia.

Meconium aspiration. Asphyxia during birth will provoke mature infants to make vigorous efforts to breath in. If there is meconium in the amniotic fluid, or if the baby's head is in the birth canal surrounded by vernix, meconium and blood, these tenacious materials may be drawn into the upper airway and then into the respiratory tree. They may result in patches of lung collapse, and other areas of over-inflation, due to a ball valve effect of the meconium plug allowing air in but not out. The infants may have severe respiratory difficulties for some days, and complications like pneumothorax and pneumomediastinum are common and may be fatal. Oxygen will be needed, and any tension pneumo-thorax must be drained. Supportive ventilation is difficult. It is better to try to prevent the meconium reaching the lungs by clearing the airways promptly at birth. If meconium is seen around the larynx, the baby is intubated and suction applied directly to the endotracheal tube as it is withdrawn. In skilled hands this can be repeated.

Milk aspiration. It is quite a challenge to the newborn infant to separate in the pharynx the air breathed in through the nose and milk sucked in through the mouth. They often get it wrong and swallow air; and they occasionally get it wrong and inhale milk. Obviously the latter is the more dangerous and every effort must be made to anticipate and avoid it. Aspiration of feeds is quite a common occurrence in preterm babies and in full term babies with a neurological or cardiorespiratory problem. Those with structural anomalies of the nose, mouth and oesophagus are particularly at risk, for example cleft palate, choanal atresia and oesophageal atresia. Management of these babies requires considerable nursing skill and judgement. A nasogastric or nasojejunal feeding tube may be needed, or even total parenteral nutrition for a while.

Transient tachypnoea of the newborn. This is not so much an aspiration as a delay in the clearance of lung fluid which is naturally present *in utero*. The rapid breathing usually settles within a few hours of birth, and chest x-ray shows the fluid as streaky shadows spreading out from the mediastinum and in the greater fissure on the right.

Disorders due to lung immaturity

Idiopathic respiratory distress syndrome. The more immature the infant the greater is the risk of respiratory distress and the lower the survival rate. In the adult, alveolar spaces are clustered around the terminal bronchioles; in the infant at term a single, simple sac is found at the end of each bronchiole. The alveolar epithelium has two type of cells. The Type II pneumocytes secrete a complex of lipoproteins, surfactant, which has the property of lowering surface tension. In some preterm infants these cells seem unable to release or produce enough surfactant, with the result that the air sacs collapse each time the infant breathes out, and the work of breathing is greatly increased. The pulmonary capillaries ooze liquid and red cells into the interstitial space causing oedema and haemor-rhage. The protein leaked into the alveolar sacs form 'hyaline' membranes which can be clearly seen on light microscopy. This finding led to the disorder being called hyaline membrane disease, but in early severe forms membranes may not have had sufficient time to form.

The ability of the Type II cells to release surfactant can be assessed before birth by measuring the ratio in the amniotic fluid of two of the lipoproteins which make up surfactant, lecithin and sphingomyelin. Certain stimuli, including maternal ill health, uterine contractions and drugs may induce the cells to begin secreting earlier in gestation. Perinatal asphyxia, acidosis, and hypothermia have the opposite effect and inhibit surfactant synthesis. Within a few days of birth, whatever the gestation, the cells begin to function and produce adequate surfactant.

As the affected infants have difficulty forming and maintaining a functional residual capacity, they are recognised clinically by their struggle to draw in air and to hold it. Each diaphragmatic tug pulls in the lower rib cage and soft tissues of the neck. An expiratory grunt accompanies each effort. The signs appear at birth or soon after, with apparent increasing severity. If the infant survives then improvement is usually seen after the second or third day and the lungs appear to recover fully. It might be deduced from the pathogenesis that the disorder will vary in severity and this is true; at one extreme it produces an unimportant transient disturbance in the respiratory pattern, at the other it leads to increasing cyanosis, acidosis and death in the first few hours of life.

Lung disorders in the newborn

ground-glass appearance
+air bronchogram:
idiopathic respiratory
distress syndrome

patchy collapse with overinflation.
meconium aspiration

1. pneumothorax
2. pneumomediastinum
3. interstitial emphysema

The diagnosis is comfirmed by the chest x-ray which shows a diffuse ground glass appearance with an air bronchogram. The management requires considerable medical and nursing skill and involves continuous monitoring of many features of the baby (HR, RR, PaO_2) and of his environment (T, FiO_2) as guides for respiratory support, nutrition programmes, and intravenous therapy. Initially oxygen can be given in a headbox, and then as additional support is needed, by a nasal tube delivering a continuous positive airways pressure (CPAP) and finally by intermittent positive pressure ventilation (IPPV) via an endotracheal tube.

Bronchopulmonary dysplasia (BPD). Forcing the lungs open when they are not ready, interruption of natural drainage by endotracheal tubes, aspiration and infection along with the hyaline membrane disease can all contribute to the development of chronic lung disease in some preterm infants with respiratory distress. The x-ray reveals patchy collapse and cystic changes in over-inflated lungs. The infants remain dependant on IPPV, then CPAP and then added oxygen alone over a period of months. Some recover and appear to recover well, but others continue to need respiratory support and die of chronic respiratory failure, cor pulmonale or added infections.

Pulmonary haemorrhage may complicate asphyxia and atelectasis, or occasionally appear to be a primary problem. It also occurs during recovery from hypothermia.

Apnoeic attacks are a common problem in sick and preterm newborn infants. The respiration of infants at risk must be continually monitored. Physical stimuli are sufficient to provoke a gasp and the recommencement of breathing. Occasionally CPAP or intubation and supportive ventilation may be required. Respiratory stimulants like theophylline may help.

Pneumothorax may occur spontaneously but is also a common complication of respiratory distress syndrome and of meconium aspiration, especially when CPAP or IPPV are being used. The air leak can be confirmed by transilluminating the affected side with a powerful fibreoptic light or by x-ray. The air can be aspirated with a large syringe and needle, but will usually require placement of a chest drain.

Extra-pulmonary causes of respiratory distress

Three non-lung diseases may present with respiratory symptoms. Cerebral anoxia can produce bizarre respiratory patterns mimicking dyspnoea though more commonly cerebral asphyxia leads to hypoventilation. If lung expansion matches respiratory effort this possibility should be considered. Metabolic acidosis, frequently an outcome of disorders of aminoacid metabolism presents with hyperventilation, deep and effective breaths. Congenital heart disease is perhaps the most difficult to exclude. Auscultation may not help or be positively misleading; assessment of peripheral perfusion, an electrocardiograph and chest X-ray are often more helpful. Babies with cyanotic heart disease will not improve on breathing 100 per cent oxygen.

JAUNDICE IN THE NEWBORN

Many healthy normal newborn infants develop jaundice after birth. *In utero,*

The range of bilirubin concentrations in infants, and bile pigment metabolism

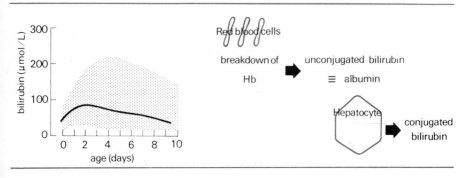

bilirubin crosses the placenta and is excreted by the mother. After birth, the infant must activate his own excretory systems but there is usually some delay and blood bilirubin concentrations rise. This 'physiological' jaundice appears at 2–3 days of age and begins disappearing towards the end of the first week; the bilirubin is largely unconjugated and the baby remains generally well. There is considerable variation from one infant to another. The condition is more severe and prolonged in preterm infants; if hypoxia and hypoglycaemia further limit bilirubin conjugation; and if the infant has an ileus or bowel obstruction then there may be increased enteric reabsorption of bilirubin. The diagnosis of physiological jaundice is made by the typical presentation, and by excluding other more serious causes.

Kernicterus

Unconjugated bilirubin is lipid soluble and travels in the circulation largely bound to albumin. It is the small fraction of free bilirubin which escapes from the vascular compartment and enters the cellular lipid fractions of the brain cells, which may cause transient or permanent damage, kernicterus. When this happens the infant behaves abnormally, feeds badly and may fit and develop opisthotonus when the back is arched and the head thrown back. If the infant recovers there is usually residual brain damage, often with severe choreoathetosis and mental handicap. High-tone deafness is common after hyperbilirubinaemia, and hearing should be tested carefully in early life.

In healthy full term infants unconjugated bilirubin concentrations above 380 umol/l are considered dangerous, but much lower thresholds apply to preterm babies and those who are sick. The risks are greater when albumin levels are low or when there is competition for albumin binding by, for example free fatty acids and drugs like sulphonamides and aspirin. Various diseases can cause unconjugated bilirubin to rise to dangerous levels, and these are best considered chronologically.

Jaundice in the first 24 hours of life

A few babies who are jaundiced at birth are suffering from one of the congenital infections which can cross the placenta and may severely damage the fetus: toxoplasmosis, rubella, cytomegalovirus, herpes virus and syphilis. The jaundice is usually mixed conjugated and unconjugated, and the babies have other abnormal signs of the infection. Most jaundice appearing in the first 24 hours is however due to excess haemolysis.

Haemolytic diseases of the newborn. Haemolysis of the newborn red cells may be caused by antibody from the mother. This will only happen if the maternal and fetal blood are incompatible. The haemolytic jaundice which causes some of the most severe problems is due to rhesus incompatibility. The problems occur after the mother has been sensitised by either a mismatched blood transfusion, or from fetal blood entering her circulation during a miscarriage or, more commonly, at the end of a previous pregnancy during labour and delivery. She reacts to the fetal blood by producing antibodies. The concentration of the antibodies are measured serially during pregnancy in affected mothers. It is these globulin antibodies which cross the placenta in increasing concentrations during the pregnancy, and which attack and haemolyse the red cells in the fetal circulation.

When the condition is mild, the fetus and newborn tolerate the small increase in haemolysis rate, although after birth the baby may become moderately jaundiced and have mild anaemia. With higher rates of haemolysis, the bilirubin levels in the fetus may still stay low because the unconjugated bilirubin passes back across the placenta and the fetus can tolerate moderate anaemia, but after birth the bilirubin concentrations rise rapidly and dangerous bilirubin levels may be reached within 24 hours. In the severe forms with high rates of haemolysis the fetus is unable to maintain his haemoglobin and becomes severely anaemic, and this with an associated general disturbance in fetal metabolism leads to severe oedema (hydrops fetalis), a condition which is usually fatal.

The aim of obstetric management is to deliver the baby before the anaemia becomes critical. A measure of the state of the fetus can be gained by serial analysis of amniotic fluid, taken by amniocentesis, for bilirubin products. If the fetus is very severely affected and too immature to be delivered, fetal blood transfusions can be given *in utero* to correct the anaemia. Rhesus incompatibility is now far less common, following the discovery that administration of anti-D antibodies to the mother immediately after birth destroys any red cells which might have leaked into the maternal circulation and so reduces the risks of the mother producing antibodies.

Incompatibility of the ABO system is more common, and produces a similar but usually milder clinical picture. The mother is usually group O and the baby A or B. There is a marked rise in the titres of the naturally occurring anti-A or Anti-B haemolysins, but these drop back to normal levels after the pregnancy, and the next pregnancy is not at greater risk, unlike rhesus disease.

Haemolysis may also be due to a deficiency of one of the red cell enzymes. Many Asian and Negro babies have relative lack of glucose-6-phosphate dehydrogenase. This can be found with a screening test. Those affected have to avoid a number of drugs which precipitate haemolysis. Finally abnormalities of the red cell shape, such as spherocytosis, can result in increased osmotic fragility and haemolysis.

Jaundice beginning on the 2nd to 5th day
Before jaundice at this age is labelled 'physiological', the baby has to be examined carefully to exclude any infection. Bruising, especially in forceps or breech deliveries, may be exacerbating the jaundice. The urine is checked for reducing sugars to exclude galactosaemia, and sent for a metabolic screen if the baby is acidotic and ill.

Jaundice from the end of the 2nd week onwards
Many babies who are being breast fed have a prolongation of their jaundice. This does not rise to harmful levels, and the mother is encouraged to continue breast feeding, but the diagnosis can only be made by exclusion. Thyroid function tests are needed to exclude cretinism. Distinguishing between neonatal hepatitis and biliary atresia is both difficult and important, because early surgery is essential in the atresia but would exacerbate hepatitis (p. 163).

Causes of neonatal jaundice, by time of appearance

Early neonatal	Prolonged neonatal
Haemolytic disease of newborn	Liver disease
Bruising and petechia, haemorrhages due to asphyxia and birth trauma	Infection
Glucose G6PD deficiency	Infants of diabetic mother
Inherited red cell anomalies	Hypothyroidism
E. coli septicaemia.	Galactosaemia
	Breast milk jaundice
	Biliary atresia

Management of neonatal jaundice

Having established the cause of the jaundice, bilirubin levels can be measured serially. This is especially important in the haemolytic diseases since the bilirubin level may rise rapidly. Good hydration and an adequate calorie intake help the liver to conjugate the bilirubin efficiently. The hyperbilirubinaemia can be treated by using phototherapy. Light of wavelength 450 nm from the blue-band of the visible spectrum (*not* ultraviolet) converts unconjugated bilirubin by photodegradation to a biliverdin-like pigment which is water soluble and harmless. Light of the correct wavelength is produced by fluorescent tubes or more specialised blue lamps. Care is needed with temperature control and fluid balance.

If there is a risk of the bilirubin rising to dangerous levels in spite of phototherapy and the measures above, then an exchange transfusion is performed. During this procedure blood is alternately withdrawn and transfused in 10 to 20 ml aliquots via a catheter in the umbilical vein, until 60 to 70 per cent of the infant's red blood cells have been replaced. In rhesus incompatibility an exchange transfusion is often needed shortly after birth, even before bilirubin levels have had time to rise, in order to remove from the baby's circulation the antibodies which are causing the haemolysis.

Haemorrhagic disease of the newborn

This coagulation disturbance arises from vitamin K deficiency and the resulting impairment of hepatic production of factors II, VII, IX and X. It characteristically develops between the second and fourth days of life and presents with gastrointestinal bleeding. Breast fed infants, premature infants and those exposed to perinatal asphyxia are most at risk. The occasional tragedy due to this readily preventable condition merits the prophylactic use of vitamin K_1 in all newborn infants shortly after birth (oral or intramuscular dose 0.5 to 1 mg).

GASTROINTESTINAL PROBLEMS

Oesophageal atresia

Oesophageal atresia (incidence 1:2500) is usually associated with a tracheo-oesophageal fistula. In every infant born to a mother with hydramnios, it should be excluded by passing a firm, large-bore (12 G) tube through the mouth into the stomach. After birth, the affected infant is unable to swallow his own saliva and bubbles fluid from the mouth, another sign requiring investigation. It is always a sad event when the diagnosis is made only after the child has choked over his first feed. It is the condition of the lungs as well as the extent of the abnormality which dictates the success of surgical correction.

The diagnosis is confirmed radiologically by passing a firm, radio-opaque tube into the upper pouch and taking a lateral film of the chest, and an antero-posterior film of the chest and abdomen. Air in the stomach confirms the presence of a fistula. Associated anomalies may include ano-rectal agenesis and cardiac defects, particularly Fallot tetralogy.

Oesophageal atresia with diaphragmatic hernia

tracheo-oesophageal fistulae

85%　8%　4.5%　diaphragmatic hernia

Congenital diaphragmatic hernia

Congenital diaphragmatic hernia (incidence 1:2200) is due to a defect of the hemidiaphragm, usually the left. Where the diaphragmatic defect is the only anomaly, the baby may appear well at birth, but observation will show a deep chest and a scaphoid abdomen. Respiratory distress develops as the child swallows air, which passes into the small bowel within the chest cavity. The resulting mediastinal shift leads to compression of the previously unaffected lung. The diagnosis is confirmed by x-rays of chest and abdomen. A nasogastric tube should be passed to empty the stomach and small bowel. Endotracheal intubation and ventilation may be necessary pre-operatively.

Babies with diaphragmatic hernias may also have bilateral pulmonary hypoplasia so that even initial resuscitation is impossible, or a major heart defect, which in itself may be incompatible with survival.

All cases of diaphragmatic hernia are associated with abnormalities of gut rotation.

Small bowel obstruction

The most common form of organic obstruction of the small bowel is meconium ileus. Other causes of small bowel obstruction in the neonatal period include atresia, stenosis and diaphragms of the duodenum, jejunum or ileum, midgut volvulus 'volvulus neonatorum', Ladd's band associated with failure of caecal descent, enterogenous cyst and milk curd obstruction. Meconium ileus and atretic lesions will present very early with distension and vomiting within hours of birth. The other lesions may not produce symptoms for some days or even a week or two after birth.

B – The higher up the gut the lesion
⇒ the earlier the symptoms present!

Duodenal atresia and small bowel atresia

duodenal atresia	'double bubble'	ileal atresia	fluid levels

Vomiting of green rather than yellow bile-stained material is suggestive of organic obstruction. Meconium may or may not have been passed in the early hours of life. The area of distension will depend on the level of the obstruction; in duodenal obstruction it is confined to the upper abdomen, in ileal obstruction it is generalised. Erect X-rays of the abdomen should be taken, and may be diagnostic, for example, the double-bubble of duodenal atresia, the ground glass appearance of some cases of meconium ileus, and the calcification of an ileal atresia with prenatal perforation. In other cases fluid levels may be present but these do not necessarily indicate mechanical obstruction. They will be present in functional ileus, and in a baby with ileus secondary to septicaemia.

May be present in the 1st few days of life!

Large bowel obstruction

In the neonate there are two main causes of large bowel obstruction, Hirschsprung's disease and ano-rectal agenesis. The former is the more common, and it is suggested by delay in the passage of meconium beyond 24 hours. The baby may appear otherwise well for a few days but is liable to become suddenly and acutely distended, with peripheral circulatory collapse, a feature of a 'Hirschsprung's enterocolitis'.

Ano-rectal agenesis is an all embracing name for a very large number of anatomical anomalies. Basically there are two types of ano-rectal agenesis, high

Anorectal agenesis

normal	'High' agenesis with or without fistula into urogenital tract	'Low' agenesis—covered or anterior ectopic anus, both usually with stenosis

and low, depending on whether the bowel ends above or below the pelvic floor. All low anomalies are easily treated at birth by a perineal procedure. High anomalies require a temporary colostomy; in boys there is always a fistula into bladder or urethra; in girls there may be a fistula into the vagina.

Most babies with ano-rectal agenesis have no visible anus at birth: it is extremely rare for the anal canal to be present but not communicating with the upper bowel (rectal atresia).

Exomphalos and gastroschisis

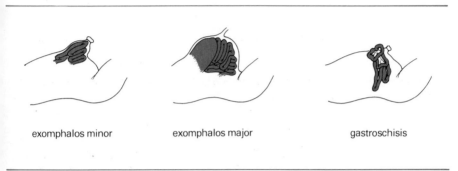

exomphalos minor   exomphalos major   gastroschisis

Exomphalos
Exomphalos is a persistence of the herniation of the gut into the extra-embryonic part of the umbilical cord which is normally present between the sixth and fourteenth weeks of intrauterine life. Occasionally complete return of the gut into the abdominal cavity does not occur, the bowel which remains outside will be obvious at birth. In its mild form one or two loops of bowel are seen in the base of the cord, exomphalos minor; at its most severe a huge swelling occurs in the centre of the abdomen containing most of the abdominal contents (exomphalos major). The gut is covered by membrane. In gastroschisis there is a defect in the abdominal wall to the right of a normal umbilical cord. Gut prolapses through the defect and has no covering.

NEURAL TUBE ANOMALIES

The neural tube should be completely formed and closed throughout its entire length by the end of the third week of intrauterine life. The process starts at the 14th day with thickening of the dorsal ectoderm to form the neural plate. The neural plate starts folding into a groove and by about 22 to 23 days complete fusion of the groove has occurred to form the neural tube. Fusion commences in the mid dorsal region and extends towards the head and tail of the embryo.

Catastrophies at this very early stage of development may cause severe neural tube anomalies and result in intra-uterine death. Despite this fetal loss, two to three per 1000 liveborn infants have a neural tube defect of some sort, about half are due to anencephaly.

The normal development of the spinal cord

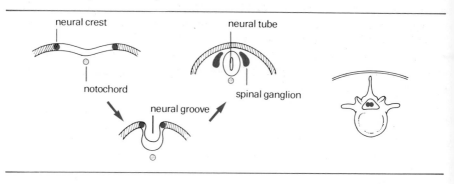

Anencephaly

Anencephaly is a tragic deformity in which most of the infants are stillborn, but if liveborn survive only a few hours.

Cranium bifidum defects

Cranium bifidum defects are relatively uncommon. The minor lesions are eminently treatable; all that is required is a good skin cover, and the prognosis is excellent, for there is no associated spinal neurological lesion, and the incidence of hydrocephalus is low. An occipital meningocele, even when very large, is also treatable, although hydrocephalus is more likely. The overall prognosis is still good. On the other hand, a large encephalocele is not open to treatment, for surgery usually means either excision of a mass of brain tissue or a closure which results in raised intracranial pressure.

Cranium bifidum

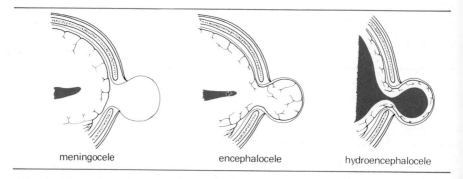

meningocele   encephalocele   hydroencephalocele

Spina bifida

Spina bifida defects are common. The number of infants born with major 'open' defects has fallen considerably in the last few years due, in part, to the widespread introduction of screening procedures.

   Spina bifida cystica defects vary from a meningeal sac full of cerebrospinal fluid with a normal placement of the spinal cord (a meningocele), to the exposure and complete unfolding of the spinal cord on the surface of the child's back (a myelomeningocele).

Spina bifida cystica

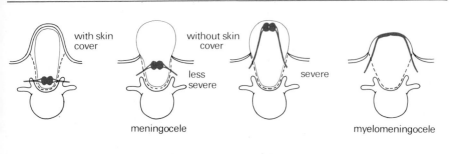

Meningocele is less common and has a good prognosis. Neurological problems with the lower limbs and hydrocephalus are rare, but partial neurological deficit affecting the bladder is not uncommon. Virtually all babies with a meningocele will be treated surgically in the first days of life. During infancy they may develop minor foot problems and bladder dysfunction but they usually can cope well. Children with meningoceles should be followed up throughout the whole of their growing period since neurological problems may develop with growth of the spine.

Myelomeningocele is both more common and more serious. It is usually located in the lumbo-sacral region. The range of severity varies considerably. A child with a small lumbo-sacral myelomeningocele, which is closed on the first day of life, may with careful attention have good mobility, normal bladder function and intellect. On the other hand, a baby with an extensive thoraco-lumbar myelomeningocele is likely to have no functioning motor or sensory nerves distal to his nipple line. His skin will be completely anaesthetic and therefore at risk of trauma; his trunk and limbs will be paralysed and either completely flaccid or deformed as a result of reflex activity. Involuntary movements may be seen. The bladder and bowel will be paralysed and insensitive. Hydrocephalus is present in 80% of infants with myelomeningocele.

Early management. Every baby with spina bifida cystica should have full and expert assessment as soon as possible after birth to determine the extent of neurological deficit; the presence or otherwise of hydrocephalus, the extent of bony deformity of the spine; and the coexistence of any other congenital abnormality. This will permit an estimate to be made of his potential. The decision to operate can only be taken after a full and open discussion between surgeon and parents. Many babies with extensive defects will die within a short time whether their lesions are covered with skin or not. In these instances, early surgery would not

Survival of children with myelomeningocele — effect of surgery (after Lorber)

Age at death	No surgery	Surgery
0–1 month	37.5%	20%
1–12 months	37.5%	20%
1–5 years	10%	10%
Survival over 5 years	15%	50%

seem to be justified. On the other hand, a baby with a lesser lesion is still at risk of infection and the complications of hydrocephalus even after surgery. It is a mistake to think that all babies will survive if operated upon and that those with uncorrected lesions will always die. One can only say that the majority of babies with minor lesions and a good prognosis will survive with treatment to adult life, and that most babies with very major lesions will die without treatment.

Long term management. Once active treatment is commenced the child's management should be directed by a team consisting of an orthopaedic surgeon, a paediatric surgeon, and a physiotherapist. The facilities of an assessment unit are useful, and close contact with local schools for the physically handicapped is essential. Orthopaedic problems are particularly common in those children with unbalanced lower limb function. Urinary tract infections, urinary obstruction, ureteric reflux and urinary incontinence are common. The latter in girls may necessitate ileal loop diversion. A ventriculoperitoneal or atrial shunt is usually required to control hydrocephalus. The complications of these shunts are blockage and infection, and they may be very troublesome. The anaesthetic skin

The treatment of hydrocephalus

is also a problem especially in the more mobile child; pressure sores and accidental burns are likely to occur. Learning and psychological problems may add to the child's troubles in the school years but their unhappiness may be most profound when they begin to realise the full meaning of their handicap, with regard to job prospects, sex and marriage.

The quality of life in children over five after surgery for myelomeningocele (after Lorber)

18% mild/moderate physical handicap and normal IQ
49% severe physical handicap and normal IQ
33% severe physical handicap and borderline or subnormal IQ

Spina bifida occulta is a common anomaly, said to occur in up to 20% of normal individuals. Most people with an occult deficit are asymptomatic. Occasionally the bony defect is associated with a hairy patch or a birth mark on the back. A few children with spina bifida occulta develop a mild spastic gait, or bladder problems with spinal growth due to tethering of the cord, a split notochord syndrome, or an associated intraspinal dermoid or lipoma. Myelography may be necessary.

Spina bifida occulta and the split notochord syndrome

spina bifida occulta

split notochord syndrome
(diastematomyelia) with
meningocele

Hydrocephalus without spina bifida

This may result from a congenital abnormality of the brain, for example aqueduct stenosis, or it may follow an intracranial bleed, or early neonatal infection. It depends to some extent on the aetiology, but on the whole the prognosis is good and all babies should be treated. They should all have a CT scan before surgery is performed. Later abilities are likely to be very reasonable, unless shunt complications occur.

CLEFT LIP AND PALATE — One child affected · Risk 1:25   ♂ > ♀.
Two   "   " 1:10   Left H.Side

The middle third of the face develops as the result of migration and fusion of mesodermal folds covered by ectoderm. The earlier or primary palate creates the olfactory pits, and failure of fusion results in unilateral, bilateral or, rarely, median cleft lip. The secondary palate originates from folds on either side of the tongue. These rise above the tongue and fuse in the mid-line to form the true palate. Cleft palates occur when tissue migration is disorganised or obstructed by the tongue. It is sometimes the result of a small mandible. (Pierre-Robin Syndrome)

Cleft lip and palate are common, 1 in 600 births. The majority are isolated abnormalities but they may be part of a chromosomal or other malformation syndrome. The family history is often positive, and most clefts are determined by polygenic inheritance which influences the threshold to ill-defined environmental factors. Occasional cases have been linked to maternal corticosteroid

etiological :
recently found Genetic Marker : Growth factor
ass. ē α. Gene?

Malformations of soft and hard palate

alveolus
hard
palate
soft
palate

uvula

| Normal | Cleft of soft palate | + hard palate | + alveolus | + bilateral alveolus |

(handwritten top margin, left):
1/3 – lip only.
1/4 – Palate only
⇒ < 1/2 – Both.

(handwritten top margin, right):
Cleft Palate only: ♀ > ♂.
-one child affected – Risk 1:50

therapy. One-third of clefts are limited to the lip, one-quarter to the palate and the remainder involve both.

(handwritten right margin): Ass. Problems: Recurring ear infec (glue drainag) Tongue tie. Mucosal pits of lip. Micrognathia.

(handwritten left margin): > Problems - feeding (sucking) - May use a "feeding plate".

Management *(handwritten):* — imp to strengthen Tongue.

The alarming facial appearance calls for prompt counselling of the parents, preferably with 'before and after' photographs to emphasise the successful outcome of corrective surgery. Feeding problems can usually be overcome by using a soft teat with an enlarged hole and by nursing the baby erect. Those with a cleft lip may cope with breast feeding.

The aims of surgery are to provide a good cosmetic result and an adequate speech mechanism. The usual practice is to repair the cleft lip at three months of age and the palate at six months or later. Too early a repair may interfere with mid-facial growth. An orthodontist may be able to provide a plate to reduce the cleft size during the waiting period.

In the later years additional specialist help is required to overcome Eustachian tube obstruction, speech delay and dental problems. *(handwritten):* (When 2nd dentition comes need further orthodontic t prevent collapse of arch

Pierre-Robin syndrome
(handwritten): If do not get adequate closure of Nasopharynx - Do pharyngoplasty @ 10-12 yrs.

Pierre-Robin Syndrome refers to severe micrognathia with a secondary cleft palate. The affected infants are susceptible to feeding and respiratory problems, and require expert nursing until the mandible grows.

Treacher-Collins syndrome
Treacher-Collins Syndrome encompasses a spectrum of ear and facial malformations caused by first and second pharyngeal arch developmental failure.

CLUB FOOT p. 252

(handwritten right): * Rule of 10.
- 10 wks
- > 10 lbs we
- 10 g Hb.

DISLOCATED HIP p. 248

NEONATAL INFECTIONS

Newborn babies can die from infections before anyone is aware that they are ill. The signs of a systemic infection are generalised and often not specific to a particular system. Apparently trivial infections can rapidly lead to systemic sepsis, especially in the preterm baby.

Systemic infections
If an infant goes 'off his feed', handles badly, has an unexpected body temperature up or down, or develops unusual respiratory patterns, fits or apnoeic spells, he should be thoroughly examined at all sites for signs of possible infection. A 'septic screen' is performed in which samples of blood, urine, and cerebrospinal fluid are taken for examination and culture, together with swabs from eyes, ears, throat, umbilicus and rectum. While awaiting the results of the investigations the ill baby should be started immediately on an antibiotic combination parenterally

to cover the common pathogens of the newborn period: *Group B streptococcus*, *Staphylococcus aureus*, *Escherichia coli*, and the Gram negative organisms pseudomonas, klebsiella, proteus. Widely used combinations are gentamicin and penicillin G in the first week of life, and gentamicin and flucloxacillin thereafter; others prefer third generation cephalosporins. When the results of the septic screen are known, the length of treatment can be decided, and the antibiotics altered to cover a particular organism more thoroughly or in accordance to the antibiotic sensitivities of the organisms grown. Serious infections include septicaemia, meningitis, pneumonia, urinary tract infections, gastro-enteritis, and osteomyelitis. Further investigations and follow-up will be needed depending on which of these is present.

Neonatal meningitis. Neonatal meningitis has high mortality and morbidity rates. Penicillin is used to cover the possibility of Group B streptococcal meningitis, and a third generation cephalosporin such as cefotaxime or ceftazidime can be combined with gentamicin to cover the other organisms. Chloramphenicol is effective but must be given in specially adjusted doses for the newborn with monitoring of blood levels in order to avoid toxic effects (the 'grey baby' syndrome). It is best avoided if at all possible. Treatment of meningitis must continue for two to three weeks. Ultrasound scanning is used to identify any developing hydrocephalus.

Superficial infections

Conjunctivitis. Sticky eye is a common problem. Usually there is no underlying infection, and after taking swabs for culture, saline washes are all that is required. However sometimes, conjunctivitis is due to a staphylococcal infection, less commonly streptococcal or pseudomonal organisms. It may also be caused by organisms acquired from the mother's birth canal, in particular *Neisseria gonorrhoeae* and *Chlamydia trachomatis*. Both are sexually transmitted diseases. The latter is also responsible for the eye disease, trachoma.

If conjunctival inflammation and pus is present then swabs should be taken into standard and into chlamydial transport medium for Gram and Giemsa staining and appropriate cultures. Scrapings should also be taken from the inside of the lower eyelid with a swab on a stick, smeared onto glass slides, allowed to dry and examined in the laboratory for chlamydial inclusion bodies.

Gonococcal eye infections can involve the cornea and damage the whole eye very rapidly, and, to prevent this, significant eye infections on the first day or two, should be presumed to be gonococcal until proved otherwise and treated vigorously with penicillin given parenterally, as well as very frequent cleaning and eye drops. Chlamydial infections are now common and must be treated with both 1% tetracycline eye drops and oral erythromycin. Ordinary bacterial infections such as staphylococci are well treated with chloramphenicol eye drops or ointment.

Septic spots. Small septic spots and blisters are not unusual, especially in the skin creases, and are commonly due to staphylococcal infections. The baby can be washed with a soap containing an antibacterial agent such as chlorhexidine.

If there are only a few lesions they can be cultured, and cleaned with a spirit swab. More extensive lesions should be treated with systemic flucloxacillin.

Umbilical infections. The umbilical cord dries and usually drops off after a few days. The residual sticky stump can be treated with local antiseptic powder but if the surrounding area becomes inflamed with an offensive discharge, swabs and a systemic antibiotic are needed.

Thrush. This is a fungal infection. Inside the mouth it is recognized by adherent white plaques on the buccal membranes and the tongue. Treatment is with nystatin oral suspension or miconazole oral gel. On the perineum the candida produces a rash with red colonies around the anus and in the groins. Nystatin cream is used. The mouth should be checked for involvement.

NEONATAL CONVULSIONS AND JITTERS

Many normal newborn babies react to minor physical stimuli or loud noises with startle responses. It can be difficult to distinguish these normal 'jitters' from intermittent focal fits (twitching) and generalised tonic spasms. If the jitteriness seems excessive a blood sample is taken to exclude hypoglycaemia, and low levels of calcium, magnesium, or sodium. If the baby also seems unwell an infection screen including a lumbar puncture must be carried out. If the cause is still not determined a search is made for less common inherited metabolic disorders, and for congenital infections and CNS malformations.

Causes of convulsions in newborn infants

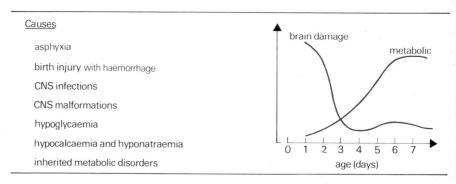

Causes

asphyxia

birth injury with haemorrhage

CNS infections

CNS malformations

hypoglycaemia

hypocalcaemia and hyponatraemia

inherited metabolic disorders

brain damage

metabolic

age (days)

Treatment. Treatment is directed at the cause. If the blood glucose is reduced below 1.7 mmol/l (1.1 mmol/l in preterms), the hypoglycaemia is corrected urgently with 25% glucose (2 ml/kg) followed by a 10% dextrose infusion. Hypocalcaemic fits are uncommon since the introduction of low phosphate milks, and normal levels vary considerably making interpretation difficult, but if fits are thought to be related to low plasma levels, 0.5 ml/kg of 10% calcium gluconate can be given intravenously, slowly and under ECG monitoring, followed up by oral supplements added to the feeds. If an infant's hypocalcaemia seems resistant to correction he may well have hypomagnesaemia as well, and this can be treated with 0.1 ml/kg of 50% magnesium sulphate intramuscularly or very slowly intravenously. Hyponatraemia responds to fluid restriction if it is dilutional, or to sodium supplements if there is a true deficiency.

If life-threatening convulsions are continuing in spite of these metabolic corrections they should be stopped with diazepam infusion 0.4 mg/kg given intravenously slowly, followed by a high loading dose of phenobarbitone 20 mg/kg and maintenance at 2 mg/kg 12-hourly. Rectal paraldehyde in arachis oil can be helpful if breakthrough fits still occur. Meanwhile meningitis must be excluded and investigations set in train to find any other underlying cause. The management is particularly difficult where the fits are due to severe birth trauma or asphyxia. The large doses of anti-convulsants required severely depress the baby's respiration. Surprisingly the prognosis in neonatal convulsions is favourable in the absence of meningitis and obvious cerebral damage, with 70% having normal development at long-term follow-up.

BIBLIOGRAPHY

Avery M E, Taeusch H W 1984 Schaffer's diseases of the newborn, 5th ed. Saunders, Philadelphia
Carter C O 1976 Genetics of common single malformations. British Medical Bulletin 32: 21–26
Chiswick M L 1983 Recent advances in perinatal medicine 1. Churchill Livingstone, Edinburgh
Davis J A, Richards M P M, Robertson N R C 1983 Parent–baby attachments in premature infants. Croom Helm, London
Fanaroff A A, Martin R J 1983 Behrman's neonatal-perinatal medicine, 3rd edn. Mosby, St. Louis
Levene M I, William J L, Fawer C 1985 Ultrasound of the infant brain. Spastics International Medical Publications, London
Lissauer T 1981 Neonatal resuscitation. Hospital Update 7: 109–126
McCracken G H, Nelson J D 1983 Antimicrobial therapy for newborns, 2nd edn. Grune & Stratton, New York
Macfarlane A 1977 The Psychology of childbirth. Fontana, London
O'Doherty N 1979 Atlas of the newborn. MTP Press, Lancaster
Office of Population Censuses and Surveys 1983 Mortality statistics — perinatal and infant: social and biological factors. Report DH3 No 9. HMSO, London
Remington J S, Klein J O 1983 Infectious diseases of the fetus and newborn infant, 2nd edn. Saunders, Philadelphia
Roberton N R C 1981 A manual of neonatal intensive care. Arnold, London
Roberton N R C 1986 Textbook of Neonatology. Churchill Livingstone, Edinburgh

Neural tube anomalies
Lorber J 1975 Ethical problems in the management of myelomeningocele and hydrocephalus. Journal of the Royal College of Physicians 10: 47–60
Stark G D 1977 Spina bifida. Problems and management. Blackwell, Oxford

5
Nutrition

15 pages.

The nutrients supplied to the young in early development are uniquely and sensitively adjusted to their requirements. During intrauterine life a mixture of water, salts, proteins, carbohydrates and fats, which are drawn from the maternal blood stream and processed by the placenta, enters the fetal circulation and determines the substrates that are available for growth and energy metabolism. After birth, the breast produces a specialised total food in an acceptable and digestable form. Breast milk production is a characteristic of mammals. The mixture of nutrients in their milk varies widely from one species to another and this is to be expected for the rates of growth of the young at birth and their motor activities are very different. In view of this it is perhaps surprising that the young of one species can be reared effectively on the milk of another. But this is so, for some decades now it has been a common practice to rear human infants on cow's milk. So successful has it been in Western Societies that the advantages of human breast milk are being questioned! Breast feeding benefits both mother and child in many ways and therefore mothers should be given every encouragement to breast feed their infants, however for those who are unable to do so it is important to reassure them that there are other ways of rearing their infant successfully.

Major constituents of various mammalian milks

Hormones involved in lactation

BREAST FEEDING

During pregnancy many endocrine agents prepare the breast for lactation. These include lactogen (human chorionic somatomammotropin), which is secreted by the placenta, and prolactin which is released by the pituitary gland and is important not only in initiating milk secretion but also in maintaining milk production after birth. Suckling is a powerful stimulus both to prolactin release from the anterior pituitary gland and to the secretion of oxytocin from the posterior pituitary gland. Oxytocin stimulates the ejection or 'let down' of milk by acting on the myoepithelial cells which surround the alveoli and ductules.

Technical problems

Even from this brief outline, it is obvious that breast feeding is a complex process which might break down at a number of stages. For example, the breast and nipple may be ill-formed, although appropriate care during pregnancy can do much to encourage adequate development. Milk production may not be initiated and maintained at a rate fast enough to suit a hungry baby or may flow too quickly for an ill or sleepy infant. If the full breast is not emptied then it may become engorged and inflamed, and the resulting pressure and pain will inhibit further milk production. Gentle manual expression of milk will avoid this complication. Finally, the unhappy, nervous, drowsy or sick mother may not be able to 'let down' her milk as she would wish or a lethargic, sick, newborn baby may not stimulate her to do so.

Breast anatomy and milk production

Breast feeding does not seem to be a basic instinct; many mothers who have not seen others breast feeding need considerable guidance initially. A simple explanation of how the breast works is often very helpful and avoids unnecessary anxiety. Should it be desirable to discontinue breast feeding, this can be achieved most simply by firm breast support and analgesia.

Constituents of breast milk

As a food, milk has some remarkable characteristics. Most of the carbohydrate is in the form of a disaccharide, lactose, which requires a specific disaccharidase for its digestion. The fats are present mainly as triglyceride in globules surrounded by lipoproteins which are probably remnants of the walls of the alveolar cells. The individual fatty acids reflect the mother's diet and her fat stores. If mothers are on low fat diets then the alveolar cells themselves make saturated fatty acid with chain lengths of 12 to 16 carbons. The protein content of human milk is surprisingly low but a large percentage is in the form of the more easily digestible whey, rather than indigestible curds. Whey contains in addition to lactalbumin, proteins which influence the infant's bowel bacterial flora, namely lactoferrin, lysozyme and IgA. Breast milk also contains vitamins, minerals, enzymes, especially lipase, and cells. The latter are predominantly macrophages and act either to keep the lacteals free from infection or to assist in the defence of the intestinal tract.

The relative amounts of the constituents vary. The first milk produced after birth, colostrum, is rich in protein and cells but the volume is small. When feeding is established, the mature milk constituents vary diurnally and from day to day. The milk at the end of a feed, hind milk, has a higher fat content than fore milk. The content of milk is also modified by the maternal diet and well-being, and by the mother's general level of nutrition.

Advantages of breast feeding

If a mother wishes and is able to breast feed then she should be supported in this and given every encouragement to do so. Human milk is an excellent nutrient mixture which also gives the baby some protection against infection. Its protein content is less likely to induce allergic reactions and the infant may be less at risk from unexplained sudden death. The process of breast feeding usually gives satisfaction and pleasure to mother and child and this in itself will be of lasting benefit to both.

Technically, breast feeding is easier than bottle feeding in as much as the mother is not required to make up the mixture according to instruction, and sterilising bottles is not a problem.

In western societies breast feeding may be economic, but elsewhere it certainly is.

Some mothers are anxious that breast feeding or, alternatively, not breast feeding may alter the contour of the breast but there is little evidence one way or the other. Under non-lactating conditions the shape of the breast is largely determined by fat cells rather than the mammary gland. However, pregnancies and age are certainly two major factors leading to change.

Approximately 9 out of 10 women who are feeding their babies do not ovulate;

Breast milk

Days after birth	colostrum 0-5	transitional 5-10	mature 10+	
g/100 ml milk	5.7	6.9	7.4	carbohydrate
	2.3	3.9	4.2	fat
	2.3	2.0	1.1	protein

but nevertheless breast feeding should not be regarded as a method of contraception.

Cancer of the breast is less common in women who have borne children and breast fed them.

Why mothers do not breast feed
Mothers give a variety of reasons when asked why they have chosen not to breast feed. Some women just do not like the thought of breast feeding and, given an alternative, they take it. Others are embarrassed or uncertain and fear that they will fail or develop sore nipples and swollen, painful breasts. Some mothers obviously believe that bottle feeding is an easier and more certain way of ensuring their baby grows well and sleeps regularly. Others feel that bottle feeding offers greater freedom by, for instance, making it possible for them to return to work and to take the contraceptive pill. They might, perhaps, feel differently if they were better informed and more carefully prepared during the antenatal period; for example, once lactation is established, the contraceptive pill can be taken without it influencing breast feeding.

Contraindications
For some mothers, breast feeding is just not possible or may be contraindicated. For example, successful breast feeding is difficult with twins and virtually impossible with triplets; and in a premature birth, neither breasts nor baby are prepared for feeding. It is possible with manual techniques to establish breast feeding for these infants who initially are unable to suckle satisfactorily, but it requires a great deal of resolve on the mother's part.

If the mother has been chronically ill, severely undernourished, subject to severe asthmatic episodes or has limited renal function, breast feeding may be an unacceptable drain on her reserves. Similarly, mothers with diabetes may find that the metabolic challenge of producing milk upsets their diabetic state. Active tuberculosis in the mother is a contraindication to breast feeding until the infant has been immunised.

Most drugs taken by the mother enter the milk. For practical purposes it can be estimated that one-tenth of the dose given to the mother enters the milk so that the possibility that a drug given to a breast-feeding mother may affect her baby must always be kept in mind.

Some babies with abnormalities of the mouth, particularly cleft palate, are unable to suckle satisfactorily and breast feeding is virtually impossible. Tongue tie, unless it is in a very extreme form with forking of the tongue, should not interfere with the baby's ability to suckle.

Babies with inherited disorders of digestion or metabolism may not be able to tolerate the nutrients in human or other natural milks and special formulae have to be prepared. The inherited mono- and disaccharide intolerances, galactosaemia and phenylketonuria fall into this group.

ARTIFICIAL FEEDING

Artificial feeding in babies who suck well is usually by the bottle, but a spoon, cup, or plastic feeding tube may be used. The currently fashionable bottle sits on its base and has a wide neck surmounted by a rubber teat or nipple. Between feeds it must be washed with cold and then warm water and sterilised. The hole in the teat must be large enough to allow the baby to take his feeds in under fifteen minutes but not so large that the feed flows so quickly as to cause the baby to splutter and choke. If a baby is unable to suck or swallow, or too weak or breathless to complete the feed, then he can be fed via a fine plastic nasogastric tube. This procedure properly performed is simple, safe and well tolerated by the infants. It has probably saved more lives than any other innovation in neonatal care. In certain situations the end of the tube may be advanced into the duodenum or jejunum.

Disadvantages of cow's milk
The feed is usually cow's milk modified in some way. Many babies have been reared successfully on ordinary pasteurised or sterilised cow's milk, reconstituted evaporated liquid, or dried powdered cow's milk, but there have been problems. Some have been due to the way cow's milk differs from human milk. Cow's milk contains more protein, in particular more curd protein or casein, and these thick curds being less easy to digest have caused bowel obstruction. Cow's milk contains more fat and phosphorus. In the early weeks of life, particularly from 5 to 15 days of age, this may lead to hypocalcaemia with subsequent fitting. Cow's milk has a relatively high sodium content and this, with the tendency of

Contents of artificial infant feeds

	Cow's Milk	Modified Cow's Milk	Highly modified Cow's Milk	Soy feed
Energy Kcal	66	65	68	60
Protein g	3.5	1.9	1.5	2.0
Casein (Curds)	80%	80%	40%	0%
Fat g	3.7	3.5	3.8	3.0
Vegetable oil	—	+++	+++	+++
Carbohydrate g	4.9	6.9	7.2	6.7
Ca mg	117	85	54	55
Na mg	50	25	18	30
Fe mg	0.05	0.5	0.5	0.6

mothers to make strong or concentrated feeds from powdered or condensed milks leads to hypernatraemia, which may cause fits and brain damage, complications which are more likely during superimposed episodes of infection, particularly gastroenteritis. Some infants are allergic to cow's milk protein; they may react to feeding with perioral rashes and oedema or by vomiting or passing frequent loose stools which usually contain blood.

Makers of infant feeds now prepare a variety of modified cow's milk formulae, which have been 'humanised' in that the mixture more closely resembles that found in average mature human milk. This has posed considerable problems for manufacturers, for milk is a complex colloid mixture and, as such, it is very sensitive to any attempts to change it. In addition, manufacturers can only modify and supplement cow's milk to resemble human milk as far as their knowledge of the constituents of human milk permits. Pyridoxine was added to formulae only after its deficiency had led to fits in artificially fed babies. They cannot of course add the 'living elements', cells and enzymes, and at the moment we do not know how important these are.

Nutritional requirements

If a breast-fed child is content and growing, one need not trouble to consider the volume and nutrient value of each feed. There are, however, many reasons why an adequately breast-fed child may not be content or may not be growing satisfactorily. The nutrient intake of artificially fed infants is as much determined by the giver as the receiver and is more easily assessed. It is this facility which tempts some mothers whose infants are not thriving on the breast to change to bottle feeding, for then she and her health advisers can at least see the feed going in! Thus, it is essential in both breast and artificially fed infants to be able to assess their nutrient intake and their nutritional status.

Nutrient intake in breast-fed babies may be assessed by weighing the baby before and after feeds, that is by carrying out a test feed. In artificially-fed babies it is advisable to watch the mother make up and give at least one feed before

Daily milk intake of healthy, thriving, free-feeding babies. Just for interest, breast milk consumption is expressed per baby, artificial feeding is given per kg body weight

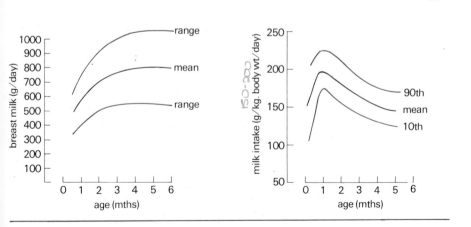

calculating a daily intake from the history of feed volume and frequency. Nutritional status is usually assessed from the infant's weight, a visual evaluation of the quality of the skin and by the amount and distribution of subcutaneous fat. More information can be gained by measuring length or height and skin fold thicknesses. Appetite and metabolic efficiency vary from infant to infant, much as they do in adults. The average intake of healthy infants can be used as a guide, but it must be remembered that the range is wide and each infant's needs must be assessed individually.

FEEDING PROBLEMS

New mothers often wish to be reassured that their babies are feeding normally. If there are problems, they may seek advice from more experienced members of the family or from shop keepers who sell milk foods, or midwives, community nurses and health visitors and it is to be expected that they will be given differing opinions. Occasionally, the problem is of such magnitude that medical advice is sought. The doctor must be aware of, or take advice about, the general abilities, approach and attitudes of the parents, the mother's feeding technique and the infant's nutrient intake, before considering the possibility of more serious underlying conditions.

Vomiting

Most babies swallow air with their milk. Gentle patting or massage of their backs helps them bring back the 'wind'. Most babies bring up a little milk as well; this is called posseting and is unimportant.

Occasionally, infants regurgitate large amounts of milk, either immediately after a feed or between feeds. It is rare for this to be sufficiently severe to affect the infant's nutrition but it does distress his mother; and, apart from other considerations, it makes all her clothes and furnishings smell and it fills her washing basket. Various strategies may be tried. By not allowing the baby to cry or become too upset before a feed and using good feeding techniques excess air swallowing can be avoided. Using agents which thicken the feed like cornflour or carob seed flour also reduces the baby's ability to bring them back. Propping the baby up after a feed may also help.

Some babies enjoy bringing their feeds back, 'ruminating' like a cow. This habit may be difficult to break but it will become less of a problem as the infant's diet, abilities and interests change.

There is no clear distinction between regurgitation and vomiting. An underlying cause must be sought if a baby suddenly starts to be sick, if the vomit contains blood or bile, if the vomiting persists to the point of dehydration or malnutrition, or is associated with other signs and symptoms. Vomiting may be the first indication of a general infection; it may be the only clue to an infected throat; it is common in pyelonephritis and is usual in meningitis and gastroenteritis. Certain disorders of the oesophagus and stomach must also be considered.

Clinical significance of gastro-oesophageal reflux

Reflux of gastric contents into the oesophagus is an exceedingly common event in early infancy for the intra-abdominal segment of oesophagus is often virtually

Oesophageal reflux (from Carré 1984)

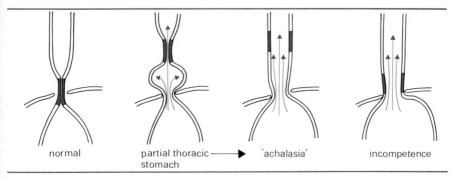

| normal | partial thoracic ⟶ stomach | `achalasia´ | incompetence |

non-existent at this age. As the abdominal segment of oesophagus lengthens over the first few months of life, so an effective anti-reflux barrier is gradually established. Gastro-oesophageal reflux in early infancy is a physiological event. Pathological reflux occurs when there is a breakdown in the anti-reflux barrier resulting from a functional abnormality of either the gastro-oesophageal sphincter or the intra-abdominal oesophagus. In clinical practice this is almost always due to displacement of the sphincter into the thorax, thus the importance of investigating children with reflux for the presence of an underlying partial thoracic stomach.

Hiatus hernia

Hiatus hernia of infancy is always sliding in type; 70 per cent are without a peritoneal sac. The congenital anomaly seems to be of the oesophageal hiatus itself which is lax, and the diaphragmatic grip is weaker than normal. The cardia of the stomach may remain competent even within the chest. Vomiting is usual from birth and eventually bleeding may occur due to ulceration of the oesophagus following persistent reflux. If untreated, this will give rise to a stricture. The clinical diagnosis is confirmed radiologically by a barium swallow.

Most infants improve if they are nursed upright in a hiatus hernia 'box' or chair, and if the feeds are thickened and alkalis given. Usually the hernia resolves spontaneously by the time the child is getting onto his feet. However, if oesophagitis is present or vomiting persists after one year of age, surgery is likely to be necessary. Hiatus hernia seems more common in children with mental handicap.

Oesophageal incoordination

Oesophageal incoordination leads to dribbling, choking and aspiration of milk as well as regurgitation and vomiting. It may be due to a wide variety of conditions all of which are rare, or sometimes it may be an isolated problem. It can be recognised by cine radiography.

Pyloric stenosis

Pyloric stenosis is due to hypertrophy and hyperplasia of the pyloric muscle mainly the circular fibres. It usually develops in the first four to six weeks of life. The condition is inherited by the multifactorial mode and is commonest in first-born, male children. Characteristically, the vomiting is projectile and may be so

Pyloric stenosis

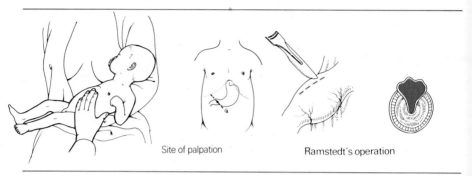

Site of palpation   Ramstedt's operation

persistent that the baby becomes undernourished or even dehydrated. Being hungry, the baby is eager to feed again soon after he has vomited. On examination, stomach wall peristalsis may be visible and a rubbery tumour is felt by gentle deep finger palpation in the area half way between the mid-point of anterior margin of the right rib cage and the umbilicus. The diagnosis is clinical and X-rays are usually not indicated. After the infant's fluid and electrolyte imbalance has been corrected, the treatment is surgical.

Failure to thrive

Mothers are naturally anxious if their infants do not appear to be growing fast enough. In most western societies now, babies are measured at regular intervals and if they fail to grow satisfactorily compared with the average for that community, further enquiry is made.

Failure to thrive can be the first indication of a serious underlying problem, such as chronic renal failure and congenital heart disease, but this is rare. More often than not, it reflects difficulties in the home, limitations in the parents, unhappiness in the relationship between mother and child or uncertain feeding methods. Many women feel 'down' after pregnancy and their unhappiness and nervousness may be communicated to their babies who in turn become irritable and restless so that a vicious spiral is begun which ultimately leaves both mother and child exhausted. Bringing one or both of them into hospital to permit both to have a good night's sleep may go a long way to easing the problem.

If a baby is undersized, and it has been established that he was of normal birth weight, that he is receiving an adequate diet in a settled home and that he has no obvious serious underlying disorder then investigation should be made for the various causes of malabsorption.

Crying and 'three month colic'

Babies cry when they are hungry. They also cry for other reasons, such as cold or discomfort and as they get older they cry when they are cross or frustrated. With experience their mothers are usually able to distinguish a cry for food and a cry in pain, but it can be difficult. Not many parents can stand a baby crying intermittently throughout the night and the temptation is to feed him, not so much for his nutrition as to keep him quiet. He may react to this by vomiting. Some babies, particularly at feeding time, but at other times as well, may have inconsolable outbursts of crying, sometimes to the point of screaming, for no obvious reason. During the attacks they may draw their knees up and go red in the face. It is difficult to believe that they are not having colic. It is possible that some infants have inflamed Peyer's patches and resulting painful bowel contractions. Drug therapy is seldom justified for they do not appear to come to any harm. This so-called 'three month colic' may last well beyond three months of age.

Diarrhoea, constipation and nappy rashes

There is no doubt that what an infant eats influences the frequency and nature of his stool and the effect the stool has on the skin of the buttocks. It is normal for a baby to have a loose yellow bowel motion with every feed, and it is equally acceptable that he has a bowel action every other day passing a firm large brown stool. But it is not acceptable that he passes frequent stools which are green and watery, or large stools which are pale and oily, or very occasional stools which are hard enough to tear the anal mucosa causing pain and bleeding. All require investigation. They may respond to simple dietary adjustments. Stool gazing is a dying art, for the information it yields is disappointingly small, but occasionally it can be instructive.

NUTRITIONAL DEFICIENCIES

Vitamin and mineral deficiencies

When unexpected symptoms or signs appear in infants and children on odd diets or with major feeding problems, the possibility of a vitamin or mineral deficiency should be considered. Clinical syndromes due to deficiency of most vitamins and many trace elements have been reported.

Xerophthalma due to vitamin A deficiency is a common serious nutritional disorder in the third world and leads to blindness. Dark green leafy vegetables are the main source of vitamin A in the developing world.

Scurvy. Scurvy is due to vitamin C deficiency. Cow's milk contains little vitamin C and most of this may disappear if the milk is stored or heated. Before artificial milks were fortified with extra vitamin C to a level similar to that in human milk, artificially-fed babies were at risk of developing scurvy. In this

Vitamin D deficiency: rickets

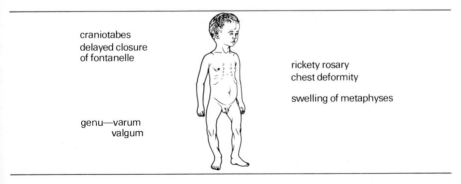

craniotabes
delayed closure
of fontanelle

rickety rosary
chest deformity

swelling of metaphyses

genu—varum
valgum

disorder connective tissues and structural membranes break down, small vessels bleed and wounds are slow to heal. The infants present with bruises, painful periosteal bleeds or persistent superficial haemorrhages.

Rickets. Rickets is due to vitamin D deficiency. The body obtains the vitamin by the action of ultraviolet light on the ergosterols in the deeper layers of the skin or from certain foods, including fish, eggs, butter and margarine. Lack of sunshine, a pigmented skin or a poor diet leaves a child at risk. It is important that lactating mothers have adequate vitamin D so that her milk will contain sufficient for her rapidly growing infant.

X-ray appearance in rickets

irregular metaphysis causing swelling of wrist

Vitamin D aids the absorption of calcium from the bowel and the formation and calcification of bone. Deficiency leads to softening and deformity, particularly of the long bones. In early life rickets may be suspected if the skull bones are soft, craniotabes; in the 3 to 6 month old child the enlargement of the ends of ribs produces a rachitic 'rosary'. In a child 12 to 18 months of age just beginning to walk, the ends of the long bones may be bowed either in or out by the strain. This is a tragedy if it occurs because the deformity is easily and cheaply avoided by vitamin D supplementation of the diet.

Classification of rickets and vitamin D metabolite levels

	Vitamin D	25 (OH) D	1,25 (OH) D
Deficient synthesis and supply — no sunlight — poor diet — immaturity	↓	↓	↓
Malabsorption	n	↓	↓
Liver disease	n	↓	↓
Chronic renal failure	n	n	↓
Vitamin D dependent rickets (recessively inherited)	n	n	↓
Vitamin D resistant rickets (sex-linked dominant)	n	n	n
Renal tubular disorders (defect of phosphate reabsorption)	n	n	n

Secondary rickets. Vitamin D deficiency may be secondary to other disorders. It occurs in the very immature when they begin to grow and can be reversed by extra vitamin D, calcium and phosphate supplements. Rarely it develops during recovery from malabsorption (rickets occurs only in the growing child) and in children with chronic liver disease when the first hydroxylation step, vitamin D to 25 (OH) D, fails. It is not uncommon in chronic renal failure when the second hydroxylation step, 25 (OH) D to 1,25 (OH) D, fails. This step is also limited in vitamin D *dependent* rickets, a rare recessively inherited disorder. In vitamin D *resistant* rickets (familial hypophosphataemic rickets, a sex-linked dominant condition) there is thought to be a defect in renal tubular transport of phosphate. Rickets also complicates more general disorders of tubular function, like Fanconi syndrome, renal tubular acidosis and cystinosis.

Dental caries

Dental caries is due to progressive decay of teeth by organic acids produced locally by bacteria that ferment dietary carbohydrate, particularly sucrose. Fluoride reduces the incidence and severity of caries, by converting the enamel mineral, hydroxyapatite to fluorapatite which is more acid resistant, by promoting remineralisation, and by antibacterial effects which reduce acid production. Thus, tooth decay may be considered to be a nutritional disorder, in part due to a deficiency of fluoride and in part due to excess of simple sugars. The risks of dental caries may be reduced by avoiding food between meals, particularly sticky sweets or sweet drinks in nursing bottles or pacifiers; by regularly cleaning the teeth; and by an adequate intake of fluoride either in the water, toothpaste or if necessary by tablet.

Dental caries

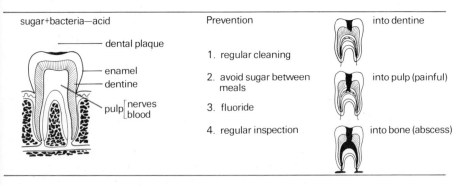

sugar+bacteria—acid

dental plaque
enamel
dentine
pulp ⌈nerves
     ⌊blood

Prevention

1. regular cleaning
2. avoid sugar between meals
3. fluoride
4. regular inspection

into dentine

into pulp (painful)

into bone (abscess)

MALNUTRITION

Protein-energy deficiency syndromes

Many children in some parts of the world simply do not get enough to eat. Following a political or natural disaster, the news media have been quick to make us more aware of the severe forms of childhood malnutrition which are prevalent during famine.

A WHO Expert Committee divided the protein-energy deficiency syndromes into marasmus, where failure to grow is associated with emaciation and a fair appetite; kwashiorkor, where malnutrition is associated with oedema and loss of appetite; and 'unspecified' where growth retardation and undernutrition are evident without frank emaciation or oedema. These terms describe the various ways by which starvation can affect the growing child.

With starvation of whatever degree comes misery and an increased risk of infections. Both add to domestic problems and increase the risk of death or permanent damage.

Marasmus. Marasmus in western societies may be seen in infants born severely undernourished, or after severe chronic illnesses, particularly affecting the bowel. In poorer communities, nutritional marasmus commonly occurs due to failure of lactation in people who just cannot afford artificial milks. Thus it is more common in low-birth-weight infants, twins and in infants after infection, particularly gastroenteritis.

The infant's survival depends on the mother's ability to maintain lactation, even if the infant is unable to suckle for a few days. If food can be found, the prognosis of these infants is good. During a famine children of all ages may become marasmic and the recovery of older children may take longer. The risk of death due to superadded infection during the recovery phase is also higher.

Malnutrition

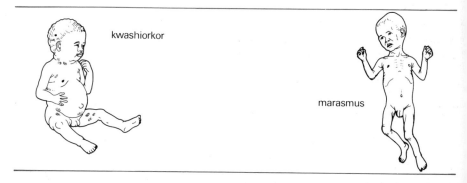

kwashiorkor

marasmus

Kwashiorkor. Kwashiorkor is a colourful word that gives the impression of a specific disease entity but it is but one end of a spectrum. Most commonly, it occurs in children 18 to 24 months old at the time of weaning. The marasmic child receives a little of a balanced diet; in the child with kwashiorkor the energy intake may be just about adequate but the protein content is insufficient for growth. As a consequence there is muscle wasting but preservation of some subcutaneous fat.

The infant is oedematous, listless and irritable. There may be a 'flaky paint' dermatitis of a depigmented skin and the hair is sparse and friable. The liver may be large due to fatty infiltration and the serum albumin concentration may be reduced.

The complications include hypothermia, hypoglycaemia, drowsiness, severe diarrhoea, cardiac failure and all these are compounded by superimposed infections.

An inadequate supply of food is not primarily a medical problem. However the health service can help in the following ways:

1. By encouraging and supporting the lactating mother; there is no reason why breast feeding should not be continued for 18 or 24 months.
2. By advising parents about weaning.
3. By recommending those local foods which will meet the protein needs of the growing child.
4. By the early recognition of children in difficulties so that limited food resources can be optimally deployed.
5. By the treatment of associated infections and vitamin deficiency states.

OBESITY

Obesity is a common health problem when food is in abundance. Fat parents tend to have fat children for there is a genetic component in the aetiology. Fat children tend to but do not invariably become fat adults. Fat people die on average at a younger age than thin people. In particular, fat adults are more likely to develop diabetes and hypertension; they weather chronic chest disease, heart failure and abdominal operations badly; and they have more problems with varicose veins, piles and skin crease ailments.

Obesity can be assessed reasonably well just by looking at the child and by plotting body weight on a centile chart. The height:weight ratio and skin fold thicknesses can be measured if more accurate analysis is required.

Prevention

As obesity is so difficult to treat it is best to avoid it. There is some evidence that bottle-fed babies are more likely to become overweight than breast-fed infants. This may be because the baby is less able to resist pressures to finish the bottle. Obesity may develop in the months after weaning when clearing the plate or emptying the cup becomes a virtue. Early weaning encourages this development. There is little virtue in commencing weaning before four or five

Skin fold thickness

Who is for dieting

months of age. One big meal a day appears to be more fattening than many small ones amounting to similar caloric value. Thus, the best prophylaxis for infants at risk of obesity because of fat parents is for them to be breast fed and weaned late; overfeeding should be avoided, particularly during the weaning period and the habit of taking regular exercise and eating small frequent meals should be established.

Treatment

Obese children may be referred for medical advice for a variety of reasons. The child may be concerned because of his appearance or the clothes he is required to wear or because he is teased. His parents may be concerned for the same reasons but also because they fear it may affect his health in other ways. His teachers may be concerned because of his lack of physical fitness. If the child really wants to be thinner and his parents are prepared to put themselves out to help him then there is some hope that a diet and exercise regimen will work. However, occasionally over-eating is an outward sign of inner confusion and unhappiness. This needs to be recognised and discussed. But in the majority of cases a detailed enquiry brings little to light except bad parental dietary attitudes and practices. One mother still gave her child aged seven years a breast feed at night; another considered that a bumper gorge was a high treat; a third used food to settle a particularly active and demanding baby.

BIBLIOGRAPHY

McClaren D S, Burman D 1982 Textbook of paediatric nutrition. Churchill Livingstone, Edinburgh.
Foman S J 1976 Infant Nutrition. Saunders
Jelliffe D B, Jelliffe P E F 1979 Human milk in the modern world. Oxford University Press, Oxford
Wood C B S, Walker-Smith J A 1981 MacKieth's Infant feeding and feeding difficulties. Churchill Livingstone, Edinburgh
Paul A M, Southgate D A T 1978 The composition of foods. H.M.S.O., London
Bond J T, Filer L J, Leveille S A, Thomson A M, Weil W B 1981 Infant and child feeding. Academic Press
Packard V S 1982 Human milk and infant formula. Academic Press
Carre I J 1984 Clinical significance of gastro-oesophageal reflux. Archives of Diseases of childhood 59: 911–912

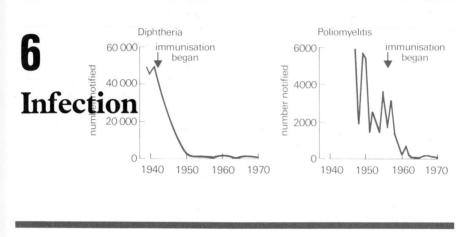

6

Infection

Diphtheria

Poliomyelitis

Infections spread readily among children. Acute respiratory infections, gastro-enteritis and the main subject of this Chapter, the infectious 'fevers' account for a very large part of childhood illness, although scourges of the past, such as diphtheria and poliomyelitis, have now virtually disappeared. Infections are most likely to occur when the child first mixes with others, at a nursery, a playgroup or at primary school, and he may bring them home to his younger siblings. Often the infectious fever is diagnosed by the mother and the child is not very ill and can usually be looked after at home. If hospital admission is required it is often for social rather than medical reasons, however occasionally complications arise which are potentially damaging or life threatening.

MEASLES

Measles is a common and very infectious viral disease. The incubation period of about ten days is followed by a prodromal illness with fever, coryza, conjunctivitis and cough. Generalized lymphadenopathy may be found, and tiny white spots on a bright red background, Koplik's spots, are present on the buccal mucosa of the checks. After three or four days a florid maculopapular rash appears, and

Measles

spreads downwards from the head and neck to cover the whole body. The earlier lesions are more numerous and become confluent and blotchy. The rash begins to fade by the third day and the child's general condition improves steadily.

Respiratory complications, particularly bronchopneumonia and otitis media are common. Encephalitis occurs in about one in 1000 affected children and is manifested by headache, drowsiness and vomiting. Convulsions and coma begin 7 to 10 days after the onset of the illness. The course of encephalitis is unpredictable but about 15 per cent of cases die, and 25 per cent suffer brain damage resulting in mental retardation, fits, deafness, or behaviour disorders. Measles may be associated with a disturbance of immune mechanisms, especially lymphopenia. Defective immune response may also be the basis of the rare late complication, subacute sclerosing panencephalitis, which occurs 4 to 10 years after an attack of measles and is characterised by slow, progressive neurological deterioration. There are very high levels of measles antibody in the blood and cerebrospinal fluid, and measles virus antigen has been demonstrated in brain tissue.

In developing countries, measles carries a high morbidity and mortality. It tends to occur in younger children than in the U.K. (median age 17 months in Nigeria, 52 months in England and Wales). Reported mortality rates range from 5.5 per cent in East Africa to between 20 and 40 per cent in a selected hospital series in West Africa. In the malnourished child, a severe form of measles may occur with a confluent rash that darkens to deep red or purple, and then desquamates. This is followed by depigmentation of the skin which lasts for several weeks and may be associated with pyodermia. A sore mouth is common during the acute illness and may lead to cancrum oris; invariably breast feeding is disturbed. Diarrhoea is common and may persist for a long time, further aggravating any underlying malnutrition. Measles mortality rate is directly related to socio-economic conditions, and there is a strong correlation with the distribution of kwashiorkor. In young, susceptible children measles itself causes loss of weight. In a village in Nigeria almost 1 in 4 of children lost more than 10 per cent of their weight following an attack of measles, and the average time to regain the previous weight was seven weeks. It is, therefore, important to maintain the child's hydration and nutrition during the illness and afterwards. Measles immunisation using a live attenuated virus has been introduced into many countries with varying success. In U.S.A. measles has been virtually eradicated.

RUBELLA

Rubella or German measles, is usually a mild illness, and may pass unrecognised. The incubation period is 14 to 21 days and there may be little or no fever or malaise before the appearance of the pink macular rash which lasts for about three days. Generalised lymphadenopathy, especially involving the suboccipital nodes may be present. A rising haemagglutinin inhibition antibody titre confirms the diagnosis. This test is seldom necessary in children but is essential when the possibility arises of rubella in early pregnancy. Complications of rubella, such as thrombocytopenia and encephalitis, do occur but they are rare. Arthritis may occur in adolescents.

Rubella

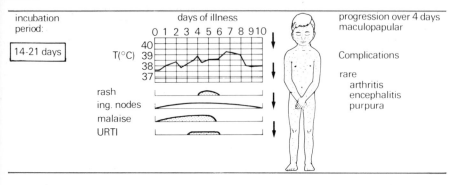

The importance of this disease lies in its devastating effect on the developing fetus if the mother contracts the infection during the first three months of pregnancy (see Ch. 3). A generalised viraemia may lead to fetal death and spontaneous abortion, or may affect the growth and development of the fetus resulting in a severely handicapped child with multiple congenital defects, classically including cataracts, deafness and congenital heart disease.

It is in an attempt to prevent this disaster that immunisation against rubella has been introduced using an attenuated virus. Some countries, including the U.K., offer it to girls before leaving school; others (e.g. the U.S.A.) offer it to all school children. In the U.K. at present only 64 per cent of girls are actually receiving it.

CHICKENPOX (VARICELLA)

Chickenpox is a common and highly infectious disease but is usually mild in children. The same virus produces herpes zoster. The incubation period is 10 to 21 days. There may be no symptoms apart from the rash and a low grade fever. Chickenpox spots appear in crops, progressing rapidly from macule to papule to vesicle. The vesicle soon dries and crusts and the scabs separate without scarring. Lesions may also occur on mucous membranes, especially in the mouth where they quickly rupture to produce shallow ulcers. Now that smallpox has

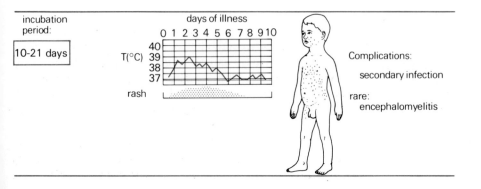

been eradicated from the world, problems of differential diagnosis are rare.

Complications of chickenpox are uncommon in healthy children. Encephalitis is rare but when it does occur there is often cerebellar involvement. The child presents with ataxia three to eight days after the onset of the rash. At least 80 per cent of affected children make a complete recovery. Pneumonia is a rare complication in children, but it may be part of the very rare severe form of the illness when the rash is haemorrhagic. This is more likely to occur in children with immune deficiency, in particular children treated for leukaemia.

HERPES SIMPLEX INFECTIONS

Infection with this virus is extremely common and usually asymptomatic, less than 10 per cent of children with primary infections becoming clinically ill.

Herpes virus Type 1 is spread by infected saliva and transmission therefore requires close personal contact. Primary infection may affect the mouth, skin or eyes. Herpes virus type 2 is a genital infection usually spread by sexual contact.

Neonatal infections
Newborn infants may be infected during delivery by maternal genital herpes infection (Type 2) or, less commonly, by the usual Type 1 virus in the postnatal period. Infection may result in a severe, disseminated disease characterised by lethargy, vesicular rash, hepatosplenomegaly, bleeding and neurological symptoms. Mortality is about 70 per cent and there is a high morbidity rate among the survivors. The risk of this severe illness is about 40 per cent if the mother has active genital herpes at the time of delivery, and an elective Caesarean section should be considered.

Mouth infections
Acute gingivostomatitis is common, particularly in preschool children from poor socio-economic circumstances. It is characterised by high fever, swelling and bleeding of the gums and extensive ulceration of the buccal mucosa, tongue and palate. The cervical glands are enlarged. Eating and drinking are painful, and the child may become dehydrated. The illness lasts about 10 to 14 days. A vulvovaginitis may result from transfer of the infection from the mouth by the child's finger.

Eye and skin infections
Keratoconjunctivitis is associated with severe oedema of the eyelids and dendritic ulcers of the cornea which may lead to scarring and loss of vision. Primary infection of the skin with vesicular lesions tends to develop in older children, often at the site of trauma. In children with eczema, an extensive vesicular rash which later scabs may occur on the eczematous skin. The child may be febrile and sometimes there is generalised infection due to blood stream spread, which is potentially fatal. Secondary infection of skin lesions is a complication.

The diagnosis of local infection is not difficult, as the vesicular lesions are characteristic. Rapid confirmation can be obtained by culture of the vesicular fluid or microscopic examination of scrapings for inclusion bodies. Topical treat-

> erythema multiforme.

ment with idoxyuridine is partially effective.

Cold sores

Recurrent herpes simplex infection is common and usually occurs as 'cold sores' round the mouth. The recurrence rate is very variable and though the lesions may be associated with respiratory infections, they may also be related to nonspecific factors such as sunshine, menstruation and emotional stress.

Meningo-encephalitis

Herpes simplex virus is a relatively common cause of meningo-encephalitis. It may occur during the primary infection or due to the activation of a virus lying dormant after an earlier infection. It develops in apparently normal children and it can occur in the absence of skin lesions. The illness may be very severe and the mortality rate is high. Frontal and temporal lobe abnormalities are found on the electroencephalogram and a brain scan may demonstrate a 'space-occupying' lesion. A rising titre of antibody in the blood or cerebrospinal fluid confirms the diagnosis. Treatment with acyclovir, if given early, is of some benefit but the improvement in survival with active treatment has not been accompanied by a reduction in the very high rate of chronic neurological handicap.

MUMPS

Mumps is caused by a paramyxovirus. Subclinical infection is common. A long incubation period of 16 to 21 days is followed by fever, malaise and enlargement of one or both parotid glands, which develop over a period of 1 to 3 days. The child may complain of earache and difficulty in swallowing, and the glands may be painful and tender. The submandibular glands may also be affected. The swellings settle in 7 to 10 days and there is no specific treatment. Other causes of parotitis are rare in children and the distinction from cervical lymphadeno-pathy should not be difficult after careful examination.

Meningitis is a common complication, but is usually mild and characterised by headache, photophobia and neck stiffness. The cerebrospinal fluid contains an increased number of lymphocytes and a raised concentration of protein. Recovery is almost always complete. Epididymo-orchitis is a rare complication before puberty; pancreatitis is a recognised but uncommon complication.

Differential diagnosis of mumps and cervical adenitis

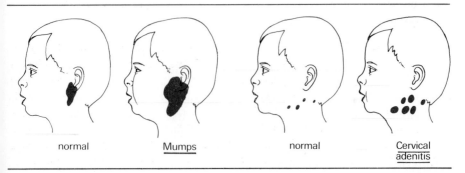

| normal | Mumps | normal | Cervical adenitis |

GLANDULAR FEVER

In developed countries glandular fever, infectious mononucleosis, occurs most often in adolescents and young adults, but is not uncommon in children. Infection is usually sporadic, though epidemics can occur in schools or residential homes. The Epstein-Barr virus is the cause of the infection and is excreted in nasopharyngeal secretions. Close contact is necessary for infection to be transmitted.

The onset of glandular fever is usually insidious and occurs after an incubation period of four to 14 days. The clinical features are anorexia, malaise and fever and they are usually accompanied by a sore throat and enlarged glands in most affected children. The tonsillitis may be very severe with a thick white exudate covering the tonsils and surrounding areas. Petechiae may be seen on the palate. Cervical lymph nodes are enlarged, and the spleen is often palpable. A macular rash occurs in 10 to 20 per cent of cases, especially if ampicillin has been given. Hepatitis, often with jaundice is common, but other complications such an pneumonitis and neurological disturbances are rare.

The diagnosis is supported by the presence of atypical mononuclear cells in the blood film. These large cells have an irregular nucleus and pale-staining cytoplasm containing vacuoles, and may account for 10 to 25 per cent of the total white cell count. The Paul-Bunnell test for antibodies is positive in about 60 per cent of patients during the first week of the illness but the agglutinins may disappear by two to four weeks. These antibodies agglutinate sheep red blood cells and are not absorbed by guineapig kidney cells as are similar antibodies occurring sometimes in normal people. Horse red blood cells are also agglutinated, and this is the basis of the monospot test. Liver function tests are abnormal in over half the patients.

Glandular fever is a self-limiting disease for which there is no specific treatment. The lymphadenopathy and splenomegaly may persist for weeks or months, and there may be a long period of debility. The differential diagnosis when tonsillitis is severe includes streptococcal tonsillitis and diphtheria; when lymphadenopathy is prominent it includes leukaemia, toxoplasmosis and cytomegalovirus infection; and when jaundice or a rash are present, infectious hepatitis, measles or rubella may be suspected. However, the diagnosis is not difficult if the clinical features are characteristic and the appropriate laboratory tests are obtained.

KAWASAKI DISEASE (MUCOCUTANEOUS LYMPH NODE SYNDROME)

First described in Japan, this condition has now been reported from many other countries. The majority of patients are under 5 years of age and present with an acute febrile illness associated with conjunctivitis, pharyngitis and a generalised polymorphous rash. The hands and feet are typically red and oedematous, with peeling of the fingers and toes as the child recovers. Cervical lymph nodes are usually enlarged. Arthritis, urethritis and hepatitis may occur. The fever persists for 1–2 weeks and then settles. A neutrophil leucocytosis, very high ESR and raised platelet counts are found but no organisms have been cultured and autoantibodies are negative. The most important complication is cardiac involvement with clinical evidence of myocarditis or conduction defects in 20 per cent in especially infants, and death in 1–2 per cent. Coronary artery aneurysms may develop and are detectable by echocardiography, but fortunately slowly resolve in the majority. Post mortem studies show a widespread vasculitis always affecting the coronary arteries.

No infective agent has been isolated and there is no evidence of person-to-person transmission, even in apparent epidemics. Treatment with aspirin in full anti-inflammatory dosage is recommended in the acute stage, and it is reasonable to continue with a small dose to reduce platelet aggregation for some weeks.

ERYTHEMA INFECTIOSUM (5TH DISEASE)

This condition is characterised by an erythematous maculopapular rash which often begins in the face giving a typical 'slapped cheek' appearance. The rash spreads to the trunk and limbs with central fading of the eruption giving a lacy or reticular appearance. It lasts about a week. There are usually no other symptoms at all, though arthralgia of the small joints may occur. Investigation of a recent school epidemic showed that all the affected children had specific IgM to human parvo-virus in their serum, so this condition seems to have found a cause.

ROSEOLA INFANTUM (EXANTHEM SUBITUM)

The patient is usually under two years of age. He develops a high fever, often without appearing particularly ill, though convulsions may occur. Examination reveals only a mild pharyngitis and lymphadenopathy. After three or four days the temperature drops suddenly to normal, and a macular rash appears which lasts for a few hours or a day or two. The child then makes an uneventful and rapid recovery.

POLIOMYELITIS

The introduction of successful immunisation against poliomyelitis has been one of the greatest success stories of modern medicine. A dreadful disease has been virtually eradicated.

In most people, the poliomyelitis virus produces a mild illness with fever, sore throat, headache and vomiting, lasting up to three days. In about one third of affected children this is followed by improvement for one to seven days and then a recurrence of more severe symptoms with pain and stiffness in the neck, back and legs. As in other types of viral meningitis, the cerebrospinal fluid contains increased lymphocytes and protein. Paralysis may develop in association with muscle pain and tenderness. This is due to anterior horn cell damage, is usually asymmetrical, and varies considerably in extent, in the severe forms causing respiratory failure and bulbar paralysis. Once the fever subsides, the spread of weakness and paralysis is halted and there is then a slow improvement over a period of about 18 months. After this time any residual paralysis is likely to be permanent.

The clinical course of poliomyelitis

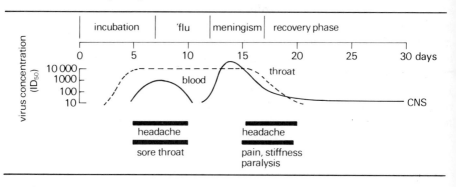

DIPHTHERIA

Diphtheria is now very rare in countries where vaccination is practised. It is caused by one of three strains of *Corynebacterium diphtheriae*. The infection usually in the throat, is spread by droplets and may be caught from infected individuals or healthy carriers. The incubation period is 2–7 days. The child presents with a sore throat and inflamed tonsils. The pharyngeal exudate may spread with epithelial destruction and membrane formation leading to upper airway obstruction. Exotoxin released by the bacterium may cause myocarditis (second week) and neuritis with paralysis (third to seventh week).

The vaccine, a modified exotoxin, gives protection. The Schick test detects immunity to diphtheria. Treatment of the disease itself requires diphtheria antitoxin to counteract its effects and erythromycin to eradicate the organisms.

PERTUSSIS (WHOOPING COUGH)

Bordetella pertussis is the cause of a prolonged respiratory illness which is particularly dangerous in infancy. After a seven-day incubation period, there is a 'catarrhal' stage lasting one to two weeks, during which the child is unwell, with signs of upper respiratory tract infection. A cough develops which becomes increasingly severe and paroxysmal. Spasms of coughing may be followed by an inspiratory 'whoop', especially in older children. Vomiting may occur, and the child can become cyanosed or apnoeic during coughing spasms and be left exhausted afterwards. Between spasms there may be no obvious respiratory difficulty and the lungs are clear on examination. This phase lasts four to six weeks, and the cough gradually improves over another two to three weeks. The causative organism is cultured in early cases from a nasopharyngeal swab using Bordet-Gengou medium, but is difficult to isolate once the cough is established. A striking lymphocytosis supports the diagnosis.

The most common complication is bronchopneumonia which is especially common in infants and accounts for most of the deaths. Bronchiectasis used to be a well-recognised sequela but is now very uncommon. Convulsions may occur due to asphyxia from severe spasms, intracranial bleeding or encephalopathy. Subconjunctival haemorrhages and facial petechiae due to raised venous pressure during spasms may be alarming but resolve spontaneously.

The treatment of pertussis is largely symptomatic and careful nursing is required. Oxygen, suction and tube-feeding may be necessary. Erythromycin given in the catarrhal stage may abort or modify the illness but the result is often disappointing. Its use in infant contacts is justifiable. No drugs prevent the spasms once the disease is established.

Immunisation against pertussis became the subject of considerable controversy in the mid 1970s, following well-publicised reports of neurological damage associated with reactions to the triple vaccine. The frequency of such reactions and the incidence of natural pertussis and its complications were not known and varying figures were reported. The debate led to a considerable fall in uptake of pertussis immunisation in the U.K. to 31 per cent in 1978 and as a consequence there was a bad epidemic in 1978–80. It became clear that pertussis is still a serious disease especially in infants. There were at least 30 deaths in England and Wales. At the same time the efficacy of the vaccine in protecting against pertussis, which had been questioned, was clearly demonstrated.

In the U.K. in an attempt to establish the incidence of neurological complications associated with the vaccine, a nationwide prospective study of all encephalopathic illness and prolonged convulsions in children aged 2 months to 3 years was made. At this age encephalopathic illness occurs in many forms, and the cause is often difficult to establish. Only 36 of the first 1000 children reported, occurred in the week after immunisation. Thus 3.6 per cent had had triple vaccine within 7 days of the onset of symptoms and this compared with 1.7 per cent in controls. The majority of these children made an uneventful recovery: 1 year later two were dead and nine developmentally retarded. The study concluded that the estimated attributable risk of serious neurological disorders occurring within 7 days of immunisation was 1 in 110 000 injections and that for previously normal children the risk of neurological sequelae 1 year later was 1 in 310 000 injections. These figures included children with alternative explanations for their problems.

It still remains to be shown that the pertussis vaccine itself causes brain damaging disease in man. The risk of precipitating an encephalopathic illness has to be balanced against the risks of natural pertussis which statistically is some ten times greater.

The pertussis vaccine is a soup of killed organisms of several serotypes. Mild local reactions are common. It is contraindicated if a previous dose caused a

Incidence of whooping cough in the UK. In 1974 immunisation rate fell but is now rising again

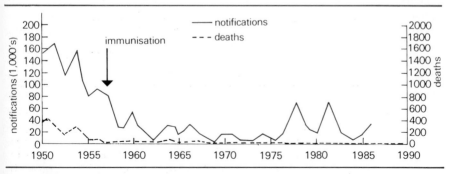

severe local or a general reaction. It is also recommended that it is not given to children who are known to have had convulsions or a neurological disorder or where there is a history of epilepsy in first degree relatives. However there is no evidence that such children are at particular risk, and they are children who need protection from the natural illness. Possibly because of the recent epidemics the immunisation rate has risen, but it is still only a little above 60%. As maternal antibody does not cross the placenta, the protection of young infants depends on the state of immunity of their older siblings. If parents refuse pertussis immunisation, it is important to ensure that the child receives immunisation against diphtheria, tetanus and polio which are normally given at the same time.

SCARLET FEVER

Group A haemolytic streptococci are responsible for a variety of problems in children, especially tonsillitis. Sequelae such as rheumatic fever and acute glomerulonephritis are important, but have become rare in western societies. Scarlet fever results from infection with a strain of the organism which produces an erythrogenic toxin. After an incubation period of two to four days, the child develops tonsillitis, fever, headache and malaise. The rash develops within 12 hours of the onset and rapidly becomes generalised. It consists of a fine punctate erythema which blanches on pressure. The face is spared, but the cheeks are flushed so that the child is indeed 'scarlet', apart from the area around the mouth. The tongue has a thick white coating through which the inflamed papillae project, the 'white strawberry tongue'. By day four or five the tongue peels, leaving a 'red strawberry' appearance. The skin rash fades after a few days, or sooner if penicillin is given, followed by desquamation, especially on the hands and feet. This may persist for some time and is useful in making a retrospective diagnosis. Scarlet fever may also follow infection of wounds or burns. Treatment with penicillin leads to a rapid recovery, but a ten day course is necessary to eradicate the streptococci.

Scarlet fever

TUBERCULOSIS

Tuberculosis is no longer the 'captain of the Kings of Death' in Europe, but remains a major problem in many developing countries. The incidence of TB in Europe fell steadily as a result of better social conditions and nutrition, and with the advent of effective chemotherapy. Most children with the disease are now identified because they are contacts of infected adults, who may be asymptomatic. In the U.K. children of Asian families are at special risk of infection from recent adult immigrants. They account for 40% of the 488 children reported with TB in 1983 in England and Wales.

The incidence is declining in all groups, at an average annual rate of 19% for Indian children, 17% for Pakistanis and 5 per cent for whites since 1978/9. Only 4% of Welsh schoolchildren were found to be tuberculin positive on routine testing in 1980, indicating that they had had a primary infection or BCG vaccination.

Children with TB in England and Wales 1983

Racial Group	Rate/100 000 popn
White	2.9
Indian	34
Pakistani/Bangladeshi	56
Children from Indian subcontinent born there	67
Children from Indian subcontinent born in U.K.	39

Primary infection

Mycobacterium tuberculosis is spread by droplets, and primary infection may occur in the lung, skin or gut. A recent outbreak in Nottingham occurred in tooth sockets following dental extractions by a dentist with pulmonary TB. Sensitivity to tuberculin develops 4–8 weeks after infection, as shown by a positive Mantoux or Heaf test. Tuberculin tests may be negative if there is severe malnutrition or overwhelming infection. Hypersensitivity reactions such as erythema nodosum (red shiny lumps on the shins) or phlyctenular conjunctivitis occur in a few instances. Only about 1 in 20 of those infected develop disease.

In these, the local infection spreads locally and to the lymph nodes; together these constitute the primary complex. Most such lesions heal slowly by fibrosis and may calcify, the process taking 12–18 months. Complications may arise from the local progression of the primary complex, especially in the lungs. An area of bronchopneumonia develops, or enlargement of the hilar nodes leads to bronchial obstruction, sometimes with rupture of the node into a bronchus. Pleural

Primary tuberculosis

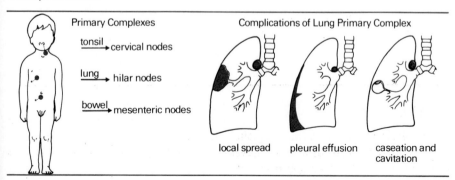

Primary Complexes

tonsil → cervical nodes

lung → hilar nodes

bowel → mesenteric nodes

Complications of Lung Primary Complex

local spread   pleural effusion   caseation and cavitation

Lung complications of tuberculosis. Miliary lesions are due to blood spread. The tubercles might be seen in the retina. Always suspect tuberculosis meningitis

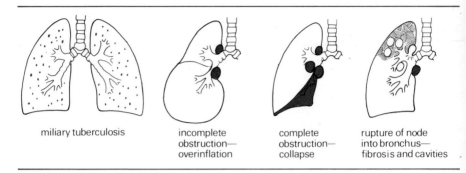

| miliary tuberculosis | incomplete obstruction— overinflation | complete obstruction— collapse | rupture of node into bronchus— fibrosis and cavities |

effusions occur in older children as a hypersensitivity reaction. Empyema, caseation and cavitation are seen more often in malnourished children from developing countries. Unless the lesion cavitates into a bronchus, children with primary TB do not cough up sputum and are not infectious. They may have no cough at all, but a general malaise and vague ill health. Adult pulmonary TB, characterised by cavitation results either from new infection or a breakdown of the primary complex. Tubercle bacilli can persist in a dormant form and cause disease many years later.

Gastrointestinal lesions
A primary focus in the tonsillar region may present with cervical adenitis and progress to a 'cold' abscess. This is usually due to human TB but may follow infection with a bovine strain after drinking unpasteurised milk. A similar infection in the small bowel occasionally leads to malabsorption, stricture formation and peritonitis. Cervical adenitis may also occur with infection due to atypical mycobacteria.

Miliary TB and meningitis
Blood stream spread is the most serious complication of primary TB and accounts for at least 70% of childhood deaths due to TB. The risk is greatest in young children especially in developing countries, and almost always occurs within one year of infection. The child presents with fever, anorexia and loss of weight. Enlargement of the liver and spleen is common and choroidal tubercles may be seen on examining the fundi. Scattered crepitations may be heard over the lungs, and the chest X-ray shows generalised mottling. There is often associated meningitis, which develops insidiously with gradual progression of lethargy, headache, convulsions and coma. Cranial nerve lesions may develop. A tuberculoma of the brain is much commoner in developing countries than in Europe and presents as a space-occupying lesion.

In TB meningitis the CSF is opalescent with increased lymphocytes and protein but low sugar concentrations. A few organisms may be seen on microscopy of the deposit. A culture may take some weeks to grow so treatment should not be delayed. Unfortunately hydrocephalus and other long term neurological damage are common in survivors.

Tuberculosis of the bones and joints can develop as a result of blood stream spread within 3 years of the primary infection. Renal infection may not become apparent for 5 or more years.

Treatment

Active tuberculous infection requires prompt effective chemotherapy. The current practice is to give quadruple therapy with rifampicin, isoniazid, ethambutol and pyrazinamide for 2 months, followed by 4 months rifampicin and isoniazid. Children found to have an asymptomatic primary complex and children who are known to have recently converted their Heaf test from negative to positive should also be treated, mainly to prevent blood stream spread. In this situation isoniazid alone is given for 6–12 months. Older children with a strongly positive tuberculin test and clear chest x-ray should be kept under regular supervision and only treated if the lesion progresses.

If rifampicin causes jaundice it has to be discontinued and alternatives sought.

Prevention

TB is a notifiable disease. It is essential to trace contacts of newly diagnosed patients and perform a Heaf test and chest x-ray. If the Heaf test is negative, it should be repeated after six weeks. If still negative BCG vaccination should be given.

The aim of BCG vaccination is to produce a highly modified primary infection with attenuated organisms. It has been shown to give 80% protection against TB and to protect completely against miliary spread.

In the U.K. BCG vaccination is currently offered to all 12-year-old school children who are Heaf negative, and to the newborn infants of Asian families. In countries with a high incidence of TB routine neonatal vaccination is advisable after an initial campaign to reach as many of the population as possible. In some countries with a low incidence of TB, vaccination has been discontinued. Initial Heaf testing is not essential; BCG can be given safely to positive reactors, they will produce an accelerated response. Following BCG, the Heaf test becomes positive, though not strongly so, and it may revert to negative after some years. Natural infection gives a strongly positive reaction so difficulties with diagnosis are rare.

MALARIA

Malaria is endemic in many parts of the world. As a consequence of the increase in international travel more children suffering from malaria are seen in non-endemic countries. 'Where have you been?' is now an important question to ask of children presenting with an unexplained high fever.

Characteristically, the fever is intermittent and the spleen enlarged, but these signs are not always present. There may be associated vomiting and rigors. The treatment is chloroquine by mouth in the appropriate dose. In certain parts of the world *Plasmodium falciparum* strains may be resistant to chloroquine. If the illness is due to *Plasmodium vivax*, a two-week course of primaquine should also be given to eliminate the parasites from the liver and to prevent a subsequent relapse — unless the patient has a glucose-6-phosphate dehydrogenase deficiency.

IMMUNISATION

Protection against some of the infectious diseases is available in the form of immunisation which is given at various stages throughout childhood and early adulthood. Immunisations for different diseases are scheduled in an attempt to balance the risks of the disease with the child's ability to produce a good immunological response. Immunisation should not be given if the child is unwell, and at least three weeks should elapse between each immunisation.

Living attenuated vaccines, that is poliomyelitis, measles, rubella, BCG, should not be given to children with immune deficiency states, including those on corticosteroids and cytotoxic drugs, because of the risk of severe generalised infection.

Recommended immunisation programme for U.K.

Age	Immunisation	
Neonatal	BCG	Infants of Asian mothers or with family history of tuberculosis
3 months	Diphtheria Pertussis DPT Tetanus Poliomyelitis , Hib.	1st dose
5 months	DPT Poliomyelitis	2nd dose
10 months	DPT Poliomyelitis Hib	3rd dose
>1 year	Measles mmR	
5 years	DT Poliomyelitis	
11 years	Rubella (girls) +Boys!!	
	BCG	(Heaf negative)
15–19 years	Tetanus toxoid Poliomyelitis	

(handwritten annotations: "2" beside 3 months, "3" beside 5 months, "4" beside 10 months, "15/12" above >1 year, "6/12 – Hib." beside 10 months row)

IMMUNE DEFICIENCY

Contact with infecting organisms is one of the major challenges that face the newborn infant as he establishes an independent existence. Cellular immunity is present at birth, and although the neutrophil count is relatively low the infant is able to respond to bacterial infection with a leucocytosis. Humoral immunity is not well developed in infancy, but the infant is protected initially by maternal IgG antibodies which cross the placenta, and IgA which he receives in colostrum and breast milk. IgM does not cross the placenta, but the infant is capable of producing it in response to infection.

Maternally provided IgG globulins are progressively catabolised so that the infant's circulating immunoglobulins fall to a minimal level at two to three months. The subsequent rise parallels endogenous production as a result of exposure to environmental antigens. IgM concentrations reach normal adult levels earliest followed by IgG and then IgA.

Sometimes there is a delay in synthesis of immunoglobulins, especially in preterm babies. Low levels of IgA are particularly common and may persist for years. IgA is important in the protection of mucosal barriers and its absence predisposes to recurrent respiratory infection.

Most children with recurrent infections are normal, but immunological investigation should be undertaken when recurrent bacterial or fungal infections occur.

Examples of diseases due to defects in the body defences

Immune deficiency	Pathogens	Disease	Treatment
Humoral	Bacteria, pneumocystis	Agammaglobulinaemia	Gammaglobulin
Cellular	Viruses, tuberculosis, candida	DiGeorge syndrome (absent thymus)	Thymus graft
Stem cell	Bacteria, pneumocystis, viruses, tuberculosis, candida	Combined immune deficiency syndrome	Bone marrow graft
Complement deficiency	Bacteria		Antibiotics
Neutrophil disorders	Bacteria	Chronic granulomatous disease	Antibiotics

There are a number of rare inherited disorders of the immune mechanisms, the immune deficiency syndromes. However, immunological deficiencies may also occur in association with systemic illness, for example transient immunosuppression occurs during viral infections, especially measles, and the resulting susceptibility to infection contributes to malnutrition which in turn impairs defence mechanisms. Susceptibility to infection also occurs in relapsed nephrotic syndrome which limits the available immunoglobulins. Corticosteroid and cytotoxic therapy also reduces immunological competence.

BIBLIOGRAPHY

Jelliffe D B, Stanfield J P 1978 Diseases of children in the sub-tropics and tropics. Arnold, London
Krugman S, Ward R, Katz S L 1977 Infectious diseases of children. Mosby, St Louis
Morley D 1973 Paediatric priorities in the developing world. Butterworth, London
Christie A B 1981 Infectious diseases, 3rd edn. Churchill Livingstone, Edinburgh

7

Hazards

Accidents are by far the commonest cause of death in children over the age of a year. Recently in the U.K. the number of deaths due to accidents has declined but still approximately 900 children between the ages of one and 14 years die each year as a result of an accident. Road accidents are by far the commonest cause of childhood accidental fatalities, followed by choking, drowning and burns. For every child who is killed, many are seriously injured and many more receive minor injuries. Again in the U.K. about 150 000 children each year have to be admitted to hospital following an accident; this represents nearly a fifth of all paediatric admissions and one child in 80 of the whole child population. As many as one child in six attends a hospital casualty department each year with an injury and a similar number seek advice from their general practitioner. As well as killing and injuring children, accidents are also expensive!

How do accidents in childhood differ from those affecting adults? Three factors are important in any accident: the causative agent or situation, for example a car or a swimming pool; the circumstances in which it took place, for example the degree of parental supervision; and most important of all, the child himself. The type of accident is related to the age, sex, intelligence, social

Accident rates in England and Wales, 1983

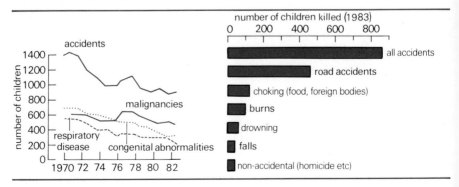

Causes of accidents at home

circumstances and personality of the child. Physical and mental development is particularly important. The toddler is fearless and inquisitive, but spends most of his time indoors, so that he is susceptible to falls, burns and self-poisoning. The child who has just started school is impulsive but inexperienced, and therefore likely to be knocked down by a car. The older school child is vigorous and adventurous, he is likely to fall and injure himself while climbing or to drown in a quarry or canal.

An understanding of the cause of accidents may lead to prevention. A young toddler cannot be reasoned with and therefore he must be protected by those around him and by those who design his house and its contents. The young school child can be actively taught about the dangers of traffic, but equally those who design schools, playgrounds and streets must take account of his inexperience. The older child can scarcely be prevented from taking risks and resents adult interference. He must learn to come to terms with himself and the amount of risk he can safely take. Most minor accidents are unavoidable and it is both unrealistic and possibly undesirable to seek ways of avoiding them altogether for they are all part of a child's experience, part of his education. But it is surely the duty of planners and educators to try to reduce the number of *serious* accidents which cause death or severely damage children to an absolute minimum.

INJURIES

Road traffic accidents
Over half of all accidental deaths are a result of road accidents. As in most accidents, it is predominantly boys who are killed or injured. Most road accidents occur when the child is on foot and is hit by a moving vehicle. In a minority of instances the child is either riding a bicycle or a passenger in a car. The management consists of dealing with the multiple injuries in order of priority.

Falls
Children frequently suffer slight head injury as a result of falling out of beds, cots or windows, down stairs or from trees, climbing frames and so forth. While such injuries are not usually fatal, they are a common cause of hospital admission.

Head injury
Injury to the brain is a common cause of death in childhood accidents, and many

Road accidents

child as pedestrian 71% child as passenger 14% child on bicycle 15%

of the survivors are left with permanent damage. However, of all the children admitted to hospital for observation after head injury, only 5 per cent will prove to have major brain trauma.

Management. Most head injuries are minor. Hospital admission is necessary if the injury was severe or associated with loss or alteration of consciousness. It is also necessary if there is blood or cerebrospinal fluid oozing from the nose or ears, if a scalp wound overlies a fracture, or if a fracture crosses the groove of the middle meningeal artery. A skull fracture is not itself an indication of the severity of injury — many serious brain injuries occur in the absence of a fracture. Pallor and vomiting are very common after minor head injury in young children and result from vagal stimulation. Many children can be allowed home if instructions regarding observations are given to the parents.

Complications. Cerebral oedema is the commonest serious complication of head injury in children, because the soft skull transmits the injury force to the brain rather than acting as a shock absorber as the harder adult skull does. Pallor, vomiting and impaired consciousness result which may last hours or days. Adequate ventilation is important, since a high $PaCO_2$ increases intracranial pressure still further.

Intracranial bleeding is less common. It may be extradural, usually from the middle meningeal artery and therefore rapid in onset, or else subdural from cerebral veins and of slower onset. The head injury observations are intended to

Profile of head injuries

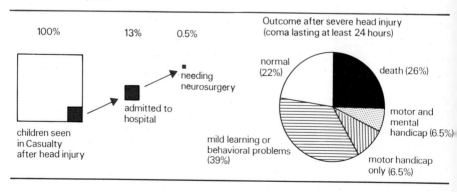

100% 13% 0.5%

Outcome after severe head injury (coma lasting at least 24 hours)

needing neurosurgery

admitted to hospital

children seen in Casualty after head injury

normal (22%)

death (26%)

motor and mental handicap (6.5%)

mild learning or behavioral problems (39%)

motor handicap only (6.5%)

Assessment of level of consciousness

Glasgow Coma Scale Best motor response		Verbal response		Eye opening	
Obeys	6	Orientated	5	Spontaneous	4
Localises	5	Confused conversation	4	To speech	3
Withdraws	4	Inappropriate words	3	To pain	2
Abnormal flexion	3	Incomprehensible	2	Nil	1
Extensor response	2	Nil	1		

make early detection of bleeding possible. Increasing intracranial pressure is assessed by a diminishing level of consciousness as measured on the Glasgow Coma Scale, a falling pulse rate and rising blood pressure, and alteration in size and reactivity of the pupils. A computerised tomography (CT) scan will distinguish between cerebral oedema, cerebral contusion and intracranial haemorrhage, both extradural and subdural. In the case of bleeding, surgery is necessary to decompress the brain, remove the clot and stop the bleeding source. In the case of worsening cerebral oedema, hyperventilation and drugs such as mannitol, dexamethasone and phenobarbitone can be used to reduce brain swelling.

DROWNING

Most drowning accidents occur in inland waters, swimming pools and baths. About a quarter occur in the sea. Again, boys are more commonly involved than girls. Swimming and life saving lessons at school, wearing life-jackets on boats and having supervision at pools and beaches are important preventive measures. Occasionally, children play the game of hyperventilation before a dive so that they may stay under the water for a long time. This can be dangerous and should be discouraged.

Children die during drowning either as a result of laryngeal spasm, when the cause of death is cerebral anoxia (dry drowning), or else water may enter the lungs, rapidly leading to respiratory failure with cardiac arrest (wet drowning). In either situation, the child may respond well to immediate cardiac massage and artificial ventilation once the airway has been cleared. Sometimes, if the water is muddy or polluted, the child may be revived only to die later with progressive pneumonia and pulmonary oedema (secondary drowning).

CHOKING

Over a hundred children die each year by choking on foreign bodies or food. An affected child is distressed, making violent respiratory efforts and becoming progressively cyanosed, but making no noise as the obstruction lies at the level of the larynx, wedged between the vocal cords. Death results if the child is unable to remove the obstruction by his efforts. The traditional first aid measure of violent slaps on the back is often unsuccessful, but abdominal compression (the Heimlich manoeuvre) can be life-saving. The rescuer stands behind the child with his clenched hands in the epigastrium — a short sharp squeeze directed inwards and upwards compresses the residual air in the lungs and may dislodge the obstruction.

BURNS AND SCALDS

Most accidents involving burns and scalds occur at home, particularly in poorer families. The inquisitive toddler is fascinated by matches and by flames. He knocks over paraffin heaters, goes too close to the open fire and sets light to his clothes, grasps a saucepan of boiling water by the handle and pulls it over himself or pulls a boiling electric kettle by the flex. Burns outside the home involving bonfires and fireworks tend to happen to older children.

The immediate treatment is to relieve the pain, ensure an adequate airway, and then assess the extent of the burns. If more than 10 per cent of the child's surface area is burned, intravenous fluids (plasma and saline) are necessary. If more than 50 per cent of the child's surface area is affected, the chances of survival are poor. Large quantities of fluid, blood and protein are lost from the burned areas and have to be replaced. A careful eye must be kept on the child's urine output and haematocrit. Tetanus toxoid and antibiotics are frequently used. Skin grafting may well necessary at a later date. Children who have been burned are often also psychologically scarred.

Supervision of toddlers in the home is the most important aspect of prevention of burns and scalds. The decreasing use of open fires and paraffin heaters, and the increased use of central heating has resulted in a decline in the incidence of burns in children in the last 20 years.

POISONING

Few children die as a result of poisoning, but many thousands attend hospital each year for treatment. Occasionally a child may intentionally ingest a poison, but in most cases the self-poisoning is accidental. Children may also be poisoned deliberately by their parents or inadvertently by their doctors. Most children who ingest a poison are fearless, inquisitive toddlers attracted by the appearance of tablets, medicines, household and garden substances, berries, seeds or fungi.

Some poisonous berries

woody nightshade   deadly nightshade   laburnum   henbane

Common poisons and age distribution of accidental poisoning (Nottingham 1984)

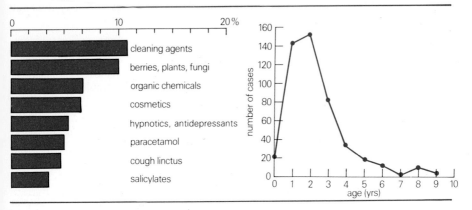

They will eat almost anything, regardless of taste. It has been shown that a child is particularly likely to ingest a poison when the family is under some sort of stress, presumably because of decreased supervision.

The management of a poisoned child consists of removal of the poison, followed by observation for the expected symptoms and signs. Treatment is generally symptomatic and nonspecific. Vomiting is induced to remove the poison from the stomach by giving the child syrup of ipecacuanha. Gastric lavage is rarely necessary, but emetic administration is obviously inappropriate for the unconscious child and in such cases the stomach should be emptied by lavage, but only after intubation with a cuffed endotracheal tube. Induced vomiting serves little purpose if more than four hours have passed since the ingestion, although there are exceptions, for example in cases of ingested aspirin and atropine, which delay gastric emptying. Vomiting is also to be avoided after ingestion of corrosive substances, or volatile agents such as paraffin or turpentine which are likely to be inhaled and may cause lung damage.

If the side effects of a poison are not known, information can be obtained at any time of day or night from one of the regional poison centres. Children likely to have ingested a toxic agent are admitted to hospital for observation. If respiratory failure develops, mechanical ventilation is necessary. If cardiovascular shock occurs, intravenous plasma or saline should be given.

Aspirin

Aspirin is a respiratory stimulant and a cell poison. When taken in large quantities it produces nausea, vomiting, tinnitus and dehydration. Hyperventilation with deep sighing respirations is a consequence of both metabolic acidosis and respiratory alkalosis. Hypoglycaemia, hyperglycaemia and an increased prothrombin time may occur in cases of severe poisoning. Fortunately children do not usually ingest sufficient amounts of aspirin to develop symptoms. If they do, then active steps should be taken to hasten the excretion of aspirin. When blood levels of salicylate are high, excretion should be enhanced by inducing a diuresis and reducing tubular reabsorption of the drug by making the urine alkaline. As with most poisons, there is no specific antidote.

Iron tablets

Iron tablets are frequently swallowed by toddlers because they are likely to be available (for example, iron tablets may be prescribed during pregnancy) and because they look like sweets. A small child can be fatally poisoned by as little as 2 grams of iron. The progress of a poisoned child can be divided into four phases. Firstly, within an hour of the ingestion the child develops severe gastro-intestinal symptoms, diarrhoea, vomiting, haematemesis and melaena. These symptoms may gradually subside so that the child seems well. However, some hours later, the serious third phase may develop with iron encephalopathy manifested by coma and fits, liver damage and circulatory collapse. Finally, a child who survives this may develop scarring of the stomach and pylorus as a consequence of local irritation. Iron ingestion is an indication for gastric lavage. The iron chelating agent desferrioxamine is useful. It can be left in the stomach to prevent further absorption of iron and it can be administered parenterally to enhance iron excretion and lessen the severity of the poisoning.

Tricyclic agents

Tricyclic agents such as amitriptyline and imipramine are among the commonest and most dangerous drugs consumed by young children. They may be available because one of the parents is taking them for depression or because a child in the family is being treated for bed-wetting. The effects of poisoning include respiratory and cardiovascular depression, as well as cerebral stimulation leading to irritability, excitation, hallucinations and fits, with exaggerated tendon reflexes. They have a marked atropine-like action, with fixed dilated pupils, a dry, red skin, sinus tachycardia, urinary retention and paralytic ileus. Finally, their most serious effect is on heart rhythm, resulting in atrial and ventricular tachycardias, fibrillation or heart block. There is no specific antidote, but after removal of the poison the atropine-like symptoms may be improved by anti-cholinesterase drugs and the cardiac arrythmias may respond to β-adrenergic blocking agents.

Alcohol

Alcohol is a dangerous acute poison in young children who drink it accidentally or older school children who drink it experimentally. The acute encephalopathy is often enhanced by severe hypoglycaemia which is particularly common in children and occasionally causes death. Blood glucose must be carefully monitored at the bedside and i.v. glucose given if it falls to low levels.

Important recent developments have led to a decrease in the incidence of severe accidental poisoning in children. Child-resistant containers have been developed which can only be opened by lining up an arrow on the lid with an arrow on the bottle or by pushing the lid down and twisting it open at the same time. In the U.K. it is compulsory for all aspirin and paracetamol tablets to be prescribed in this way, and pharmacists are encouraged to dispense other dangerous tablets in this form too. 'Blister packs' are also helpful. It takes the child a long time to eat sufficient tablets to cause symptoms, and he frequently loses interest or is discovered in the act.

Child-resistant containers

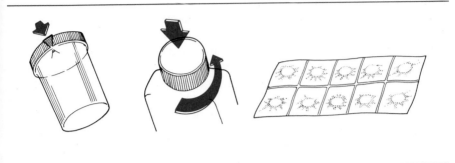

OTHER HAZARDS

The risk of a noxious agent producing permanent damage is highest in the earliest phase of development, embryogenesis. A number of such agents have been identified as being associated with a high incidence of congenital abnormalities.

Harmful environmental factors after birth are less easy to identify because so many children are exposed to potential hazards, and the ill effects may be quite subtle, making an association difficult to prove. Two hazards will be considered here, one physical, the other chemical.

Smoking

The harmful effects of smoking on those who actually smoke are well known. Chronic bronchitis, lung cancer and coronary heart disease are three common conditions whose incidence is greatly increased in smokers. Many school children now smoke regularly and are therefore at risk. It is obviously important to try to dissuade children from taking up smoking by appropriate health education in schools. It is also known that the children of smoking parents have a higher incidence of bronchitis and pneumonia; this applies particularly to babies and young children. Presumably the passive inhalation of tobacco smoke by the children at home is the important factor.

Lead

Lead is an environmental element which is undoubtedly harmful. If it is ingested or inhaled in large quantities it can produce a serious illness which may be lethal or result in brain damage. It is probable too, that chronic exposure to environmental lead has a harmful effect on mental development. There are several sources of lead. It used to be present in paint, so that children who chewed painted surfaces were liable to be poisoned. Water in lead pipes may contain sufficient lead to cause poisoning. Lead fumes produced by burning car batteries may produce toxic symptoms. Asian families use lead salts ('surma') in cosmetics applied regularly to the conjunctivae of the child and this may cause poisoning. More recently, there has been concern about atmospheric lead. Lead is present in exhaust fumes from vehicles and blood lead levels are higher in urban children and in those living close to major motorways. It has been suggested that this chronic exposure to moderate amounts of atmospheric lead may produce permanent intellectual impairment.

A child who has ingested lead may show symptoms of encephalopathy, with irritability, drowsiness, convulsions and eventually coma. Papilloedema may be present. Colicky abdominal pain is common and an abdominal x-ray may actually show radio-opaque lead fragments in the gastrointestinal tract. The diagnosis is made on the clinical picture, a history of exposure to a source of lead and investigations. Blood lead levels can be measured and are a guide to severity of poisoning. Lead affects many enzyme systems, but particularly those involved in haem synthesis. Measurement of blood levels of haem precursors forms the basis of a screening test for early lead poisoning which can be carried out in children who are at risk. In chronic poisoning, lead interferes with the growing ends of bones producing the x-ray sign 'lead lines'.

The treatment of a poisoned child is directed at removing lead from the body. This is achieved by using lead-chelating agents which increase lead excretion. In severe cases with encephalopathy, calcium edetate (EDTA) and dimercaprol (British Anti-Lewisite, BAL) are given parenterally. In less severe cases oral D-penicillamine is used. If there are signs of raised intracranial pressure, cerebral oedema can be lessened by intravenous mannitol or dexamethasone. The source of the lead must obviously be identified and removed. Severe lead poisoning carries a high mortality and survivors are often neurologically handicapped.

BIBLIOGRAPHY

Dreisbach R H 1977 Handbook of poisoning, 9th edn. Lange, California
Eason J M, Lovejoy F H 1979 Efficacy and safety of gastrointestinal decontamination in the treatment of oral poisoning. Pediatric clinics of North America. Saunders, Philadelphia, vol 26, no. 4
Gillis S S, Kagan B M 1980 Current pediatric therapy, 9th edn. Saunders, Philadelphia, Ch 20, pp 653–686
Hanenson I B 1980 Quick reference to clinical toxicology. Lippincott, Philadelphia
Kilham H A 1980 Hospital management of severe poisoning. Pediatric clinics of North America. Saunders, Philadelphia, vol 27, no. 3
Matthew H, Lawson A A H 1979 Treatment of common acute poisonings, 4th edn. Churchill Livingstone, Edinburgh

8
Airway and Lungs

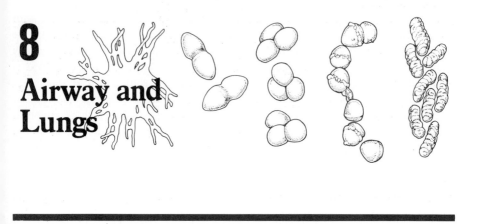

Acute respiratory problems are the commonest reason for a child visiting a doctor and are responsible for approximately 50 per cent of all patient-doctor contact. More serious respiratory illness leads to about 30 per cent of hospital admissions and respiratory disease appears to be an important factor in some 30 per cent of children who die. The preschool child has on average, six to eight respiratory infections per year, ranging from mild colds to severe bronchiolitis. Lower respiratory infections are commonest in the first year of life and then fall in incidence, presumably because of increasing resistance.

These impressive statistics are not surprising as the need to breathe air in and out of the lungs makes the respiratory tract particularly susceptible to infection. In the upper airways there are elaborate defence mechanisms and most of the infections that do occur are confined to this area. The majority of infections are viral with rhino, respiratory syncytial, influenza, para-influenza and adenoviruses being most prevalent. Though less common, bacterial infections still produce serious illness sometimes with residual damage. The bacteria which invade the respiratory tract include the β-haemolytic streptococcus, the pneumococcus, *Haemophilus influenzae* and the coagulase positive staphylococcus. In infants and those with impaired resistance the gram negative bacilli including *E. coli* and pseudomonas are also found.

Incidence of disease in childhood

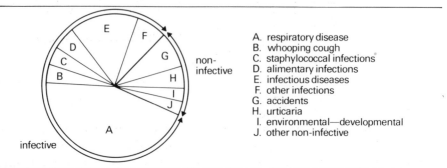

A. respiratory disease
B. whooping cough
C. staphylococcal infections
D. alimentary infections
E. infectious diseases
F. other infections
G. accidents
H. urticaria
I. environmental—developmental
J. other non-infective

non-infective

infective

UPPER RESPIRATORY TRACT

Coryza (common cold)

Coryza is usually a mild illness characterised by nasal obstruction and discharge usually due to one of the many rhinoviruses. There may be associated constitutional symptoms. It can be troublesome in infants under three months of age who are obligate nasal breathers, when feeding can become a major problem. There is also a suggestion that mild viral upper respiratory tract infections may be an important factor in some infants who die suddenly at home, cot deaths. Treatment with nasal decongestants and anti-pyretics may help feeding and reduce irritability. Antibiotics are not indicated unless there is good evidence to suggest secondary bacterial infection.

Pharyngitis and tonsillitis

These infections can occur at any age but are seen most frequently in children aged 4 to 7 years. The majority are caused by one of the many viruses which invade the respiratory tract but β-haemolytic streptococcal infections do occur and may have important systemic reactions, for example scarlet fever, rheumatic fever and acute glomerulonephritis. On examination, the feverish child will have swelling and inflammation involving his tonsils and pharyngeal mucosa. If an exudate is not visible, the infection is almost certainly viral. The presence of pus suggests, but is by no means diagnostic of, bacterial infection. Confirmation by culture of throat swabs is an ideal which is seldom possible in general practice but it does provide a scientific basis for eradicating streptococcal infection in the child and close contacts. Streptococcal infections require treatment with oral penicillin for 10 to 14 days. If, as is often the case, the tonsillitis is associated with abdominal pain and vomiting, the initial dose should be given parenterally. The other disease which regularly produces an acutely inflamed throat with exudate is glandular fever. In this condition there are often punctate haemorrhages at the junction of the soft and the hard palates.

Upper airway infections

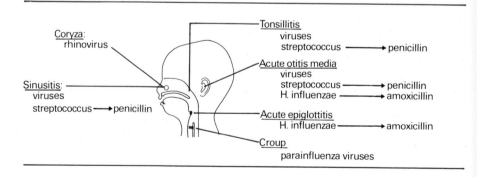

Coryza:
  rhinovirus

Sinusitis:
  viruses
  streptococcus ⟶ penicillin

Tonsillitis
  viruses
  streptococcus ⟶ penicillin

Acute otitis media
  viruses
  streptococcus ⟶ penicillin
  H. influenzae ⟶ amoxicillin

Acute epiglottitis
  H. influenzae ⟶ amoxicillin

Croup
  parainfluenza viruses

Tonsillectomy and adenoidectomy

Children who have recurrent infections in the upper respiratory tract are often considered for adenoidectomy and tonsillectomy. These operations are not without their problems and occasionally lead to death. As children on average get six to eight infections per year, recurrent tonsillitis alone is not sufficient reason for proceeding to operation. The indications for tonsillectomy are frequent attacks of tonsillitis which interfere with development or schooling, and peritonsillar abscesses. Enlargement of the tonsils is not of itself an indication unless they are so massive that they obstruct the airway. Tonsillar tissue shrinks spontaneously in later childhood. The adenoids should be removed if they are so large as to obstruct the Eustachian tubes with resultant recurrent otitis media, if there is persistent nasal obstruction or if they interfere with speech.

Otitis media

Earache is very common in children and is often associated with upper respiratory tract infection. This does not necessarily mean that the infection involves the middle ear, for the pain may be due to pressure changes resulting from obstruction to the Eustachian tube. The diagnosis of acute otitis media is based on ear pain with fever, associated with a bright red, bulging drum. Infants too young to complain of earache are irritable, restless and scream. Examination of the tympanic membrane is an essential part of the routine examination of any child with fever. The pathogens include viruses, the pneumococcus, the β-haemolytic streptococcus, and *Haemophilus influenzae*. Treatment with a 7- to 10-day course of penicillin is indicated in the older child. Those under the age of three years should be given a broad spectrum antibiotic (amoxycillin) as at this age *Haemophilus influenzae* infections predominate. Relief of pain can be accelerated by giving analgesics and decongestants to help drainage through the Eustachian tubes. Myringotomy is rarely required.

The right middle ear

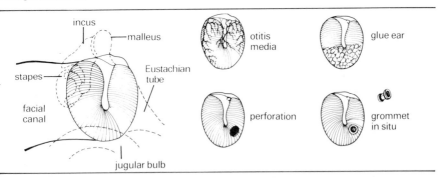

Before antibiotics, otitis media was followed by many complications including acute mastoiditis. Fortunately these are now rare, but recurrent ear infections still lead to a chronic exudative otitis media ('glue ear'), with subsequent conductive hearing loss. The parents may not be aware how much the child's ears have been involved in respiratory infections and his problems only come to light because of inattention at school. If this condition does not respond to simple treatment with decongestants, surgical drainage of the middle ear may be required.

Acute sinusitis

Viral infections may spread to the para-nasal sinuses. There may also be secondary bacterial infection in the maxillary sinuses, associated with fever, local tenderness and pain. As the frontal sinuses are not fully developed in early childhood, sinusitis is rarely a cause of frontal headache in the first ten years of life. On x-ray, the maxillary sinuses are usually completely opaque due to the presence of pus. The antibiotic of choice is penicillin but broad spectrum antibiotics such as amoxycillin should be prescribed if the child fails to respond. Recurrent or chronic infection can lead to post-nasal drip and a recurrent chronic cough with little or no evidence of local tenderness over the sinuses.

Acute laryngo-tracheobronchitis (croup)

Croup tends to occur in epidemics particularly in autumn and early spring. It is almost exclusively viral in origin, commonly the infleunza, para-influenza or respiratory syncitial virus. The larynx, trachea and bronchi are all involved in the inflammatory process. Symptoms start with a mild fever and runny nose. In the older child this progresses to sore throat, dysphagia and a dry, irritant cough. The younger child has a relatively small laryngeal airway and the resulting oedema and secretions can cause severe upper airway obstruction. The clinical features include a barking cough and a respiratory noise, particularly on inspiration (croup) which often start in the middle of the night. The natural tendency for the laryngeal airway to collapse on inspiration is increased by the child's desperate attempts to overcome the obstruction, thus exacerbating the situation. This effect is likely to be greater if parental anxiety is added to that of the child.

All children who are cyanosed or who have intercostal recession need to be admitted to hospital for observation. Many improve rapidly when they reach a warm, confident atmosphere but the occasional child has progressive airways obstruction which can only be relieved by intubation or tracheostomy. This intervention may be essential to prevent hypoxial brain damage or death. There is no evidence that putting the child in a cold mist tent or prescribing antibiotics or corticosteroids are of any value. It is of greater importance to reassure the child and to observe him carefully for signs of deterioration, measuring pulse rate, respiratory rate and looking for signs of hypoxial restlessness, cyanosis and deterioration in level of consciousness. If the child is showing evidence of these features or is becoming exhausted the obstruction must be relieved, preferably by tracheal intubation. This is a difficult procedure when the larynx is swollen and considerable skill will be required. If this fails, the obstruction must be relieved by tracheostomy. May spontaneously recover in 2-7 Days.

Some children get recurrent attacks of croup over a number of years, usually whenever they have a cold. They appear to have abnormally labile airways, closely akin to asthma but do not benefit from antiasthmatic drugs.

Acute epiglottitis 651.0

This is a rare specific infection caused by *Haemophilus influenzae* Type B and produces sudden rapid oedema of the epiglottis and aryepiglottic folds. Lethal airway obstruction can develop within hours. The children are likely to be toxic and may, by the time they come into hospital, be semiconscious. The throat will

F. Body: Small > lungs (not radio-opaque).

D.Dx - Diptheria
A. anaphylaxis
Retropharyngeal Abscess (V. Toxic child).

be intensely sore and swallowing is very painful, so the child keeps still and often drools saliva. Occasionally the swollen, cherry red epiglottis can be seen welling up into the pharyngeal space. Attempts to get a good view with the help of a tongue depressor have led to fatal acute total obstruction and this examination should only be performed when facilities for immediate intubation or tracheostomy are available.

Once the diagnosis is suspected the child must be admitted to intensive care in a humid atmosphere, propped up on pillows and given intravenous cefotaxime (200 mg/kg/day).

Despite adequate antibiotic therapy, 60% of these children develop such severe obstruction that intubation is unavoidable.

Airway collapse occurs during inspiration in children with upper airway obstruction

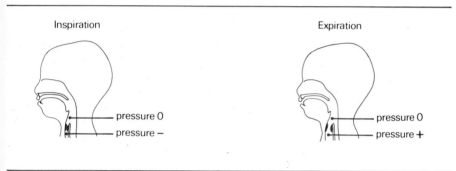

Inspiration — pressure 0 / pressure −

Expiration — pressure 0 / pressure +

Persistent stridor

There is a small group of children who have inspiratory stridor at birth which persists for many months. When this presents in the first weeks of life and follows a benign course, it is referred to as congenital floppy larynx, laryngomalacia or congenital laryngeal stridor and is presumably an exaggeration of the normal tendency for the larynx to collapse on inspiration. These infants often only have signs when excited or upset. No treatment is effective and fortunately intubation is rarely required. The stridor becomes less noticeable as the child grows and usually disappears by the age of one to two years. Symptoms are likely to get worse whenever the infant has an upper respiratory tract infection.

Persistent stridor may also be produced by pressure on the trachea from without, either by a mediastinal tumour or by a vascular ring due to a double aortic arch or anomalous origin of a large artery. This will be shown on barium swallow x-rays as the oesophagus also lies within the area of compression. Stridor can also result from lesions within the trachea including papillomas, haemangiomas and tracheal stenosis. Occasionally, a stridor present from birth is due to vocal cord palsy usually secondary to birth trauma but may also result from abnormality of the central nervous system including hydrocephalus.

If the child has stridor and recession while at rest, the investigations should include a barium swallow and direct laryngoscopy.

LOWER RESPIRATORY TRACT

Acute bronchitis

Upper respiratory viral infections frequently spread down the airway to involve the mucosa of the bronchi. The child has a troublesome cough which is initially dry but becomes productive after a few days. There is little to find on examination apart from a mild pyrexia. Towards the end of the attack the increased production of secretion may result in coarse rales and low pitched rhonchi. If the child is obviously wheezing, this is almost certainly an asthmatic attack precipitated by a viral infection in a susceptible subject. Primary bacterial bronchitis, with the exception of whooping cough, is rare in childhood and antibiotics are not indicated unless secondary infection is suspected. Night time cough suppressants, for example, linctus codeine, are useful particularly in the early stages of the illness.

Acute bronchiolitis

This is the commonest of the severe acute infections and, like laryngotracheobronchitis, occurs in epidemics, usually in the winter months. It affects infants and toddlers. The respiratory syncitial virus is responsible for the majority but outbreaks can also be caused by the para-influenza, influenza, rhino- and adenoviruses.

The inflammation predominantly affects the bronchioles whose calibre ranges from 75 to 300 μm leading to loss of cilia with oedema and necrosis of the epithelial cells and obstruction of the lumen by cellular debris and thick secretions. Typically, the child begins with coryzal symptoms and develops an irritable cough with rapid breathing and feeding difficulty within the next two to three days. If the illness is mild the child may then improve but in some it progresses with increasing breathlessness and cyanosis. In addition to the rapid, laboured respirations, the babies have tachycardia and often gross hyperinflation of their lungs, producing a barrel-shaped chest, prominent neck veins and downward displacement of the liver. Widespread crepitations can be heard over the lung fields, often with high-pitched rhonchi, particularly on expiration. The chest x-ray confirms the marked hyperinflation of the lungs but the picture is often complicated by areas of collapse produced by retained secretions.

The virus responsible can usually be identified by treating nasopharyngeal

Bronchiolitis

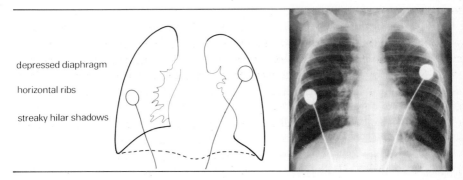

depressed diaphragm

horizontal ribs

streaky hilar shadows

aspirates with flourescent labelled antibodies (immunofluorescence) and then scanning the slide under the uv light microscope for evidence of viral aggregates in the epithelial cells.

The principles of management are similar to those of acute laryngo-tracheobronchitis; there is no specific measure that will alter the course of the disease. Confident supportive care with added oxygen in a carefully monitored setting is currently the best approach. Antibiotics are not indicated unless there is evidence of secondary bacterial infection which occurs rarely, and extensive clinical trials have demonstrated that bronchodilator drugs and corticosteroids do not modify the course of the disease. Physiotherapy should not be used in the early phase. Preliminary studies suggest that the antiviral agent, ribavirin, may be useful if given as a continuous nebulised inhalation. Monitoring for apnoea and bradycardia are important as some of these children have recurrent attacks of apnoea even when not critically ill and appropriate stimulation early in the attack is usually successful. Should the baby's breathing become critical, artificial ventilation can be given but this requires considerable skill and inexperienced staff may do more harm than good attempting the exercise.

Pneumonia

Consolidation of the lung due to secondary infection is common in any child who is seriously ill. Patches of collapse and consolidation are not infrequent in a wide range of respiratory infections but should not influence the overall management of the child. Babies with feeding problems not infrequently inhale and produce patchy collapse and consolidation. In these instances physiotherapy is probably more important than seeking an organism which might be responsible for a secondary infection.

Viral pneumonias

Primary viral infections can spread down the respiratory tract and into the lungs and should be suspected in any child, particularly those in the first year of life, in whom a respiratory infection has produced a serious illness with marked constitutional effects and circulatory failure. Respiratory syncitial virus, influenza, para-influenza and adenoviruses are among those most commonly implicated. Clinical examination of the child's respiratory system often gives little clue to the patchy shadowing which is demonstrated on a chest x-ray. Although the infection is suspected to be viral, a broad spectrum antibiotic such as amoxycillin is likely to be given.

— recover Spontaneously

Pneumococcal pneumonia   *>1yr.   20% -> Pl. effusions.*

Streptococcus pneumoniae is a common secondary pathogen in the lung but occasionally produces a dramatic primary disease characterised by lobar or segmental consolidation. The child often appears very ill and drowsy and gives no clue to the site of the infection. Indeed, the headache and drowsiness with associated neck stiffness may lead to the child having a lumbar puncture before a chest x-ray. If the pneumonia involves the lower segments of the lung then referred abdominal pain may be the presenting symptom and the child is seen first by the surgeons. Localising signs, dullness to percussion, bronchial breathing and fine crepitations, are easy to miss in the young child even when

pA Strep — Similar to pneumococcus.
Do Antisteptolysin titre.
*yr.   * Can go from throat Swab.*

Klebsiella *newborns + older children.*
debilitated c̄ other LRT problems.
Destructive → pneumatocoele.
Rx Cs + Aminoglycoside.

AIRWAY AND LUNGS 115

Features seen on chest X-ray

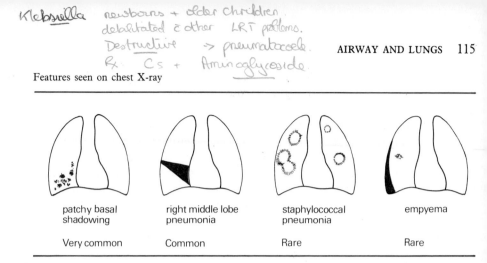

patchy basal shadowing	right middle lobe pneumonia	staphylococcal pneumonia	empyema
Very common	Common	Rare	Rare

the diagnosis is known but a chest x-ray will resolve the problem showing segmental or lobar consolidation. If the diagnosis is suspected a lateral x-ray is necessary in addition to an antero-posterior view to avoid missing consolidation at the posterior segment of the upper lobes. The organism may be grown on blood culture as well as from the upper respiratory tract. Parenteral penicillin remains the antibiotic of choice. *10 Days*

Haemophilus influenzae type B pneumonia   *3-5yrs   O. Media, A pro*
This is the second commonest bacterial pneumonia in the world. The chest x-ray usually shows the scattered pattern of bronchopneumonia rather than a lobular shadow. Most respond to oral amoxicillin but i.v. ampicillin should be given if necessary. *onset more insidious,   or Chloramphenicol*

Staphylococcal infections   *80% Unilat   R>L*
In debilitated children or weakly infants the coagulase positive *Staphylococcus aureus* can invade the lungs, producing widespread consolidation with abscesses. Affected babies are usually under 12 months of age and present with an acute illness often with peripheral shock due to an associated septicaemia. They have been colourfully described as 'near cot deaths'. Other infants have less constitutional reactions despite showing massive lung involvement on x-ray. The children sometimes have signs of lung over-inflation. More striking are the widespread coarse crepitations often with areas of dullness to percussion and bronchial breathing. The chest x-ray may show scattered areas of consolidation throughout the lung fields. More commonly there is a large dense area with one or more abscess cavities. Pleural effusions or empyemas also occur. These children need careful monitoring, as respiratory failure and circulatory collapse can occur with frightening rapidity, often secondary to a tension pneumothorax. Active treatment with circulatory and respiratory support and parenteral antibiotics effective against the coagulase positive staphylococcus, for example cloxacillin and gentamicin can give gratifying results. *± Chest drain.*

? P. c̄   underlying cd (1) primature ? Synd Risk premature

c̄ Pl. effusion - Do a Mantoux Test !   (> Neonate → Throat Culture

Mycoplasma pneumonia
Mycoplasma pneumonia affects older children, particularly those between 5 and 15 years of age and can produce a wide range of respiratory tract infections. The picture most commonly seen is that of generalised malaise, anorexia with head-

Colder months of the year

ache, fever and sore throat, followed by the development of a cough producing mucoid sputum occasionally tinged with blood. Fine crepitations may or may not be heard on examination. The chest x-ray may show either widespread diffuse shadowing or, on occasions, lobar or segmental consolidation. The diagnosis is made by culturing the organism or finding specific antibodies in the serum. The infection responds most readily to erythromycin. , tetracycline (if > 10 yrs)

Other organisms including β-haemolytic streptococcus group A can cause pneumonia. In the newborn period *E. coli*, pseudomonas and klebsiella infections may also occur and for this reason gentamicin is probably the antibiotic of choice.

Bronchiectasis

In bronchiectasis there are cystic changes involving the bronchi particularly in the lower segment of the lungs leading to chronic abscesses with purulent smelly sputum, often complicated by haemoptyses. This used to be a common complication of respiratory illnesses particularly whooping cough, measles and bacterial pneumonias. Fortunately, with improvements in general nutrition and wider use of antibiotics, it is now rarely seen except as a complication of cystic fibrosis and in children with immune deficiency states. Regular physiotherapy with courses of antibiotics for exacerbations of infection provides the best means of control.

ASTHMA

Asthma is a disorder characterised by hyper-reactivity of the airways leading to paroxysmal attacks of airways obstruction which produce coughing, respiratory distress and wheezing. It is by far the commonest chronic respiratory disease of childhood affecting up to 12% of children. There is a wide spectrum of disease ranging from single mild wheezing episodes to continuous asthma with episodic severe exacerbations. The airways obstruction is a combination of muscle spasm, mucosal oedema and increased secretions.

Clinical features

Usually episodes of coughing and wheezing appear in the latter months of the first year and as at this age the attacks are almost exclusively brought on by viral upper respiratory tract infections, a diagnosis of recurrent, wheezy bronchitis is often made. Frequently there is a history of eczema and a family history of allergic disorders. Over the next two years the pattern remains unchanged with wheezing attacks lasting several days whenever the child gets a cold. Nocturnal cough and sleep disturbance are conspicuous complaints by the parents.

If the child is over the age of three years the parents may have noticed that prolonged exercise results in attacks of coughing and wheezing lasting for 10 to 20 minutes. Exercise induced bronchoconstriction may be an isolated disorder in a child who is otherwise free from asthmatic attacks. In others, the attacks are also induced by a variety of inhaled allergens. These foreign proteins react with IgE antibody on the surface of mast cells within the respiratory tract, leading to release of histamine, leukotrienes, serotonin and other substances which produce smooth muscle constriction and local oedema, the so-called Type I immunological response. Many of the important allergens can be identified by taking a careful history; for example grass pollen sensitivity produces symptoms

Allergens

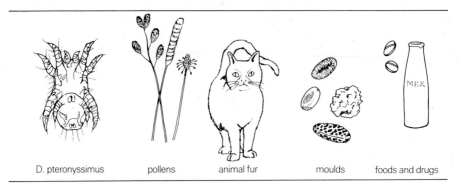

| D. pteronyssimus | pollens | animal fur | moulds | foods and drugs |

from May to June, and fungal sensitivity in the autumn. The house dust mite, *Dermatophagoides pteronyssimus*, feeds on shed skin and is found in greatest concentrations in the bed. This is probably the single most important allergen in childhood asthma and is responsible for the troublesome nocturnal symptoms. Other common sensitising substances include cat and dog fur, feathers and occasionally foods and drugs. Skin tests may be helpful in providing additional evidence of suspected allergens, but many otherwise healthy children have positive skin tests; they are also often negative in food allergies. Nasal or bronchial provocation tests are probably more significant but are also more dangerous. Emotional factors are also important and enquiry about the home and school is essential in children whose asthma is difficult to control. In many children symptoms are exacerbated when the weather changes.

Children with asthma may be graded into three groups:

1. The mild group includes children whose occasional attacks are usually precipitated by infection but who have no symptoms between attacks and whose growth and pulmonary function tests are normal apart from exercise-induced bronchoconstriction.
2. The intermediate or moderate group consists of those with severe, recurrent episodes but, again, they are symptom-free between attacks apart from exercise-induced bronchoconstriction.
3. In the severe group, the asthmatic attacks may vary in severity but the child is never free from symptoms and the illness affects his general growth and development. Lung function tests remain abnormal at all times in this category. These children have chest wall deformity and chest X-rays show the presence of over-expanded lungs even when they are at their best.

Management

The best results are achieved by a single doctor paying attention to detail and giving the correct therapy at the appropriate time, in the optimal amount for that particular child within the particular family.

General management. The amount an asthmatic suffers from his disease is often related as much to the advice of his medical advisor and the anxiety of his parents as to the reactivity of his bronchial tree. Parents should be given a simple

Peak expiratory flow rates measured by a Wright's Peak Flow Meter. Normal values are related to height rather than age. The serial measurements are those of a child with exercise-induced bronchospasm who responded to salbutamol

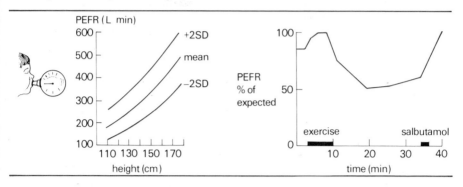

explanation of the nature of the disease and the purpose of the various treatments recommended. They are often the best judge of the most effective approach. In children who have recurrent severe episodes, direct admission to a ward not only allows the child to have immediate and appropriate care but it is also very reassuring to his parents. Children should be encouraged to lead a normal, outgoing existence and the parents should be encouraged to help their children to be independent and to avoid over-protection. Many who were asthmatic as children have turned out to be outstanding athletes. Indeed the prognosis for mild and moderate asthma in childhood is very good. Unfortunately severe chronic asthma tends to persist, although there may well be improvement as they enter adolescence.

Out-patient therapy. Where possible, allergens should be identified and avoided. For example, the number of house dust mites can be reduced by frequent washing of bedclothes and vacuuming of the mattress and bedroom in order that the child sleeps in a relatively allergen-free environment. The child with only occasional wheezing attacks can usually lead a virtually normal life with the help of oral bronchodilator drugs like salbutamol. Immediate relief can be

> 20'/. ↓ PEFR on Exercise Test!

Forced expiratory volumes measured by spirometry. In children the volume exhaled in the first 0.75 of a second is used, rather than the full second which is preferred for adults. The serial values are those of a child showing response to salbutamol after bronchial provocation with house dust mite.

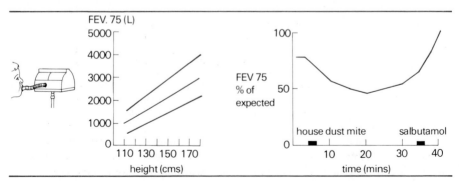

obtained if the drug is inhaled from a pressurised aerosol or as a dry powder. Those who have symptoms which are troublesome despite adequate broncho-dilator therapy should be tried on sodium cromoglycate. This compound, inhaled on a regular basis either by spinhaler or, in the young child, as a nebulised solution, interferes with the IgE mediated process and prevents or reduces the frequency of asthmatic attacks in about 70% of children with asthma. If the child fails to obtain sufficient benefit and is missing school, an inhaler delivering a topically active steroid, for example beclomethasone, should be prescribed. Long-term systemic steroids should be avoided wherever possible because of the side effects, in particular growth suppression. Short sharp courses of prednisolone given infrequently do have a part to play and may avoid the need to admit the child to hospital.

In-patient management. Admission to hospital with severe asthma indicates that the drugs used have failed. Despite this, inhalation of nebulised salbutamol respirator solution can be very effective if this has not already been used. Aminophylline, preferably given intravenously, is also beneficial but an overdose can lead to vomiting, convulsions and collapse. Particular care is need if the child is already on oral theophylline therapy. If the child has not responded well, intravenous hydrocortisone is indicated. In status asthmaticus the airways are often blocked with plugs of thick exudate and desquamated cells leading to gross hyperinflation. By this stage the patients are usually dehydrated so that they need intravenous fluids and controlled humidified oxygen therapy. If respiratory failure develops, artificial ventilation for a period will help. Experts agree that sedatives are contraindicated in children with status asthmaticus.

Drugs in asthma

Type of drug	Drug	Mode of administration	
β₂ adrenergic stimulants	Salbutamol	oral, i.m., i.v., inhalation	
	Terbutaline	oral, i.m., i.v., inhalation	
Xanthines	Aminophylline	i.v.	
	Slow release theophyllines	oral	
Prophylactic	Sodium cromoglycate	inhalation	powder or nebulised solution
Corticosteroids	Beclomethasone	inhalation	powder or aerosol
	Betamethasone isovalerate	inhalation	aerosol
	Prednisolone	oral	
	Hydrocortisone	i.v.	

CYSTIC FIBROSIS

Cystic fibrosis is now the commonest cause of chronic suppurative lung disease in the U.K. It is an inherited condition (autosomal recessive) affecting about 1 in 2000 live births in European population; it is much less common in Asians or Africans. Many tissues are affected, particularly those with exocrine glands. Abnormally viscid secretions cause duct obstruction resulting in pancreatic insufficiency, biliary cirrhosis and male infertility. The sweat has a high salt content which appears to be due to an abnormally low Cl⁻ permeability of the duct epithelium.

Clinical features

The majority of patients present with diarrhoea and failure to thrive due to malabsorption, or recurrent or persistent chest infections, or both. While most are infants, the severity of symptoms and age of diagnosis are quite variable. A small group of patients with mild disease and little, if any, malabsorption, present late. The diagnosis is made by finding high concentrations of sodium and chloride in sweat obtained by pilocarpine iontophoresis, the sweat test.

Meconium ileus. Meconium ileus is a form of neonatal small bowel obstruction due to viscid meconium. A gastrografin enema establishes the diagnosis and may relieve the obstruction. More severe cases will need surgery. The most severely affected bowel is resected, viscid meconium removed and a temporary ileostomy made.   Poor Prognostic feature!

The lungs. The lungs are normal at birth, but a persistent cough may soon develop, or recurrent cough and wheeze occur with colds. The symptoms are initially intermittent but gradually become more persistent, the cough becomes chronic and sputum is produced. Clubbing of the fingers and chest deformity develop relatively early, later there is growth impairment, limitation of activity and eventual respiratory failure. The rate of progression of the lung disease is variable, lung disease at different stages may be found at all ages. Progression in an individual child tends to be episodic, punctuated by acute exacerbations of symptoms with intercurrent infection. Chest x-rays show either overdistension of the lungs or may appear normal. Later generalised peribronchial thickening develops, followed by obvious dilatation of the bronchi and mottled shadows. Larger opacities appear with acute illness, but in general lobar or segmental pneumonia is uncommon. Initial sputum cultures usually reveal *Haemophilus influenzae* or *Staphylococcus aureus* organisms, but these pathogens are eventually

Mode of presentation and age at diagnosis of children with cystic fibrosis

Postural drainage

drainage of lower parts of lung

drainage of upper parts of lung

drainage of lateral parts of lung

replaced by *Pseudomonas aeruginosa* in most patients.

Treatment is aimed at minimising symptoms and delaying the progression of the disease. Regular physiotherapy and physical activity are very important. Antibiotics are given for exacerbations depending on sputum cultures. High doses are given for prolonged periods if necessary. Hospital treatment with i.v. antibiotics such as azlocillin and tobramycin maybe needed for pseudomonas infections. It is impossible to eradicate it. The value of prolonged oral antistaphylococcal antibotics is unproven. Inhalation of bronchodilators, mucolytics or antibiotics may benefit some patients. Immunisation, especially against pertussis and measles, is essential.

Malabsorption. Malabsorption is due to pancreatic insufficiency. The stools are frequent, loose and offensive and the child fails to thrive, often despite a large appetite. Rectal prolapse may occur. Microscopy of the stool for fat globules and testing for chymotrypsin is a useful screening tests. Detailed investigation of pancreatic function is usually unnecessary. Symptomatic liver disease is uncommon, though portal hypertension may occur. Abdominal pain is common. In older children it is sometimes associated with a palpable faecal mass in the right iliac fossa and subacute obstruction.

The malabsorption is improved by taking a pancreatic enzyme preparation with meals. Some dietary fat restriction is usually needed but should be tailored to the individual's tolerance. The diet should contain a high calorie and protein content with added vitamins.

Some older children have a very poor appetite and may benefit from dietary supplements.

Outlook

The longterm outlook for survival has improved considerably in recent years, and there are now many adult CF patients. The disease is, however, very variable and it is difficult to give an accurate prognosis for an individual child. There are now many older children with little lung disease, attending normal schools and able to undertake full activity. The longterm nature of the disease, uncertainty of prognosis and the demands of regular treatment put a considerable strain on the family. Compliance, especially with physiotherapy, may be poor. Older patients have an increasing incidence of pneumothorax, haemoptysis, diabetes

Survival figures for cystic fibrosis

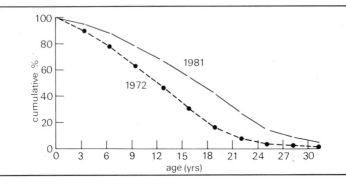

and liver disease as well as problems getting jobs and becoming independent. Almost all males with CF are infertile due to obstruction of the vas but females may have successful pregnancies.

Genetic counselling is essential as one in four siblings will be affected. The gene mutated in cystic fibrosis has now been identified and holds promise for prenatal diagnosis and carrier screening. Neonatal screening is undertaken in some areas by estimation of immunoreactive trypsin using the Guthrie blood specimen. This test has proved to be a reliable screening test but it has not yet been shown convincingly that early diagnosis improves the longterm prognosis.

RARE LUNG DISEASES

Occasionally children present with respiratory problems which do not fit into the categories already described. The typical picture is that of an infant who has a persistently raised respiratory rate with respiratory distress, cough and failure to thrive. There are a number of causes which need to be considered which include antenatally acquired infections such as rubella, chlamydia and cytomegalovirus pneumonia or respiratory problems secondary to an underlying congenital abnormality. These include clefts of the larynx, a persisting tracheooesophageal fistula, congenital lung cysts and abnormalities of the diaphragm. Infants who have difficulty in coordinating their swallowing or those with hiatus hernias may also present with chronic respiratory infection due to recurrent chronic aspiration of milk and food. Infants and children with an immunological deficiency state frequently have severe respiratory tract infections, often due to organisms such as *Pneumocystis carinii* which are not pathogenic to the healthy child. Occasionally, an acute viral infection, particularly an adenoviral bronchiolitis can produce severe lung damage resulting in a condition known as obliterative bronchiolitis. Some infants present with respiratory distress due to congenital lobar emphysema, the aetiology of which is often obscure. Finally, there is a group of rare respiratory diseases including fibrosing alveolitis and pulmonary haemosiderosis which occur in the young as well as the old. Severe lung disease can be regarded with rather more optimism in the infant than in the adult, as alveolar budding occurs up to the age of eight years so that remarkable improvements can occur even after the most devastating illnesses.

BIBLIOGRAPHY

Clark T J H, Godfrey S 1983 Asthma, 2nd edn. Chapman & Hall, London
Colley J R T 1976 The epidemiology of respiratory disease in childhood. In: Hull D (ed) Recent advances in paediatrics — 5. Churchill Livingstone, Edinburgh, ch 9, p 221–258
Godfrey S 1974 Exercise testing in children. Saunders, Philadelphia
Kendig E L 1983 Disorders of the respiratory tract in children. Saunders, Philadelphia
Leer J A, Green J L, Heimlick E M, Hyde J S, Moffett H L, Young G A, Barron B A 1969 Corticosteroid treatment in bronchiolitis. American Journal of Diseases of Childhood 117:495
Miller F J W, Court S D M, Walton W S, Knox E G 1960 Growing up in Newcastle Upon Tyne. Oxford University Press, Oxford
Phelan P D, Landau L I, Olinsky A 1982 Respiratory illness in children, 2nd edn. Blackwell, Oxford
Williams H E, McNichol K N 1969 Prevalence, natural history and relationship of wheezy bronchitis and asthma in children. An epidemiological study. British Medical Journal 4:321

9
Heart

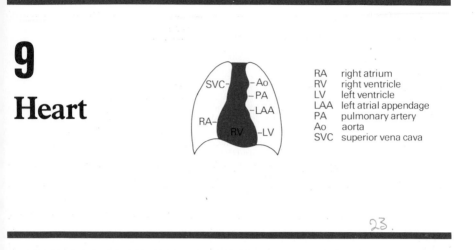

RA	right atrium
RV	right ventricle
LV	left ventricle
LAA	left atrial appendage
PA	pulmonary artery
Ao	aorta
SVC	superior vena cava

23.

Now that rheumatic fever is rare, congenital abnormalities have become the main cause of heart disease in children. Acquired heart disease still occurs but it is not common; congenital heart defects, however, occur in approximately seven to eight infants per thousand live births and congenital heart disease thus forms the commonest single group of serious congenital abnormalities. Less than a quarter of affected children will die in the first year of life, the majority within the first month. These children have severe cardiac abnormalities which, in many cases, are complex and inoperable. However, the number of children with severe lesions who are now surviving beyond the first year is increasing, a tribute to the skill and ingenuity of cardiac surgeons. Ten to 15% of children with congenital heart disease have more than one cardiac abnormality. Ten to 15% have an associated non-cardiac abnormality; the skeletal, gastrointestinal and genito-urinary systems are the most commonly involved. There are nine common congenital heart lesions which together make up 90% of all cases. The remaining 10% consists of numerous rarer, more complex anomalies.

Aetiology
As with most congenital defects, the precise aetiology is unknown but both genetic and environmental factors have been identified. Family studies suggest that the mode of inheritance is polygenic, although occasionally single gene mutations occur. If a mother has a child with a congenital heart defect, the

The nine commonest congenital heart defects

Acyanotic	Cyanotic
Ventricular septal defect	Transposition of the great arteries
Atrial septal defect	Tetralogy of Fallot
Patent ductus arteriosus	
Pulmonary stenosis	
Aortic stenosis	
Coarctation of aorta	
Hypoplastic left heart	

124

Congenital heart disease in chromosome disorders

Chromosomal Abnormality	Clinical syndrome	Type of lesion commonly seen
Partial deletion of chromosome 5	Cri du chat	VSD
Trisomy 13–15	Patau syndrome	VSD, PDA Dextrocardia
Trisomy 18	Edward syndrome	Complex lesions
Trisomy 21	Down syndrome	VSD, ASD, Fallot tetralogy
XO	Turner syndrome	Coarctation, and aortic stenosis

chances of a second child being affected are about three times higher than if her child had no heart defect. Children with chromosomal abnormalities have a greatly increased incidence of congenital heart disease; nearly half of all children with Down syndrome have a cardiac lesion. Maternal rubella in the first trimester of pregnancy, maternal diabetes and drugs in pregnancy (like thalidomide, alcohol, phenytoin) are environmental factors associated with an increased incidence of congenital heart disease.

Presentation

Congenital heart disease usually presents in one of the three following ways:

Heart murmur. This is the commonest mode of presentation. Most murmurs are detected in the first year of life, either on routine examination in the newborn period or in the child health clinics. A minority are not discovered until the child starts school.

Heart failure. A number of lesions will cause heart failure, commonly in the first year of life. The symptoms and signs are similar to those found in an adult. The baby becomes breathless, particularly after the exertion of feeding or crying. He may have difficulty completing feeds and as a consequence fails to thrive. Sweating is often a prominent symptom. On examination, the baby has a rapid

Heart failure in infancy

Symptoms

breathlessness on exertion
(especially feeding and crying)

sweating

failure to thrive

Signs

rapid respiratory rate
(often with recession)

increased heart rate

enlarged heart

murmur (± thrill)

enlarged liver

respiratory rate and a rapid pulse rate. Heart enlargement is usually present and can be detected clinically; a thrill or murmur may be present and there is often a gallop rhythm due to a third heart sound. Invariably, the liver is enlarged due to venous congestion. Oedema of the dependant parts of the body is rarely seen, although infants in failure frequently show rapid weight gains suggesting fluid retention. Fine moist sounds of pulmonary oedema are less easily heard in babies than in adults. If frank pulmonary oedema is present, the baby may be centrally cyanosed and the cyanosis will disappear when oxygen is given.

Cyanosis ('blue baby'). If the heart defect results in unsaturated venous blood by-passing the lungs, central cyanosis will be present and is not corrected while breathing 100% oxygen. This lack of response to oxygen helps to distinguish cyanosis due to heart disease from cyanosis due to severe lung disease, especially in the newborn period when this distinction can be difficult. Long-standing central cyanosis results in clubbing of the fingers and toes and secondary polycythaemia. A child with cyanotic congenital heart disease often has a reduced exercise tolerance and fails to grow normally.

Investigations

Investigations must be carried out urgently in symptomatic infants. A chest x-ray and electrocardiogram are essential investigations in the assessment of a child with suspected heart disease. Echocardiography using ultrasound, is a non-invasive investigation which gives detailed information about the anatomy of the heart and great vessels. Almost all lesions which cause heart failure or cyanosis in infancy, and many of those which produce a murmur, can be confidently diagnosed by echocardiography, and the infant referred for surgery. Cardiac catheterisation is an invasive investigation, only performed in specialist units — it enables the pressures and saturations within the cardiac chambers to be measured and, with angiocardiography following injection of radio-opaque dye, permits precise anatomical and physiological diagnosis. It is particularly useful for estimating the severity of a lesion, and judging the need for surgery in asymptomatic patients.

The innocent murmur

Many babies and children have heart murmurs without any structural abnormality of the heart. Indeed, in one reported series, a cardiologist detected a heart murmur in the majority of healthy school children on routine examination! Such murmurs are termed innocent, or functional. They are diagnosed as being innocent on the basis of their characteristics and are associated with a normal chest x-ray, cardiac ultrasound and ECG. If a murmur is obviously innocent, the parents need not be told and no follow-up is necessary. If there is uncertainty, an expert opinion should be sought as soon as possible, before the seeds of cardiac neurosis are sown. There are three types of innocent murmur:

1. Venous hum. This is a blowing, continuous murmur heard at the base of the heart, often just below the clavicles. It varies both with respiration and the position of the head, and disappears when the child lies down. It is due to blood flow through the systemic great veins and is sometimes confused with a patent ductus arteriosus.

Innocent murmurs

[handwritten annotations: Low f. / Low intensity ≤ Grade III / Δ c̄ Posture / Δ c̄ Respiration. / Apex./L Sternal Border./ Ao Area. / Ejection Murmur = (= vibratory) / α turbulent flow]

[diagram labels:] venous hum
pulmonary flow murmur
vibratory murmur *= Still's Murmur*

2. Pulmonary flow murmur. This is a soft, systolic ejection murmur heard in the pulmonary area (the second left intercostal space). It is due to rapid flow of blood across a normal pulmonary valve and is especially prominent when the cardiac output is high, for example after exercise, in febrile children or in cases of anaemia.

3. Vibratory murmur. This is a short, buzzing murmur heard in systole at the left sternal edge or at the apex of the heart. It is variable and changes with position. *↳ STILL'S MURMUR !*

If a murmur is pansystolic, diastolic, loud or long, associated with a thrill or with cardiac symptoms, it is not innocent.

Classification of congenital heart disease
Congenital heart disease can conveniently be classified into two groups: (1) acyanotic due to either a left to right shunt or obstructive lesion, and (2) cyanotic with either increased or diminished pulmonary flow.

ACYANOTIC LESIONS WITH A LEFT TO RIGHT SHUNT

A common type of congenital heart defect is a hole between the two sides of the heart, at the level of either the atria, the ventricles or the great arteries. In fetal life, pulmonary blood flow is small and the pressure in the right ventricle and pulmonary artery is high. With the onset of regular respirations, the pulmonary vascular resistance falls, with a consequent fall in the pressures on the right side of the heart. Since the pressure on the left side of the heart now exceeds that on the right side, blood will start to flow from the left side to the right side through the hole. The fall in pulmonary vascular resistance occurs rapidly in the first few days after birth and then more slowly over the next few weeks, so that by the age of about three months the left to right flow of blood reaches a maximum. There is therefore an additional circulation of blood from the left side of the heart to the right side, thence to the lungs and back to the left side of the heart again. This is termed a shunt. If the hole is small, the shunt may be trivial, but if it is large, it may represent the majority of the cardiac output, so that the blood flow through the pulmonary artery may be several times greater than the flow through the aorta. A large shunt imposes an added burden on the heart, with consequently hypertrophy, dilatation and sometimes failure. Because of the high pulmonary vascular resistance immediately after birth, frequently a murmur is not heard and in babies with a simple left to right shunt, heart failure is uncommon in the first few weeks of life.

A left to right shunt, if appreciable, will give rise to a number of consistent findings, regardless of the site of the hole. Clinical examination may show an enlarged heart with hypertrophy of one or both ventricles. Signs of ventricular hypertrophy will be present on the electrocardiogram. A chest radiograph will reveal an enlarged heart with a prominent pulmonary artery and an increase in vascular markings (pulmonary plethora) due to the high pulmonary blood flow.

ATRIAL SEPTAL DEFECT (OSTIUM SECUNDUM)

In the majority of atrial septal defects, the hole is in the atrial septum in the region of the fossa ovalis, the site of the foramen ovale: this is the ostium secundum defect. Because the right ventricle is less muscular and easier to fill with blood than the left ventricle, blood will flow from the left atrium to the right atrium through the defect, thence to the right ventricle and the lungs. The right side of the heart therefore takes the whole of the added burden of the shunt.

Natural history. Symptoms are rare in infancy and uncommon in childhood, even if the shunt is large. However in the third or fourth decade, heart failure, pulmonary hypertension or atrial arrhythmias may occur.

Clinical features. Because symptoms are unusual in childhood, most children with atrial septal defects present as a heart murmur. The murmur is often quite soft and frequently not detected until the child is at school. If symptoms do occur, they are of breathlessness or tiredness on exertion, or recurrent chest infections.

Examination. The child is well, pink and has normal pulses. The right ventricle may be easily felt. There is a systolic murmur at the second left interspace. This is due not to flow of blood across the defect,

Atrial septal defect (ASD): anatomy, presentation, examination and investigations

CXR — Chest X-ray	1 — first heart sound
ECG — Electrocardiogram	A2 — Aortic component of the second heart sound
RAD — Right axis deviation	P2 — Pulmonary component of the second heart sound
RBBB — Right bundle branch block	
PA — Pulmonary artery	

but to a high flow of blood across a normal pulmonary valve. If the shunt is large, a mid-diastolic tricuspid flow murmur may be heard too. The aortic and pulmonary components of the second sound are widely separated because the excessive filling of the right ventricle delays closure of the pulmonary valve. Furthermore, the time interval between these two sounds does not vary with respiration ('fixed splitting') because the two atria function as a single unit and respiration affects them both equally.

Investigations. The chest x-ray shows cardiomegaly with a prominent right atrium and pulmonary artery, and pulmonary plethora. The electrocardiogram shows right axis deviation, right ventricular hypertrophy and in most cases right bundle branch block. The diagnosis is confirmed by echocardiography.

Treatment. If the defect is moderate or large, closure is advisable, using cardiopulmonary by-pass. Repair is by simple suture or by insertion of a patch.

ATRIAL SEPTAL DEFECT (OSTIUM PRIMUM)

Although less common than secundum defects, ostium primum defects are more serious. The hole is situated low down in the atrial septum and represents a failure of development of the septum primum in fetal life. The defect is just above the atrioventricular valves, and usually extends to the insertion of the anterior leaflet of the mitral valve, so that the latter is cleft and frequently incompetent. An ostium primum atrial septal defect represents the mild end of the spectrum of developmental abnormalities involving the central portion of the heart, endocardial cushion defects. In the most severe form, the defect extends from the atrial septum, through the origin of both atrioventricular valves into the ventricular septum. This is described as an atrioventricular canal defect and gives rise to a large left to right shunt and both mitral and tricuspid incompetence. The endocardial cushion defects are particularly common in children with Down syndrome.

Clinical features. Heart failure commonly develops in infancy and childhood and there is a high mortality without surgery. The development of severe pulmonary hypertension is common, especially in Down Syndrome.

Examination. There are commonly signs of heart failure with marked cardiac enlargement. The child is often breathless at rest, with deformities of the lower ribs (Harrison's sulci). He is pink, with normal pulses. Clinically, the heart is large with increased activity of both ventricles. In addition to the auscultatory signs of an atrial septal defect there may be an apical pansystolic murmur signifying mitral regurgitation.

Investigations. The chest x-ray shows marked cardiomegaly, prominent pulmonary arteries and pulmonary plethora. The electrocardiogram is frequently diagnostic, showing left axis deviation and right bundle branch block. Catheterisation is required to assess the size of the shunt and the degree of mitral incompetence.

Treatment. Early surgery is usually advised for children with ostium primum defects. The defect is closed and the cleft mitral valve repaired. It is a more difficult and risky operation than that for a secundum defect.

VENTRICULAR SEPTAL DEFECT

This is the commonest of all congenital heart lesions. Usually a single defect is found in the membranous portion of the ventricular septum, adjacent to the tricuspid valve, or below the aortic valve. Less commonly, single or multiple defects are found in the muscular part of the septum. In 25 to 30% of affected children other heart defects are also present.

Natural history. There are four possibilities,
1. The hole may close spontaneously. This occurs in perhaps as many as 50% of cases, usually in early childhood but sometimes in later childhood, adolescence or adult life.
2. The hole may remain the same size. Since the heart is growing throughout childhood, the defect becomes relatively smaller.
3. Stenosis of the outflow tract of the right ventricle (the infundibulum), may occur. This raises the pressure in the right ventricle and steadily reduces the size of the left to right shunt. Eventually the shunt may reverse and the child will become cyanosed. The child in effect develops Fallot's tetralogy.
4. Progressive pulmonary hypertension may develop. If the left to right shunt is large, the torrential pulmonary blood flow irreversibly damages the smaller pulmonary vessels, giving rise to pulmonary hypertension. This makes the defect inoperable and considerably reduces the child's life span.
   Clinical presentation depends on the size of the defect and whether pulmonary hypertension is present.

Small ventricular septal defect ('maladie de Roger')
Since the shunt through the defect is small, the child is symptom-free and the heart murmur is often picked up on routine examination. The child is well, pink and has normal pulses, and the heart is not enlarged. Frequently there is a thrill at the lower left sternal border. On auscultation a harsh, pansystolic murmur is heard at the same site due to flow of blood through the defect. The heart sounds are normal.

Investigations. The chest x-ray and electrocardiogram are usually normal. Catheterisation is unnecessary.

Treatment. There is a risk of bacterial endocarditis and antibiotic prophylaxis is therefore necessary at the time of dental extractions, etc.

Moderate ventricular septal defect
Symptoms usually occur in infancy, with breathlessness on feeding and crying, failure to thrive and recurrent chest infections. As the child gets older, the symptoms tend to improve and may disappear altogether, because of actual or relative closure of the defect.

Examination. The baby is breathless at rest but is pink, with normal pulses. The heart is enlarged clinically with prominent activity of both ventricles. There is a systolic thrill at the lower left sternal border. On auscultation there is a loud, harsh pansystolic murmur, maximal at this site but heard all over the chest. There is frequently an apical mid-diastolic murmur, caused by an increased flow

Ventricular septal defect

of blood across a normal mitral valve. The second heart sound is noticeably split and the pulmonary component may be louder than normal.

Investigations. The chest x-ray shows cardiomegaly, prominent pulmonary arteries and pulmonary plethora. The electrocardiogram shows biventricular hypertrophy, since both ventricles are involved in the shunt. Cardiac catheterisation should be carried out if the child does not improve with age or if there is evidence of pulmonary hypertension.

Treatment. If symptoms are prominent, digitalisation will help. Surgery should be avoided because of the tendency to spontaneous improvement. Exceptions are continuing symptoms and the development of pulmonary hypertension.

Large ventricular septal defect

When the pulmonary vascular resistance falls to its lowest level at about three months of age, the shunt through a large defect is great and results in heart failure. Symptoms of breathlessness on feeding usually start earlier than this and sweating is very common. Affected babies may be severely ill with congestive cardiac failure, and they have an increased tendency to chest infections which often precipitates episodes of failure.

Examination. The baby is usually underweight, breathless and ill. If there is frank pulmonary oedema, cyanosis will be present. The heart is large clinically with increased ventricular activity and a systolic thrill. Signs of heart failure will be present. On auscultation, there is a harsh systolic murmur which is caused by increased flow across the pulmonary valve. A pulmonary systolic ejection and a mitral mid-diastolic flow murmur are usually heard and the pulmonary second sound is loud.

Investigation. The chest x-ray shows very marked cardiomegaly, large pulmonary arteries and pulmonary plethora. The electrocardiogram shows biventricular hypertrophy. Echocardiography will display the defect but catheterisation is necessary to measure the size of the shunt and the pulmonary artery pressure.

Treatment. The initial treatment is medical. The infant in heart failure is nursed sitting up, in oxygen if necessary. Digoxin, diuretics and potassium supplements are given. The success of treatment can be gauged by regular weighing and by recording the size of the liver. As the heart failure responds to treatment there will be a rapid weight loss and a progressive decrease in liver size. If the baby does not respond to treatment, surgical closure is necessary. This is best done as a single stage operation, using cardiopulmonary by-pass. Such an operation in an ill baby requires the highest medical and surgical skills. An alternative method of surgical treatment is to place a constricting band around the base of the pulmonary artery, thus reducing the size of the shunt. A second operation is required to remove the band and close the defect. If the baby's heart failure responds to medical treatment, then surgical closure is best delayed. It is necessary if repeat catheterisation suggests that pulmonary vascular disease is developing or if the child is chronically underweight and getting frequent chest infections. However, even the largest defects have been shown to close spontaneously, and since surgical closure carries a certain risk a conservative approach is favoured.

PATENT DUCTUS ARTERIOSUS

This is a common congenital heart lesion, either singly or in combination with other heart defects. It is particularly common in girls, in children whose mothers had rubella in early pregnancy and in babies who are born prematurely. In fetal life the ductus arteriosus, which is a large vessel with a muscular wall, diverts blood from the right ventricle and pulmonary artery into the aorta. Within the first 24 hours after birth, it closes in response to oxygenated blood. Spontaneous closure of a ductus arteriosus which remains patent after the first few days of life is unlikely, the only exception is the premature baby in whom closure of the ductus may still occur at any time in the first three months of life. As the pulmonary vascular resistance falls after birth, a left to right shunt of blood from the aorta to the pulmonary artery occurs through the ductus (the opposite direction to the flow in fetal life).

Small ductus
The child is symptom free and a heart murmur is detected routinely or coincidentally. He is pink with normal pulses. On auscultation there is a loud, continuous murmur heard best below the left clavicle. The murmur extends through systole into diastole because the pressure in the pulmonary artery is lower than that in the aorta throughout the whole cardiac cycle. It has a rough 'machinery' quality.

Investigations. Chest x-ray and electrocardiogram are normal. Catheterisation is unnecessary.

Treatment. Surgical ligation is recommended because of the risk of bacterial endocarditis. The operation itself carries a very low risk.

Large ductus
The severity of symptoms is related to the size of the shunt. The child may be rather underweight with a reduced exercise tolerance and increased tendency to chest infections. At the other end of the spectrum, severe heart failure may

develop in infancy. On examination the child is often small and thin. An increased respiratory rate is common. There is no cyanosis, but the pulses are easily felt, being full and collapsing in nature. The diastolic blood pressure is low and pulse pressure is wide. The heart is enlarged clinically with a prominent left ventricle and there is a systolic thrill in the pulmonary area. On auscultation, there is a harsh systolic murmur which may extend through the second sound into early diastole. The length of the murmur depends on the pulmonary artery pressure. This is high in large shunts so that blood only flows from left to right during systole. The pulmonary second sound is loud. A mitral (mid-diastolic) flow murmur may be heard.

Patent ductus arteriosus (PDA). LVH = left ventricular hypertrophy

Investigations. The chest x-ray shows the typical features of a left-to-right shunt. The electrocardiogram shows left ventricular hypertrophy. Catheterisation is unnecessary since the diagnosis can be made clinically.

Natural history. If the duct is small, the only risk to the patient is from bacterial endocarditis, or more accurately, endoarteritis. This is appreciable. If the duct is larger, heart failure may occur in infancy, or may occur for the first time in adult life. Pulmonary hypertension and shunt reversal can occur.

Treatment. If heart failure is present, medical treatment is necessary. Surgical ligation should be carried out as soon as the child's condition allows.

PULMONARY HYPERTENSION

A large left to right shunt with a high pulmonary blood flow may produce an elevation of pulmonary artery pressure simply because of the increased flow (hyperdynamic pulmonary hypertension). Following surgical closure of the defect, the pulmonary artery pressure returns to normal. Persisting high pulmonary blood flow may result in permanent damage to the smaller pulmonary vessels with consequent narrowing and irreversible pulmonary hypertension. If the defect is closed under these circumstances, the pulmonary artery pressure remains elevated. When the pulmonary artery pressure reaches systemic levels the left to right shunt ceases and may actually reverse.

Clinical features. The child becomes mildly cyanosed, with clubbed fingers and toes, but otherwise may appear remarkably well. However, exercise tolerance is usually considerably reduced. On examination, the right ventricle is prominent and heaving, and the pulmonary second sound is palpable. On auscultation there is usually a systolic ejection murmur in the pulmonary area due to blood flow through the huge pulmonary artery, not through the shunt, and sometimes an early diastolic murmur signifying pulmonary incompetence. The pulmonary component of the second sound is very loud.

Investigations. A chest x-ray shows an enlarged heart with a prominent right atrium. The pulmonary artery is greatly increased in size but its smaller branches are not seen. The electrocardiogram shows right axis deviation, right atrial hypertrophy and right ventricular hypertrophy. Cardiac catheterisation is needed to demonstrate the site of the shunt and to measure the pulmonary artery pressure.

The development of severe, irreversible, pulmonary hypertension as a result of a large left to right shunt is called the Eisenmenger syndrome. Although it was originally described in association with a ventricular septal defect (Eisenmenger complex), it may occur with a left to right shunt at any site. It is particularly likely to occur in cases of large ventricular septal defects, atrioventricular canal defects and transposition of the great arteries where there is a large shunt. No surgical treatment is possible and the life expectancy of affected children is considerably reduced.

OBSTRUCTIVE LESIONS

The most common examples of obstructive lesions are aortic stenosis, coarctation of the aorta and pulmonary stenosis. The chamber of the heart proximal to the obstruction hypertrophies in an attempt to overcome it. If the obstruction is severe, heart failure may result.

AORTIC STENOSIS

This is a common congenital heart lesion which may occur in isolation or in combination with other heart defects. In the majority of cases the aortic valve itself is narrowed by congenital deformity. The deformed valve may be bicuspid instead of tricuspid and the cusps are frequently fused at the edges. The degree of stenosis may worsen as the child gets older, with thickening and calcification of the cusps. A biscuspid aortic valve may open normally in childhood, but becomes thickened and narrowed in adult life. If the aortic valve is particularly narrowed and rigid, a degree of aortic incompetence is common too.

Occasionally, aortic obstruction may be above or below the aortic valve. In supravalvular stenosis, the ascending aorta above the valve is narrowed. This is often a familial condition, associated with an unusual facial appearance, mental retardation and hypercalcaemia in infancy. In subvalvular aortic stenosis, there may be a fibrous diaphragm below the valve obstructing the flow of blood from left ventricle to aorta, or there may be excessive hypertrophy of the left ventricle and interventricular septum which obstructs the outflow tract of the left ventricle during systole, that is, a hypertrophic obstructive cardiomyopathy.

Clinical features. In very severe aortic stenosis, heart failure in infancy results. In most other instances a heart murmur is detected routinely. A minority of older children with severe aortic stenosis may feel faint or dizzy on exertion, and lose consciousness. This is an indication for urgent treatment. Bacterial endocarditis is a complication of aortic stenosis of any degree.

Examination. The child appears well and is pink. The pulses are often small in volume, and of the slow rising, plateau type. The systolic blood pressure may be low. On palpation, the left ventricle is prominent and a thrill may be palpable at the lower left sternal border, in the suprasternal notch and in the neck over the carotid arteries. On auscultation there is a systolic ejection murmur heard at the apex and lower left sternal edge, which is conducted upwards into the neck. There is usually an ejection click immediately before the murmur. The aortic second sound is soft and delayed. If the stenosis is severe the aortic second sound may actually occur later than the pulmonary component so that there is apparent paradoxical splitting of the second sound with respiration.

Aortic valve stenosis. ec = ejection click

Investigations. A chest x-ray may show a prominent left ventricle with post-stenotic dilatation of the ascending aorta. An electrocardiogram shows varying degrees of left ventricular hypertrophy relating to the severity of the stenosis. If there is clinical evidence of moderate or severe stenosis cardiac catheterisation is required to measure the pressure gradient across the aortic valve.

Treatment. If the gradient across the valve exceeds 70 mmHg an aortic valvotomy is indicated. Residual stenosis and incompetence are common but severe stenosis producing heart failure in infancy requires urgent surgery. Aortic stenosis is the *one* congenital heart lesion in which strenuous activity should be avoided because of the risk of sudden death. Prevention of bacterial endocarditis is important.

COARCTATION OF THE AORTA

This is a localised narrowing of the descending aorta, close to the site of the ductus arteriosus and usually distal to the left subclavian artery. Arterial blood by-passes the obstruction reaching the lower part of the body through collateral vessels which become greatly enlarged. The left ventricle hypertrophies to overcome the obstruction and heart failure may result. The systolic blood pressure in the upper part of the body is usually elevated.

Clinical presentation. If the narrowing is severe, heart failure may occur in the first few days or weeks of life. In most cases, however, the diagnosis is made on routine or coincidental examination, either because a murmur is heard, or the femoral pulses cannot be felt or because of the discovery of hypertension. Occasionally, a child or adult may present with a complication such as a subarachnoid haemorrhage from rupture of a berry aneurysm or bacterial endarteritis.

Examination. The child is well and pink. The brachial and radial pulses are normal but the femoral pulses are either absent or weak and delayed. There is usually systemic hypertension and the left ventricle may be prominent. On auscultation, a systolic ejection murmur is usually heard over the left side of the chest, especially at the back. Collateral arteries are often palpable over the scapulae.

Coarctation of the aorta

Investigations. A chest x-ray may show a prominent left ventricle. In older children rib notching may be seen where the enlarged intercostal arteries have eroded the under side of the ribs. An electrocardiogram may show left ventricular hypertrophy.

Treatment. In most cases surgery is recommended when the child reaches school age. The narrowed segment of aorta is resected and the two ends sewn together. In infants, the proximal portion of the left subclavian artery can be used to repair the aorta after excision of the narrowing. Earlier surgery is more effective in permanently treating the hypertension but as the child grows there is a risk that relative narrowing at the site of the coarctation will occur again, requiring further surgery.

HYPOPLASTIC LEFT HEART

In this condition, the left ventricle is underdeveloped, frequently with hypoplasia or atresia of the mitral valve, aortic valve and arch of the aorta. The ductus arteriosus is patent and blood therefore by-passes the left-sided obstruction. Affected babies present in the first few days after birth with severe progressive heart failure. They are pale and shocked, with very weak pulses. Unfortunately it is a relatively common condition for which there is no treatment. Diagnosis is made by echocardiogram and death occurs within the neonatal period.

PULMONARY STENOSIS

In this condition the pulmonary valve is congenitally deformed, thickened and narrowed. The right ventricle hypertrophies in an attempt to overcome the obstruction. The muscular outflow tract of the right ventricle, the infundibulum, also hypertrophies and this may increase the degree of obstruction.

Clinical presentation. If the stenosis is severe, the infant presents with right-sided heart failure. There may be cyanosis from a right to left shunt of blood through the foramen ovale. In mild and moderate cases a heart murmur is heard on routine examination. Symptoms are rare in childhood. However, in cases of moderate stenosis, dysfunction of the right ventricle and arrhythmias are liable to occur in adult life.

Examination. In mild to moderate cases the child is well, pink, and has normal pulses. Right atrial hypertrophy produces a large 'a' wave in the jugular venous pulse. The right ventricle is heaving and a systolic thrill is palpable in the pulmonary area. On auscultation, there is usually an ejection click followed by a systolic ejection murmur caused by blood flowing across the narrowed valve. The murmur is heard in the upper part of the left chest anteriorly and is conducted to the back. The pulmonary component of the second sound becomes softer and more delayed as the stenosis increases.

Pulmonary stenosis (PS). RA = right atrium; RVH = right ventricular hypertrophy

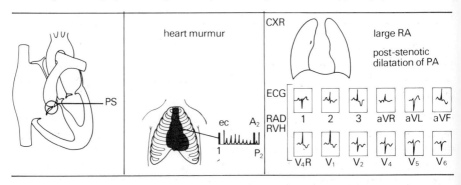

Investigations. A chest x-ray shows post-stenotic dilatation of the pulmonary artery. An enlarged right atrium and right ventricle are seen in severe cases. An electrocardiogram shows varying degrees of right axis deviation, right atrial hypertrophy and right ventricular hypertrophy, according to the severity of the stenosis. Catheterisation is indicated to measure the gradient across the pulmonary valve if signs suggest that the stenosis is moderate or severe.

Treatment. If the gradient across the valve exceeds 70 mmHg, a pulmonary valvotomy is indicated.

CYANOTIC CONGENITAL HEART DISEASE

A minority of babies or children with congenital heart disease are centrally cyanosed because unsaturated blood is by-passing the lungs. An affected child may be quite well at rest, even though he may be very blue. However, when the body's demand for oxygen increases during exercise, he becomes very easily tired and breathless. Even though the arterial oxygen saturation may be very low, the child's intelligence is usually normal. Secondary polycythaemia follows chronic hypoxia. This is to the child's advantage at first since it increases the actual amount of oxygen that can be transported in the blood. However, when the packed cell volume exceeds a certain limit, the viscosity of the blood increases with a resultant tendency to thrombosis, particularly in cerebral vessels. Embolism from thrombosis and haemorrhage from consumption coagulopathy are also well recognised complications of cyanotic heart disease.

Cyanotic heart disease can be subdivided into two types. In the first type the lungs are under-perfused as blood shunts from right to left by-passing the lungs. Fallot's tetralogy is the commonest example. In the second type, the lungs are normally filled or even over-perfused with blood, but cyanosis results because there is inadequate mixing of the systemic and pulmonary circulations. Transposition of the great arteries is the commonest example.

FALLOT TETRALOGY

The two essential features of this condition are a large ventricular septal defect, usually sited high up in the membranous part of the septum beneath the aortic valve, and stenosis of the pulmonary valve or infundibulum. There is therefore resistance to the flow of blood through the pulmonary valve with a consequent shunt of blood from the right to left ventricle and thence to the aorta. In fact, since the septal defect is just below the aortic valve, the aorta appears to override the right ventricle and the shunt is directly from the right ventricle to the aorta. Pulmonary or infundibular stenosis leads to right ventricular hypertrophy. The overriding of the aorta and right ventricular hypertrophy, in combination with the ventricular septal defect and pulmonary stenosis make up the tetralogy originally described by Fallot. The main pulmonary artery is small and in the most severe cases may not be patent (pulmonary atresia with a ventricular septal defect).

Clinical features. Affected children are usually pink in the newborn period, although a heart murmur due to blood flow through a narrowed infundibulum or pulmonary valve may be detected. Cyanosis develops and increases over the next few weeks or months. Sometimes the baby may be quite pink when at rest, only becoming cyanosed with the exertion of crying or feeding. Sometimes cyanotic 'attacks' or 'spells' occur. An affected baby is relatively well most of the time but is prone to attacks during which he becomes extremely cyanosed and pale often with loss of consciousness. Such spells result from reduced systemic vascular resistance, increasing the right to left shunt and preventing blood from reaching the lungs. As the children become older, cyanosis at rest becomes more obvious, exercise tolerance is reduced and the typical squatting may occur. The latter is a manoeuvre to gain symptomatic relief after exercise in which the child squats down on his haunches with his knees up to his chest. It traps unsaturated venous blood in the legs preventing it from returning to the heart and also raises aortic pressure by obstructing the femoral arteries, with consequent reduction in size of the right to left shunt.

Heart failure is extremely rare in Fallot tetralogy but the thromboembolic complications of polycythaemia, bacterial endocarditis and cerebral abscess may occur.

Examination. The affected child may be cyanosed at rest with clubbing of the fingers and toes. The heart is not enlarged clinically but the right ventricle is easily felt and there may be a systolic thrill in the pulmonary area. On auscultation, there is a systolic ejection murmur in the pulmonary area and a single second heart sound. No murmur arises from blood flow through the septal defect because the pressures in the two ventricles are similar.

Fallot tetralogy. RAH = right atrial hypertrophy

Investigations. The chest x-ray shows a normal size heart with the apex above the left diaphragm but the left heart border is concave because the main pulmonary artery is small and the heart is said to look like a boot. The lung fields are oligaemic. The electrocardiogram shows right axis deviation, right atrial hypertrophy and right ventricular hypertrophy.

Treatment. This is usually surgical. β-adrenergic blockers such as propranolol may increase peripheral vascular resistance thereby reducing right to left shunting and lessening cyanotic spells. Severely affected infants require a palliative operation to improve their symptoms until they are old enough to have a total repair of their defect. A shunt operation is performed, creating a communication between the aorta and pulmonary artery, so that sufficient blood can enter the lungs. A Blalock operation, in which the subclavian artery is joined to the pulmonary artery on either the left or right side, or a Waterston operation, in which the ascending aorta is joined to the right pulmonary artery, are the most commonly used procedures. Alternatively, pulmonary valvotomy and infundibular resection (Brock operation) may give symptomatic improvement. When the child approaches school age, total correction of the defects is carried out using cardiopulmonary by-pass. The results of such surgery are excellent.

1. No Murmur.
2. Single S₂ (loud).
3. Cyanosis Early.
4. Failure to △ c̄ 100% O₂.

TRANSPOSITION OF THE GREAT ARTERIES

In this heart lesion, the aorta and pulmonary arteries are 'transposed' so that the aorta arises from the right ventricle and the pulmonary artery from the left ventricle. This means that there are now two isolated circulations, pulmonary and systemic, working in parallel. Obviously this would not be compatible with life were it not for the fact that there must be some mixing between the two circulations. In fetal life, the baby is in no difficulty because the pulmonary blood flow is very small. After birth however, as the ductus arteriosus and foramen ovale begin to close, progressive cyanosis develops. The severity of the symptoms depends on the degree of mixing of the two circulations through these fetal channels. In some cases, a large ventricular septal defect or a large patent ductus arteriosus may be present, in which case there is a high pulmonary blood flow and only slight cyanosis. In the simple form however, progressive cyanosis develops in the first hours or days after birth. Without treatment, few children survive the first year of life.

Clinical features. Progressive cyanosis develops within the first few hours or days of life. The affected baby becomes increasingly blue and acidotic. Breathlessness and heart failure may follow.

Examination. Cyanosis is the major physical sign and persists even if the baby is given 100% oxygen. There are usually no heart murmurs but the second sound is loud because the transposed aorta lies anteriorly, close to the chest wall.

Transposition of the great arteries

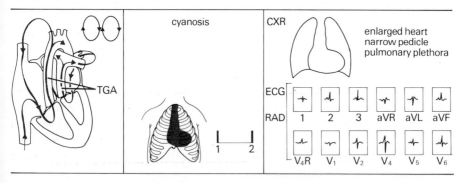

Investigations. The chest X-ray is often typical. The heart is slightly enlarged and is said to look like an egg lying on its side. The vascular pedicle of the heart is narrow because the aorta and pulmonary artery lie one in front of the other. The lung fields are normally filled or plethoric. Diagnosis is made by echocardiography.

Treatment. A shunt between the systemic and pulmonary circulations is urgently needed. This can be created without recourse to surgery by performing a balloon atrial septostomy (Rashkind procedure). A special double lumen catheter is passed via the inferior vena cava, right atrium and foramen ovale into the left atrium. A balloon near the tip of the catheter is then inflated using contrast medium and the catheter and inflated ballon are pulled sharply back through the atrial septum, tearing it and creating a large septal defect. The effect is usually dramatic; the baby, who is often desperately ill, becomes moderately pink. The shunt is usually large enough to enable him to thrive until a definitive procedure can be performed, usually at about the age of one year. The commonest definitive procedure is the Mustard operation which provides a physiological, although not anatomical, correction. The atrial septum is excised and the two venous returns diverted using a patch of pericardium or Dacron. The systemic venous blood from the venae cavae is diverted into the left ventricle and the pulmonary artery. The pulmonary venuous blood is diverted into the right ventricle and thus to the aorta. Sometimes an anatomical correction is possible, whereby the aorta and pulmonary arteries are re-attached to their appropriate ventricles.

L.T. Complications

Poorer S.T. Survival
Better L.T. ?

CARDIAC ARRHYTHMIAS

Children often have cardiac arrhythmias which are of no clinical significance; sinus arrhythmia is the most common example. A number, however, have symptoms which are a direct result of an abnormality of heart rhythm. *1 in 1000*

Paroxysmal supraventricular tachycardia

This is a regular, rapid rhythm at the rate of 240 to 300 beats per minute. It is due to impulses originating in the atrio-ventricular node re-entering the atria via an accessory pathway and thus exciting the atrio-ventricular node prematurely. Since the heart rate is so rapid, diastolic filling of the ventricles is impaired and cardiac failure arises. The younger the patient, the less well is the rapid heart rate tolerated and the earlier heart failure develops. The tachycardia is paroxysmal and frequently recurs. About a quarter of the children with this disorder have an underlying cardiac defect, either congenital or acquired.

Clinical features. Paroxysmal tachycardia may be noted *in utero* or occur at any time in infancy, childhood or adult life. As the heart rate suddenly becomes rapid, the baby may go pale, start to breathe quickly and vomit. After a few hours, symptoms of heart failure occur and death may result if no treatment is given. Older children can usually recognise the onset of the tachycardia by describing palpitations. Paroxysms may occur spontaneously or be precipitated by illness. Return to sinus rhythm produces a diuresis.

The ECG of supraventricular tachycardia

supraventricular tachycardia
(rate 280/minute)

sinus rhythm
(rate 140/minute)

[Handwritten margin notes at top: "Do NOT give VERAPAMIL. — long acting .↓BP — Adenosine — V. Rapidly metabolised → Complete H. Block. May → Asthma attack"]

Examination. The child looks pale but may be otherwise well. A baby is more likely to show obvious signs of heart failure. The pulse is weak, rapid, regular and does not gradually slow when carotid sinus or eyeball pressure is applied.

Investigations. The electrocardiogram shows a heart rate in excess of 240 per minute. The P waves may be present, abnormal, or absent, and the QRS complexes are normal. Between paroxysms, the electrocardiogram shows normal sinus rhythm. A number of children show the Wolff-Parkinson-White syndrome, an electrocardiographic abnormality comprising a short P-R interval and slurring of the beginning of the QRS complex. *[Handwritten: δ wave]*

Treatment. In some cases an attack can be terminated by vagal stimulation. Carotid sinus or eyeball pressure may be tried in older children. Ice packs applied to the face may be effective in babies. If this fails, digitalisation is effective but may take some time to work even if given intra-muscularly. Conversion to sinus rhythm using DC shock may be necessary if the baby is desperately ill. Recurrent attacks can be prevented or suppressed by regular digoxin or propanolol.

[Handwritten: Maintenance — Flecainide]

Complete heart block

Complete heart block with atrio-ventricular dissociation may occur in otherwise normal children or in children with underlying congenital or acquired heart disease. It is usually congenital and is sometimes suspected before birth. The ventricular rate of contraction is in the region of 50 per minute and may increase with exercise. Many affected children lead normal, healthy lives and remain symptom-free. A minority have classical Stokes Adams attacks in which they fall to the ground and lose consciousness. The latter require treatment and this can either be given with drugs, such as long-acting isoprenaline, or by insertion of an artificial pacemaker.

SUBACUTE BACTERIAL ENDOCARDITIS

This is a well recognised complication of congenital as well as rheumatic heart disease. The risk is highest with those lesions which result in a turbulent jet of blood, such as a ventricular septal defect, coarctation, patent ductus and aortic stenosis. The endocardium becomes infected in the presence of a bacteraemia which may occur during dental treatment or cardiac surgery. As in adults, *Streptococcus viridans* is the commonest infecting organism.

Clinical features. Fever, malaise and anorexia are usually the presenting symptoms. Peripheral signs such as clubbing of the nails, splinter haemorrhages, and abscesses are common. The spleen may be palpable and the physical signs of the heart defect may change rapidly as the endocarditis damages the heart valves.

Investigations. The diagnosis is made on one or more positive blood cultures. Microscopic haematuria is common, and the white count and ESR are usually raised.

Treatment. Bacteriocidal antibiotics are given parenterally in large dose for a period of six weeks. The combination of benzylpenicillin and gentamicin is

Clinical features of subacute bacterial endocarditis

particularly useful for *Str. viridans* but frequent monitoring of serum levels for activity against the organism is necessary.

Prevention. Any child known to have a congenital heart lesion, no matter how trivial, needs antibiotic prophylaxis with dental treatment and should carry a card to show to his dentist. The card states that the child has congenital heart disease and that in the event of dental treatment (extraction, fillings or scaling) antibiotics should be given. The usual practice is to give oral amoxicillin as a single large dose one hour before the treatment. Similar prophylaxis is also necessary before surgery involving the middle ear, tonsils or adenoids.

RHEUMATIC FEVER

There has been a dramatic decline in this disease which used to cause much illness in children and permanent valvular damage in adults in the Western world. It remains common, however, in the Middle East and Africa. The decline of the disease is probably the result of diminished virulence of the β-haemolytic streptococcus, the introduction of antibiotics and improved social conditions. Rheumatic fever may represent an abnormal immunological response to the β-haemolytic streptococcus, an organism commonly responsible for sore throats and tonsillitis. It is thought that the body confuses its own antigens with those of the organism, thereby causing an autoimmune reaction.

Clinical features. One to three weeks after a throat infection, the child (usually of school age) develops a fever, malaise and an acute migratory poly-arthritis involving the medium-sized joints (knees, ankles, wrists, and elbows). Carditis is common, involving all the layers of the heart. Pericarditis produces a friction rub or a pericardial effusion. Myocarditis produces a tachycardia, cardiac enlargement and arrhythmias. Endocarditis causes heart murmurs, systolic and diastolic. Skin rashes, especially erythema marginatum, and subcutaneous nodules over the occiput or extensor surfaces of the elbows, wrists and fingers are less common. Chorea is a neurological manifestation of rheumatic fever which is rarely seen in the presence of carditis.

Investigation. There is usually evidence of a recent streptococcal infection (raised ASO titre and/or positive throat swab) with a raised white count and ESR.

erythema Marginatum — pink rings on trunk. come & go.

Clinical features of rheumatic fever

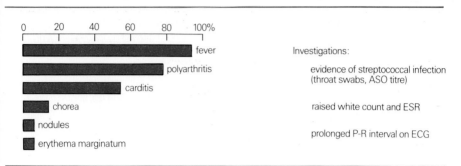

The P-R interval is commonly increased in the presence of carditis, often above 0.2 seconds.

Treatment. Penicillin is given to eradicate the streptococcus and high doses of aspirin lower the fever and relieve the arthritis. Steroids shorten the illness but do not reduce the incidence of permanent cardiac damage from the carditis — they are used in particularly severe cases of rheumatic fever. Rheumatic fever tends to recur and carditis is very common in subsequent attacks if it occurred in the initial attack. Such recurrent episodes of carditis produce severe rheumatic valvular disease and should be prevented by penicillin prophylaxis for life. On the other hand, children who have no carditis with rheumatic fever have a reduced risk of further relapses and a very low chance of carditis in future episodes.

HYPERTENSION

Unfortunately blood pressure measurement is often overlooked when assessing a child's problems. This attitude arises from the difficulties of making accurate measurements in a restless young child with equipment which is designed for adults and also because the yield of abnormal readings is very low. With attention to correct technique using suitable cuff sizes and making repeated attempts in a relaxed atmosphere, reliable measurements can be made using a mercury sphygmomanometer. In infants and young children the Doppler method is more reliable. Blood pressure increases with age, height and weight although it should be remembered that the fat arm may give an artificially high reading. Too narrow a cuff in a normal arm also causes this error. There is no precise definition of hypertension in childhood and although the figure 130/85 mmHg is often used, this overlooks those children who fall in the top 5% of the blood pressure distribution for age. A proportion of these high rankers, particularly those with a family history of hypertension, become the adult population at risk from symptomatic hypertension, ischaemic heart disease and cerebrovascular disease. It must be emphasised that no child should be regarded as having an abnormal blood pressure until this has been confirmed on several occasions.

Surveys in several countries have demonstrated that the majority of children

Causes of hypertension in childhood

	Normal blood pressure values				conditions causing hypertension

age (yrs)	mean mm. Hg systolic	diastolic	mean +2 SD systolic	diastolic
0-2	95	55	110	65
3-6	100	65	120	70
7-10	105	70	130	75
11-15	115	70	140	80

conditions causing hypertension
%0 20 40 60 80 100%
renal parenchymal disease
coarctation of aorta
renovascular disease
Cushing syndrome
phaeochromocytoma
other disorders

with mild asymptomatic hypertension fall into the primary or essential category. In contrast 70 to 90% of those with severe symptomatic hypertension have some underlying cause, most commonly renal parenchymal disease. Greater attention to blood pressure measurement will bring these underlying problems to attention more promptly and may avoid life threatening complications. Hypertension may manifest itself as persistent headache, dizziness, disturbed vision, unexplained irritability, convulsions, and other neurological signs. Naturally, blood pressure should always be measured in the presence of cardiac and renal disorders. Paroxysmal episodes of palpitation and sweating raise the possibility of a phaeochromocytoma.

HYPERLIPOPROTEINAEMIA

The morbidity and mortality arising from atherosclerosis has reached such epidemic proportions in industrial societies that paediatricians can no longer evade their responsibilities in this direction. Fatty streaks are already present in the aortas of children aged 10 to 11 years and the coronary arteries start to show involvement in the early twenties. Both genetic and environmental factors contribute towards atheroma. Currently there is great interest in preventive measures. Some measures, such as antismoking campaigns, the prevention of obesity and the provision of facilities for regular physical exercise are well validated although not always easy to implement; others such as the widescale modification of diet in infants and young children, must be approached with caution.

Hyperlipidaemia and in particular hypercholesterolaemia has been convincingly linked to the development of atheroma. The majority of serum cholesterol is transported as β-lipoprotein, a low density lipoprotein.

Hyperbetalipoproteinaemia (familial hypercholesterolaemia)
This is an autosomal dominant condition in which homozygote individuals have a severe disease. They develop tuberous and tendon xanthomata in early childhood and die of ischaemic heart disease in the second or third decade. The heterozygote condition is relatively common, affecting approximately 1 in 280 in England and Wales. Fifty-one per cent of heterozygote males and 12% of hetero-

zygote females have a heart attack by the age of 50 years. There are obviously grounds for detecting this disease in early childhood but serum cholesterol determination is not reliable in the first year partly because normal breast fed infants tend to have considerably higher cholesterol levels than those fed on poly-unsaturated fat formulae. There is certainly no basis for assuming that this is a case against breast milk! In older children, the diagnosis can be confirmed by measuring serum cholesterol and β-lipoprotein. Long term treatment schedules consisting of low fat intake and where necessary drugs such as cholestyramine are currently being assessed.

Diet and hypercholesterolaemia
The majority of hypercholesterolaemia in affluent society is not due to a single, genetically-inherited disorder but reflects the impact of a high animal fat diet on a polygenically susceptible population. Within families there is a significant correlation between the serum cholesterol concentrations of children and those of their parents. The family history should include details of the occurrence and age of onset of ischaemic heart disease so that advice can be offered in an attempt to safeguard at-risk children. It is obviously sensible to reduce the fat intake, particularly from dairy products, but there is still insufficient evidence for the radical exclusion of cholesterol. Children tend to acquire the tastes of their parents and habituation to high fat or salt diets or smoking may well contribute to the future toll of atherosclerosis.

BIBLIOGRAPHY

Graham G, Rossi E 1980 Heart disease in infants and children. Arnold, London
Jordan S C, Scott O 1981 Heart disease in paediatrics, 2nd edn. Butterworths, London
Keith J D, Rowe R R, Vlad P 1978 Heart disease in infancy and childhood, 3rd edn. Macmillan, New York
Moss A J, Adams F H, Emmanowvildes G C 1977 Heart disease in infants, children and adolescents, 2nd edn. Williams & Wilkins, Baltimore
Nadan A S, Fyler D C 1972 Pediatric cardiology, 3rd edn. Saunders, Philadelphia
Rowe R D, Freedom R M, Mehrizi A 1980 Neonates with congenital heart disease, 2nd edn. Saunders, London
Shinebourne E A, Anderson R H 1980 Current paediatric cardiology. Oxford University Press, Oxford

10
Gut

Normal function of the gastrointestinal tract depends on a carefully regulated balance between motility, sphincter tone, exocrine secretion and integrity of the absorptive surfaces. These functions begin to evolve early in fetal life: digestive enzymes and primitive swallowing movements are first detectable in the 12-week fetus and regular flow of amniotic fluid into the gut occurs from 20 weeks; by term this amounts to approximately 500 ml per day or half the total amniotic volume.

Gut function must undergo abrupt adjustment and maturation with birth and the onset of intermittent oral feeding. There is a marked increase in small intestinal mucosal surface area and this is at least partially mediated by gut hormones such as gastrin which are released in response to milk feeds. Digestive enzymes show a varied pattern of maturation, lactase activity being fully developed at term whereas trypsin takes 12 months to reach maximal levels. Although the gut is probably sterile at birth, it is rapidly colonised by bacterial entry through the mouth and anus. A normal microflora contributes to the available supply of vitamin K, folic acid and biotin. Immunological protection is provided to the newborn by secretory IgA antibodies in the maternal milk and by the transplacental passage of IgG antibodies. Endogenous IgA is produced in the first three to four weeks and is a major component of the barrier against bacteria and other antigens. Infants with immunological deficiencies are liable to develop gastrointestinal symptoms after three months of age when the reserve of maternal IgG is exhausted.

ACUTE ABDOMINAL PAIN

In children the 'acute abdomen' is a common and testing problem. Surgical conditions which require prompt diagnosis and treatment have to be distinguished from a large number of medical disorders. Careful general examination and urinalysis is essential.

Causes of acute abdominal pain

Surgical	Medical (relatively common)	Medical (rare but important)
Acute appendicitis	Mesenteric adenitis	Lead poisoning
Intussusception	Constipation	Diabetes
Intestinal obstruction	Gastroenteritis	Sickle cell crisis
Torsion of ovary or testis	Lower lobe pneumonia	Acute porphyria
Hydronephrosis	Acute pyelonephritis	Pancreatitis
Renal calculus	Henoch Schönlein purpura	Primary peritonitis
	Hepatitis	Meningitis

Acute appendicitis

Appendicitis is the commonest acute surgical emergency of childhood. Three or four children in every 1000 have their appendix removed each year. It can occur at any age but is usually seen in children over five years of age. The characteristic triad of clinical features seen in adults, abdominal pain, low grade fever and tenderness with guarding in the right iliac fossa, is seen in the older child but in infants pain may not be a feature; they are more likely to present with a history of a recent respiratory infection followed by anorexia, vomiting, irritability and a high fever. This often leads to diagnostic confusion and delay so that the incidence of perforation with resulting peritonitis or abscess formation is higher in the younger child. The course of the disease in the young child is extremely rapid: a two-year-old can progress from apparent normality to perforation in six hours. There is no place therefore for prolonged observation in the young patient.

Features which distinguish appendicitis and mesenteric adenitis

	Acute Appendicitis		Mesenteric Adenitis
	37-38°C	above 38°C	
1.	temperature		
	—	—	
2.	pharyngitis, cervical adenitis		
	—	+	
3.	headache		
	—	+	
4.	vomiting		
	+−	−	
5.	abdominal pain		
	++	+	
6.	guarding		
	+	+	
7.	shifting tenderness		
	−	+	
8.	rebound tenderness		
	+	−	

upper respiratory tract infection and appendicitis can occur simultaneously

Mesenteric adenitis

Vague central or generalised abdominal pain commonly accompanies viral upper respiratory tract infections. It is due to non-specific inflammation in the mesenteric lymph nodes which provokes a mild peritoneal reaction and stimulates painful peristalsis in the terminal ileum. It is usually possible to distinguish mesenteric adenitis from acute appendicitis, but if there is any doubt four to six hours after the child is first seen, and in all cases where there is persisting local tenderness, the child must be surgically explored.

Primary peritonitis
Primary peritonitis, usually due to pneumococcus, is considerably rarer than peritonitis secondary to appendicitis. Patients with nephrotic syndrome and immune deficiency states are susceptible.

Malrotation
The midgut loop of the developing embryo elongates by herniating out into the umbilical cord from the sixth to the fourteenth intrauterine weeks. The apex of the loop communicates with the yolk sac by the vitelline duct, and this is the site of a possible Meckel diverticulum. While still in the extra-embryonic coelom a counter clockwise rotation of 270° round the superior mesenteric artery occurs. At about 14 weeks the gut starts to return to the abdominal cavity, the proximal jejunum leading and lying in the left upper abdomen. The caecum is the last portion of the gut to re-enter the abdomen and it initially lies in the

Maldescent and malrotation

arrested caecal descent   incomplete rotation   reverse rotation
                                 90° AntiClockwise.   True Malrotation 90°

subhepatic position. This state of affairs is the most common abnormality seen clinically and to be accurate it should be called arrested caecal descent, not *mal*rotation. It can cause neonatal duodenal obstruction due to Ladd bands, and partial recurrent volvulus in the older child due to the narrow mesenteric attachment between caecum and the duodenojejunal flexure. Often it is asymptomatic but causes severe technical difficulty if the patient develops acute appendicitis.

The second anomaly causing clinical problems is correctly called incomplete rotation of the gut, and again is not malrotation. Here rotation in the extra-embryonic coelom only amounts to 90° counter-clockwise, and the colon and caecum return first to the abdomen and occupy the left side. The small bowel fills the right side. The whole small bowel is suspended by an extremely narrow 1 cm mesenteric attachment between duodenojejunal flexure and caecum, and volvulus in the early days of life is extremely likely. Total small bowel infarction can result.

A true malrotation can occur when embryonic rotation is 90° clockwise instead of 270° counterclockwise but this is rare. In this case, the duodenum will be anterior to the transverse colon. Clinical problems are unusual.

Meckel diverticulum

This diverticulum is a remnant of the vitellointestinal duct. It arises from the antimesenteric border of the terminal ileum and usually gives no trouble, but very rarely it may become inflamed and then the symptoms and signs mimic acute appendicitis. More commonly the diverticulum causes an intussusception or a volvulus. It may also contain ectopic gastric mucosa in which peptic ulceration can produce haemorrhage or perforation. A technetium scan may help to identify ectopic mucosa.

Intussusception

Intussusception is an invagination of bowel into an adjacent lower segment. The usual origin is the terminal ileum or ileo-caecal valve resulting in an ileocolic intussusception. Although uncommon (2:1000 live births), it is the most frequent cause of intestinal obstruction in the first two years of life. It presents as paroxysmal pain sometimes with reflex vomiting and a sausage shaped mass is palpable in the right upper abdomen. If there is delay in diagnosis the child will develop fever, a distended abdomen and will pass bloodstained mucus rectally. *Red currant Jelly* The diagnosis is clinical and time-consuming x-rays are not indicated in an ill child. Immediate surgery must be arranged since bowel viability is rapidly lost. If the history is for less than 24 hours and there are no signs of fever, tenderness or blood rectally, the intussusception can sometimes be reduced hydrostatically by barium enema. This only has a 75% success rate in suitable cases and the remaining 25% have to go to theatre thereafter. Surgery has the advantage of establishing underlying causes such as a Meckel diverticulum but such a cause is found in only 5 to 7 per cent. Recurrence is more frequent following barium enema reduction. A barium enema is useful in the diagnosis of chronic recurrent non-obstructive intussusception.

Intussusception

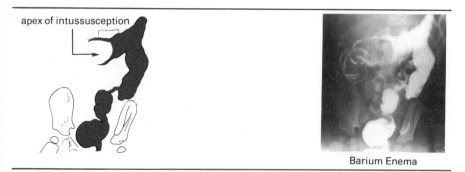

apex of intussusception

Barium Enema

RECURRENT ABDOMINAL PAIN

This is a common problem affecting at least 10 per cent of school children. Although no organic cause is found in over 90%, it is essential to identify those with an organic condition promptly. This enables specific management of the problem and confident counselling of children with functional disorders. Ideally,

Features of 200 children with recurrent abdominal pain (from Apley 1975)

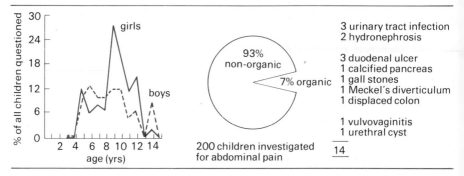

3 urinary tract infection	
2 hydronephrosis	
3 duodenal ulcer	
1 calcified pancreas	
1 gall stones	
1 Meckel's diverticulum	
1 displaced colon	
1 vulvovaginitis	
1 urethral cyst	
$\overline{14}$	

93% non-organic   7% organic

200 children investigated for abdominal pain

the children should be assessed when they have the pain as well as between episodes.

Childhood migraine
Children who go on to have classical migraine commonly present with recurrent episodes of prolonged midline abdominal pain associated with nausea or vasomotor symptoms. A positive family history of migraine is an important clue.

Renal tract infection
Renal tract infection must be excluded by urine culture and microscopy. Loin pain in the absence of urinary abnormality may still be an indication for an intravenous pyelogram, for it may reveal a hydronephrosis.

Peptic ulcers
Peptic ulcers are now being diagnosed more often in children, partly as a consequence of the wider application of endoscopy. Sleep disturbance due to nocturnal epigastric pain is a useful clue and may be reinforced by a family history of peptic ulceration. Duodenal ulcers occur more frequently than gastric

Features pointing to an organic cause for recurrent abdominal pain

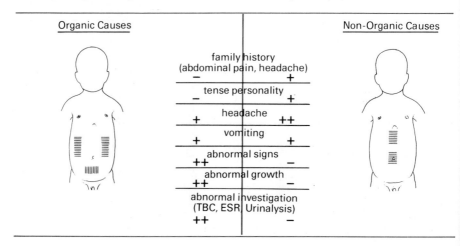

Organic Causes		Non-Organic Causes
	family history (abdominal pain, headache)	
−		+
	tense personality	
−		+
	headache	
+		++
	vomiting	
+		+
	abnormal signs	
++		−
	abnormal growth	
++		−
	abnormal investigation (TBC, ESR Urinalysis)	
++		−

ulcers. Management includes dietary advice, appropriate antacids and H2-receptor antagonists. The longterm implications of using cimetidine in childhood are being assessed.

Chronic recurrent pancreatitis
Although rare, it may be suggested by a family history and by central abdominal pain radiating through to the back. Clinical suspicion is confirmed by finding calcification of the pancreas on abdominal x-ray.

GASTROENTERITIS

Diarrhoeal illness, frequently superimposed on malnutrition, extracts a terrifying toll from the world's children, at a conservative estimate 10 to 15 million deaths annually. WHO has committed itself to 'Health for All by the Year 2000', major targets being universal availability of safe water supplies and simple but life saving oral rehydration treatment. In the developed world gastroenteritis is common and usually mild but should not be underestimated particularly in vulnerable settings such as neonatal units.

Bacterial gastroenteritis
Bacteria interfere with mucosal integrity by direct invasion, by toxin release, or by adherence to and disruption of the enterocyte brush border. Groups of *E. coli* operate by all three mechanisms, the genetic determinants of virulence being carried in chromosomes or in plasmids. Gene probes are being developed to facilitate the laboratory identification of pathogenic *E. coli*.

Fever is common in bacterial gastroenteritis and in particular in Shigella infection where pyrexial convulsions and marked meningism may precede overt enteric symptoms. Food poisoning may arise due to the ingestion of the exotoxin produced by coagulase positive staphylococcus.

Viral gastroenteritis
In developed countries viral infection is responsible for 50 to 60% of acute gastroenteritis in children under the age of five years. Rotavirus, a double stranded RNA virus, is the main agent responsible for winter epidemics of

Bacterial gastroenteritis may be due to either invasive or non-invasive organisms

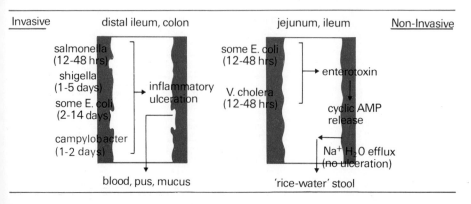

Gastroenteritis Congenital   Acquired infection < enteral > Ba
                                                        parenteral
            Disaccharidase Def.   Dietetic
            Milk (lactalbumin) Intolerance   Coeliac.
            C.F.   Structural ausg of GIT.   Temp. intolerance GUT 153
                                              Giardiosis

gastroenteritis. There are several different strains of Rotavirus, and of other agents for example Astroviruses, Caliciviruses, and this is an obstacle to the development of effective vaccines. Vomiting may be the only obvious presenting feature as diarrhoea may not occur for several hours and even then a watery stool is liable to be confused with urine in the wet napkins. Colicky abdominal pain with ill-defined tenderness and exaggerated bowel sounds is common. It is important to remember that vomiting and diarrhoea may be the presenting symptoms of surgical conditions, for example appendicitis, Hirschsprung disease and intussusception. They also result from non-gastrointestinal disorders such as upper respiratory tract infections, renal infections and meningitis.

Dehydration

The water loss associated with gastroenteritis places a relatively greater stress on the young infant for he has a higher percentage of body water (80% at term and 60% at 12 months), a higher metabolic rate and a larger surface area to volume ratio. The assessment of dehydration relies upon a series of clinical signs which reflect changes in body tissues and circulatory status. The tissue changes are more easily recognised in thin than in overweight infants. A recent reliable weight is the best guide to body fluid loss. The clinical estimate indicates the percentage of the expected body weight which requires to be replaced, so that 10% dehydration in a 5 kg infant indicates a replacement volume of 500 ml. It is also necessary to assess the type of dehydration; hypotonic, isotonic or hypertonic (also termed hypernatraemic when the serum sodium is above 150 mmol/l).

Clinical assessment of dehydration

Sign	5% dehydration	10% dehydration
Skin	Loss of turgor	Mottled, poor capillary return
Fontanelle	Depressed	Deeply depressed
Eyes	Sunken	Deeply sunken
Peripheral pulses	Normal	Tachycardia, poor volume
Mental state	Lethargic	Prostration, coma

Features which differentiate isotonic and hypertonic dehydration

lethargic : hypotonic : depressed fontanelle : sunken eyes : loss of skin turgor

irritable : hypertonic : normal or full fontanelle : normal eyes : doughy skin

dehydration recognised before circulatory failure

circulatory failure due to masking of dehydration

Isotonic Dehydration   Normal   Hypertonic Dehydration

↓ECF
↔ICF

ICF

↓ ICF
↓ EC Flu

Na⁺ and H₂O loss in proportion

H₂O loss greater than Na⁺

Dioralyte: Na - 35.   Dextrose - 200 mmol   ∴ Late Clinical Assess
             K - 20   + 200 mls H₂O
             HCO₃⁻ - 18

Day 1 — Full IV Drip / O by Mouth
2 — 2/3 IV | 1/3 Oral.
3 — 1/3 IV | 2/3 Oral.
4 — STOP IV.

Mild dehydration (under 5 per cent). Mild dehydration can be treated in the home by a regimen of clear fluids for at least 24 hours, followed by the gradual reintroduction of a normal diet. There is now a range of formulations available based on the principle that oral rehydration therapy is considerably more efficient when glucose or sucrose is added to an electrolyte solution. In impoverished cultures effective rehydration solutions can be created using cheap local ingredients for example salt and boiled rice water. It is essential to advise families how to use these solutions appropriately and to avoid unnecessarily prolonged use which places the child at risk of malnutrition.

Maintenance requirements

Age months	H$_2$O ml/kg	Na mmol/kg	K mmol/kg
0–6	150	2.5	2.5
6–12	120	2.5	2.5
12–24	100	2.5	2.5
Over 24	80	2.0	2.0

Moderate to severe dehydration (over 5 per cent). Moderate to severe dehydration requires intravenous therapy and this is especially urgent when there are signs of peripheral circulatory failure. Appropriate management demands an understanding of normal maintenance requirements as well as an assessment of the deficit. Acidosis may accompany dehydration and if severe is treated by

Principles of intravenous therapy

Total fluid requirements =
- maintenance   0.2 N saline in 4.3% glucose plus KCl
- deficit   N saline plus KCl
- ongoing loss   N saline plus KCl

Scheme	0–½ h	Treat shock immediately:	Plasma or N saline 20 ml/kg body weight
	½–4 h	Initial replacement: (awaiting serum electrolyte results)	0.5 N or N saline 10 ml/kg/h
	4–24 h	Continuing replacement: (a) Serum Na under 150 mmol/l	0.2 N saline in 4.3% Dextrose plus KCl 30–40 mmol/l Plan total correction in 24 h
		(b) Serum Na above 150 mmol/l	0.2 N saline in 4.3% Dextrose plus KCl 30–40 mmol/l Restrict fluids to 150 ml/kg in first 24 h and plan total correction over 48 h

r give K+ Until Baby Passes Urine !

Solution	Na	K	mmol/l Ca	Cl	Lactate
Normal saline (0.9%)	150	—	—	150	—
0.5 N saline in 5% Dextrose	77	—	—	77	—
0.2 N saline in 4.3% Dextrose	30	—	—	30	—
Ringer's lactate solution (Hartmann's solution)	130	5	4	112	27

providing about half the calculated deficit as sodium bicarbonate: deficit (mmol) = weight (kg) × 0.3 × (24 — observed plasma bicarbonate mmol/l). Antibiotics are not indicated unless systemic spread of bacterial infection is likely. Anti-diarrhoeal agents should also be avoided as they slow transit time and encourage the persistence of an abnormal bowel flora.

Complications

Post gastroenteritis diarrhoea is relatively common in young infants. A short period of lactose-free milk may be required. Refractory cases require careful evaluation.

Complications of gastroenteritis and its treatment

Convulsions
  fever
  hypo-, hypernatraemia
  hypoglycaemia
  hypocalcaemia

Cerebral damage
  hypotension
  vascular thrombosis

Pulmonary oedema
  fluid overload

Oliguria
  prerenal failure (urine urea ↑, urine Na⁺ ↓)
  renal failure   (urine urea ↓, urine Na⁺ ↑)
  —renal vein thrombosis
  —medullary necrosis

Protracted diarrhoea
  secondary lactose intolerance
  secondary cow's milk protein intolerance
  bacterial overgrowth

MALABSORPTION

Enzymatic degradation of the major nutrients occurs within the gut lumen, at the microvilli and in the cytoplasm of the columnar epithelial cells. Disorders in the lumen may be due to failure of exocrine secretion, for example pancreatic insufficiency in cystic fibrosis, or disrupted bile salt circulation as in cholestatic liver disease. The mucosa may suffer non- specific epithelial damage in a variety of conditions, including coeliac disease and post-gastroenteritis. Other more specific inherited disorders interfere with individual pathways in the epithelium, for example primary congenital alactasia and familial chloride diarrhoea. Malabsorption may also occur due to obstruction of lymphatics in the intestinal wall as in congenital lymphangectasia.

Investigation of malabsorption

Investigation of malabsorption is relatively complex and must not be initiated until it has been established that the child is failing to gain weight on a normal diet, does not have other systemic diseases and is being cared for in an adequate environment. Stool microscopy may reveal abundant fat globules. Three-day stool fat collections provide a more exact measure of steatorrhoea, an abnormal fat content being greater than 10 per cent of intake but it is a demanding and often unsuccessful investigation. A sweat test to exclude cystic fibrosis and a barium meal to detect anatomical malformations may be indicated. Peroral jejunal biopsy is a valuable diagnostic tool when appropriate care in patient selection is exercised.

Handwritten top margin:
nook, Bloods :- Ig's
age, Jejunal Bx:
meal ; Sweat Test
 eat Tablets
—/see lecture.

Def States
1. Calories
2. Protein
3. Anaemia - iron
4. F.A
5. Rickets (10↑), Ca²⁺
7. Vit K def.
8. Skin lesions - Eczema + Exfoliative Dermatitis.
(Ass. Cows Milk Prot Allergy → ↑↑ Eczema)

Coeliac disease

Coeliac disease is the permanent inability to tolerate dietary wheat or rye gluten. Exposure to gluten results in morphological and functional abnormality of the proximal small intestine which can be reversed by exclusion of gluten. The incidence is about 1 in 2000 in the U.K. and as high as 1 in 300 in West Ireland. It is becoming less common in Europe. There is evidence that affected children have an abnormal immune response to the gliadin fractions of gluten. The majority of children with coeliac disease present before the age of two years. The weight record may show progressive growth failure dating from the introduction of gluten-containing solids. In a few, overt malabsorption may not occur for many years. The one hour xylose absorption test in which 5 grams of xylose is given while fasting and the blood level measured after 1 hour, is of help in screening for coeliac disease. The jejunal biopsy is essential for definitive diagnosis. There are other causes of a flattened mucosa in childhood such as post-gastroenteritis, cow's milk protein intolerance and giardiasis so that repeated biopsies with and without dietary gluten are usually necessary to make a precise

Handwritten: Ig ↓ - ↑IgA, ↓ IgG, IgM Prot loss — Mimic Coeliac → Anaemia.

Normal and abnormal jejunal mucosa, and the clinical features of gluten enteropathy

Handwritten right: Pale fatty stool, Distended Abd (May occur Simul too)

normal jejunal mucosa — leaf and finger-shaped villi
— regular columnar epithelial cells
— lamina propria
— crypts of Lieberkühn
— muscularis mucosae

abnormal jejunal mucosa
irregular surface epithelial cells (increased loss)
lamina propria contains an excess of chronic inflammatory cells
— proliferating crypts

failure to thrive
vomiting — v. Common, Intermitt
diarrhoea — 75%. (10% Const)
irritability
anorexia → Try to Conserve energy
anaemia ∴ Do not want to move
hypotonia
abdominal distension — Pain ~25%
wasted buttocks
rickets
delayed bone age
short stature
delayed puberty

Handwritten: ↑ CF → ↑appetite. Wasting 1. Shoulder Girdle. Coeliac → Thighs, buttocks!

diagnosis. Coeliac disease has life-long implications. There is a risk of intestinal lymphoma which may be reduced by strict adherence to a gluten free diet. Infants with bowel upsets may display a temporary gluten intolerance.

Sugar intolerance

Sugar intolerance results from failure to absorb particular sugars, most commonly lactose. The osmotic load of the undigested sugar results in explosive watery diarrhoea and the intraluminal fermentation produces an excess of lactic acid and carbon dioxide. The fluid stools are acid (pH less than 5.5) and contain reducing substances which can be demonstrated using Clinitest tablets.

Lactose intolerance is a common sequel of gastroenteritis or coeliac disease. It also occurs in premature infants; as a rare inherited disorder in Caucasians (autosomal recessive) and as a frequent finding in non-Caucasians after early

Partial Villous Atrophy ⇒ Broadening of villi tips
└ infection or Anaemia.
S.T.V.A ⇒ flattening of villi tips
└ Coeliac (Classical)!

Digestion and absorption

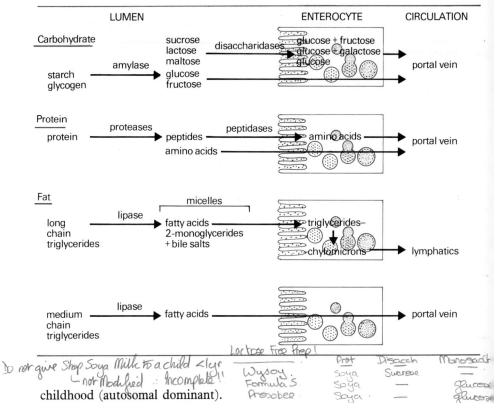

Lactose Free Prep!

Do not give Shop Soya Milk to a child <1yr
└ not Modified ∴ Incomplete!!

	Prot	Disacch	Monosacch
Wysoy	Soya	Sucrose	—
Formula's	Soya	—	glucose
Prosobee	Soya	—	glucose

childhood (autosomal dominant).

Sucrase-isomaltase deficiency. This can occur after severe mucosal damage or be inherited in an autosomal recessive mode.

Galactose-glucose malabsorption is extremely rare, and results in severe persistent diarrhoea from birth.

CHRONIC DIARRHOEA

Chronic non-specific diarrhoea *Toddlers Diarrhoea ≡ Peas + Carrots Stools*
Persistent diarrhoa in a thriving child is a very common complaint. The most frequent explanation is an exaggerated gastrocolic reflex repeatedly provoked by frequent snacks and cold drinks. Simple measures such as restricting fluid intake to meal times obviates the need for antidiarrhoeal preparations of dubious therapeutic value. *Due to ↑ Gut Motility!   May Continue for Mo*

restrict ? fluids between meals.

Cow's milk protein intolerance

This is a mainly clinical diagnosis which is made when either acute or chronic symptoms appear to be related to cow's milk ingestion. Acute reactions after small amounts of milk include vomiting, diarrhoea, urticaria, stridor and broncho-spasm, and when this happens the association with milk intake is fairly readily established. It is more difficult to confirm that chronic effects such as failure to

→ Subtotal Villous Atrophy!

onset : @ 6-8wks.
→ Diarrhoea, failure to thrive, Vomiting.

thrive, rectal bleeding, anaemia and hepatosplenomegaly are due to a reaction to milk protein. Immunological studies indicate a variety of mechanisms. Susceptible infants may have enhanced absorption of antigenic quantities of β-lactoglobulin in early infancy and this may in turn be related to transient IgA deficiency or follow gastroenteritis. Jejunal biopsy shows variable villous flat- *Subtotal Villous Atrophy* tening. The disorder is usually temporary and can be managed by dietary adjustments. Protein is given in the form of casein hydrolysate, chicken meat or soy protein.

Other food intolerance

Children may have clearly documented hypersensitivity to one or more foods, for example eggs and fish. More difficult are the claimed associations between a wide range of food substances and problems such as behavioural disturbance, headaches and even convulsions. While it is appropriate to conduct sensibly structured dietary trials, the doctor must ensure that the child is not exposed to unfounded, bizarre or deficient diets.

Acrodermatitis enteropathica

This is a rare genetic disorder recently recognised as being linked to a defect of zinc metabolism. The infants develop severe diarrhoea and failure to thrive with a characteristic rash over the mucocutaneous junctions and pressure areas. There is also alopecia and nail dystrophy. The onset is delayed if the child is breast fed. Without appropriate therapy it is a fatal condition, and until the recognition of the value of zinc supplements the disease was controlled by the use of diodoquin.

Crohn disease   *Rare ∠ 12 yrs*

Crohn disease is rare in children but its incidence is thought to be on the increase. The diagnosis is often delayed because the symptoms are confused with functional complaints. The usual features are recurrent abdominal pain with anorexia, diarrhoea, fever and growth impairment. Perianal lesions, finger clubbing, arthritis and an abdominal mass may occur. Diffuse involvement of the jejunum and ileum makes surgical resection difficult. Recurrence is common. Corticosteroids and sulphasalazine together with dietary and vitamin supplementation are used in medical treatment but up to 90 per cent require surgery. It is sometimes difficult to distinguish Crohn disease from ulcerative colitis although the latter seldom causes recurrent abdominal pain. *(Diarrhoea ; Recurr Abd pain Aphthous Stomatitis Erythema Nodosum Polyarthritis ; Clubbing*

Ulcerative colitis   *irtis, arthritis, F Clubbing, Malabsorption Aphthous Stomatitis , Malignancy*

This is a condition in which there is mucosal ulceration of the large bowel. In children, total colon involvement is relatively more common than in adults. The child usually presents with diarrhoea, the stool containing both mucus and blood. Anaemia and growth failure are common, and arthritis, erythema nodosum, recurrent mouth ulceration and pyoderma gangrenosum may also occur. In the initial stages it is important to exclude bacterial infection and to define the extent of the disease by means of endoscopy and barium enema. Ulcerative colitis is a lifelong condition and is very disruptive to the young person. Initial control of the disease is by means of dietary measures, iron supplements, sulphasalazine and corticosteroids. The long-term risk of carcinoma of the colon eventually necessitates colectomy. If possible these drastic procedures are delayed until after puberty, but disturbed schooling and growth failure favour earlier surgery. Ulcerative colitis in infancy appears to be a separate entity and has been linked to cow's milk protein allergy.

INTESTINAL PARASITES

In the developing world these provide a further threat to children's health and result in malabsorption, anaemia and chronic diarrhoea.

Enterobius (threadworm). Enterobius is a frequent cause of perianal and vulval pruritis. The mobile thread-like worms are easily recognised on separating the buttocks of the sleeping child. They are difficult to eradicate and justify treatment only when symptomatic. The entire family must be treated with, for example, piperazine. Hygiene measures are also necessary to break the cycle of self-infection.

Giardia lamblia. *Giardia lamblia* is a flagellate protozoon transmitted by contaminated food and water. Infection may be asymptomatic or result in malabsorption due to jejunal mucosal damage. Metronidazole is the treatment of choice.

Ascaris lumbricoides (roundworms). Roundworm infection follows ingestion of the eggs. The larvae migrate via the portal system to the lungs where they ascend the bronchial tree to re-enter the gut. Heavy infestation may result in pneumonitis and eosinophilia during the larval phase. Gut symptoms are rare but include pain, obstruction and appendicitis. Piperazine treats the adult phase.

Ankylostoma (hookworm). Hookworm is a major cause of iron deficiency in hot, humid climates. Bephenium hydroxynaphthoate is an effective treatment.

See over ⇒

Threadworm and roundworm

Hookworm and toxocara

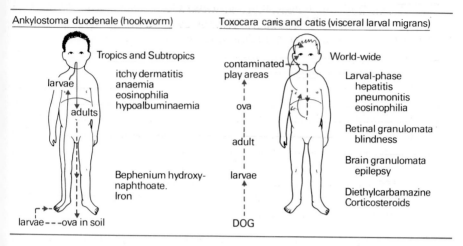

Ankylostoma duodenale (hookworm)	Toxocara canis and catis (visceral larval migrans)

Ankylostoma duodenale (hookworm)

Tropics and Subtropics

larvae

itchy dermatitis
anaemia
eosinophilia
hypoalbuminaemia

adults

Bephenium hydroxy-
naphthoate.
Iron

larvae - - -ova in soil

Toxocara canis and catis (visceral larval migrans)

World-wide

contaminated
play areas

ova

adult

larvae

DOG

Larval-phase
hepatitis
pneumonitis
eosinophilia

Retinal granulomata
blindness

Brain granulomata
epilepsy

Diethylcarbamazine
Corticosteroids

Toxocara canis and catis. *Toxocara canis* and *catis* may have their migratory larval phase in children who are in close contact with animal excreta. Infection produces eosinophilia, hepatomegaly and bronchospasm. The larvae may encapsulate in the eye producing retinal granulomata, or in the brain acting as potential epileptogenic foci.

Taenia saginata (beef tapeworm) and Taenia solium (pork tapeworm). The adult worms inhabit the intestinal canal of man. It is also possible for man to be infected by the larval phase of *T. solium* as a result of consumption of inadequately cooked pork. The larvae or cysticerci may encapsulate and calcify in the tissues. The adult tapeworms may be killed by niclosamide.

CONSTIPATION

Constipation is a frequent complaint in all age groups and reflects a common obsession with regular bowel function. It is valid to differentiate the problem of infrequent hard stools from the less worrying complaint of infrequent normal stools. Healthy infants show a considerable variation in the pattern of bowel frequency depending on their diet, and indeed mother's diet if breast fed. They may also show alarming colour changes and vigorous abdominal contractions during defaecation which may be interpreted by mother as straining. Genuine hard stools may result from an inadequate milk intake, hunger stools, or from over strength artificial feeds where the free water is diverted to facilitate renal solute excretion. The change from an artificial milk formula or breast milk to cow's milk is accompanied by production of smaller, harder and less frequent stools. Their passage may require more effort and resulting anal irritation may provoke withholding, and a pattern of behaviour which can evolve into troublesome constipation. Constipation may accompany more generalised disorders but it is seldom the chief complaint. Hypothyroidism, idiopathic hypercalcaemia and neuromuscular problems fall into this category.

In older children, acute constipation is a common accompaniment of febrile illnesses and the resulting hard stools may cause an anal tear which in turn initiates the cycle of faecal retention and chronic constipation. The prompt use of gentle laxatives and abundant fluids facilitates healing of the traumatised anal margin and helps the child to regain confidence in his toilet activities. It is sad that so many of these children are allowed to develop chronic constipation with all its attendant problems. These include abdominal pain, anorexia, vomiting, failure to thrive, and a predisposition to urinary tract infections. The accumulation of hard stool in the rectal ampulla leads to an acquired megacolon. The distension of the rectum results in relaxation of the internal sphincter so that the child must continually call on the external sphincter and the levator ani, which are voluntary muscle groups, in order to resist stool passage. Eventually this effort fails and the external sphincter is no longer able to prevent constant leakage of faecal matter. The soiling is often the dominant complaint and the families become desperate in their attempts to cope with this unsocial problem. Examination confirms the presence of the indentable faecal mass, the perianal soiling and the firm stool just within the internal sphincter.

Treatment requires an enthusiastic but relatively simple approach. The main objectives are to dislodge the faecal mass, overcome withholding behaviour and promote a regular bowel habit. Success revolves around the child regaining confidence in being capable of painless easy defaecation. A short course of a powerful liquid laxative is an effective means of dislodging the faecal mass. More refractory cases may require a brief course of enemas but the oral approach is more satisfactory for both child and therapist. This is followed by a programme of copious fluids a high roughage diet and Senokot at a dosage sufficient to amplify the gastrocolic reflex. The child must learn to take advantage of the latter by spending 5 to 10 minutes on the toilet after breakfast and the evening meal. It is worth checking that the child has firm foot support so that he can obtain the optimal mechanical advantage while sitting on the toilet. The use of laxatives and in particular liquid paraffin may cause the soiling to be worse during the initial period of treatment and parents must be warned about this. In most children, the physical and emotional problems improve in parallel with the recovery of normal bowel function. In a minority there are more profound behavioural problems which warrant a careful psychiatric evaluation.

Although chronic constipation can usually be overcome by this regimen, in some children the possibility of short segment Hirschsprung disease arises. If

Chronic constipation

Acquired Megacolon		Hirschsprung Disease
	neonate 60-70%	
3-6 yrs	later 30-40%	
soiling and constipation	constipation (occasionally diarrhoea)	
thriving	failure to thrive	
mild abdominal distension	gross abdominal distension	
loaded rectum	empty rectum	
anal tone decreased	anal tone normal or increased	
soiling	no soiling (✓ Rarely get This!)	

the problem persists in spite of anal dilatation under general anaesthetic, reevaluation is necessary.

*[handwritten: 1. fail to pass meconium in 1st 24 hours.
2. progressive abd distension.
3. Refuses feeds.
4. Bilious vomiting → Enterocolitis, - Perforation. Septicaemic]*

Hirschsprung disease

Hirschsprung disease must be considered if constipation presents in infancy. The incidence is 1 in 4500 live births. It accounts for about 10% of neonatal intestinal obstruction, but it may also present in the older child. It results from failure of migration of ganglion cells to the submucosal and myenteric plexuses of the large bowel. The aganglionic segment, which remains tonically contracted and aperistaltic, invariably involves the internal sphincter. Sometimes there is a very short segment, but 80% involve the recto-sigmoid colon and 15% extend to more proximal colon. In one large series 85% developed difficulties in the first month of life and 95% by the end of the first year. The typical infant fails to pass meconium within the first 24 hours of life, develops progressive abdominal distension, refuses to feed and finally has bilious vomiting. A severe form of enterocolitis with perforation and septicaemia may complicate this picture and has a high mortality rate. The older child suffers with intermittent bouts of intestinal obstruction from faecal impaction, failure to thrive, hypochromic anaemia and hypoproteinaemia. Soiling is extremely unusual but not unknown in Hirschsprung disease. On examination, the upper abdomen is distended with gas as well as faeces, the costal margin is flared and the umbilicus is displaced downward. Characteristically, the anal canal and rectum are free of faeces and may feel narrow and grip the finger. The diagnosis may be confirmed by barium enema of an unprepared colon, rectal biopsy and ano-rectal manometry. The latter demonstrates an absence of the normal reflex inhibition of the internal anal sphincter on rectal distension. Surgical treatment often entails an initial colostomy to relieve the obstruction. The subsequent definitive operation is designed to bypass the aganglionic segment and bring normal bowel down to the anus.

LIVER DISEASE

Hepatomegaly

Liver disease presents with hepatomegaly, jaundice, metabolic disturbance or intestinal bleeding either singly or in combination. The normal liver has a soft, smooth, non-tender edge 1 to 2 cm below the costal margin. An enlarged liver may be a transient finding accompanying acute disorders like infectious hepatitis or glandular fever, or it may be long-standing, requiring detailed investigation.

Persistent neonatal jaundice

Jaundice persisting beyond the second week is abnormal and in considering the possible cause, a distinction must be made between conjugated and unconjugated hyperbilirubinaemia.

Breast milk jaundice. Breast milk jaundice is a relatively uncommon problem, and may be due to a complex steroid in the milk which inhibits hepatic glucuronyl transferase. It is seldom necessary to advise against breast feeding in this condition as it resolves spontaneously. It is often confused with jaundice due to fluid deprivation.

Prolonged neonatal jaundice

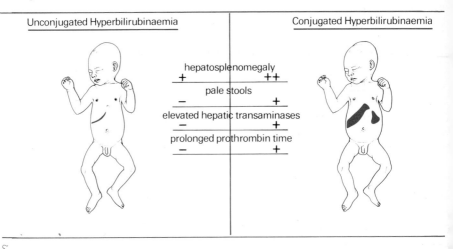

Unconjugated Hyperbilirubinaemia		Conjugated Hyperbilirubinaemia
hepatosplenomegaly		
+		++
pale stools		
−		+
elevated hepatic transaminases		
−		+
prolonged prothrombin time		
−		+

Crigler-Najjar syndrome. Crigler-Najjar syndrome is a rare, autosomal recessive condition in which hepatic glucuronyl transferase is deficient or absent. The most severe form causes neonatal kernicterus and is incompatible with life. A milder variety may respond to long-term phototherapy.

Neonatal hepatitis. Neonatal hepatitis is not a discrete entity but is the end result of a range of injurious processes which produce a similar histological picture, hepatocellular necrosis and inflammatory cell infiltrates in the portal tracts and lobules. Infants with conjugated hyperbilirubinaemia must be investigated for the known infective, genetic and metabolic causes, and it has to be appreciated that neonatal hepatitis is part of a spectrum of hepatic injury which overlaps with biliary atresia.

Biliary atresia. Biliary atresia is the end stage of a sclerosing process in an initially patent biliary tree. With few exceptions the prognosis was uniformly dismal until the introduction of early laparotomy and porto-enterostomy, the Kasai procedure. This operation is followed by bile flow in approximately 50%

1 in 10,000 live Births :   70% < 60 days old when operated o

Causes of persistent neonatal jaundice

Unconjugated hyperbilirubinaemia	Conjugated hyperbilirubinaemia
Infection, e.g. urinary tract	(a) Neonatal hepatitis syndrome.
Hypothyroidism	Congenital infection, e.g. rubella,
Haemolytic anaemia	cytomegalovirus, toxoplasmosis
High gastrointestinal obstruction	Metabolic
Breast-milk jaundice	alpha-1 antitrypsin deficiency *
Transient familial hyperbilirubinaemia	galactosaemia
Crigler-Najjar syndrome	tyrosinosis
	cystic fibrosis
	storage disorders
	(b) Duct obstruction or obliteration
	Extrahepatic biliary atresia
	Intrahepatic biliary hypoplasia
	Choledochal cyst

of children and has provided a stimulus to the early diagnosis and selection of those infants who might benefit from surgery. The longerterm outcome has still to be assessed.

Percutaneous liver biopsy and radioisotope excretion studies are useful in separating the majority of infants with biliary atresia from those with neonatal hepatitis syndrome. The latter may deteriorate if subjected to inappropriate surgery, and if no specific therapy is indicated by the investigations, a trial of phenobarbitone and cholestyramine may promote recovery. In a prospective study of the neonatal hepatitis syndrome in S.E. England, homozygous α_1-antitrypsin deficiency was the single most commonly identifiable cause but the majority of cases had no demonstrable aetiology.

Infectious hepatitis

Hepatitis A (incubation 15 to 50 days). Hepatitis A infection is the commonest cause of jaundice in older children. It spreads by the oral route and is usually mild or subclinical. Anorexia, fever, vomiting and abdominal pain may precede the jaundice. Elevation of serum transaminase levels is the first biochemical abnormality and they remain raised for up to three weeks in most cases. Passive immunisation with pooled immunoglobulin provides protection and may be indicated for family and other close contacts. Hepatitis A specific IgM is the best single marker of recent infection.

Hepatitis B (incubation 50 to 180 days). Hepatitis B is uncommon in European children, but infection and chronic carrier status are frequent in developing countries. Vertical transmission from carrier mothers to newborn babies is a major route of spread, and contributes to a new generation of chronic carriers. Infected infants are seldom symptomatic but are vulnerable to cirrhosis and hepatocellular carcinoma. Programmes to protect infants with combined passive and active immunisation schedules are showing great promise.

Non-A, non-B hepatitis. These are caused by a group of viruses showing intermediate characteristics. Their importance is emerging as specific laboratory tests for infective hepatitis evolve. Infectious mononucleosis (EB virus) and cytomegalovirus are other recognised causes of hepatitis.

Reye syndrome. Reye syndrome is an important cause of acute encephalopathy in early childhood. In addition to non-inflammatory cerebral oedema there is diffuse fatty infiltration of viscera, notably the liver. The usual history is of an apparently innocuous viral illness progressing to refractory vomiting, altered consciousness and convulsions. Liver impairment produces hypoglycaemia, increased plasma ammonia levels and disturbed coagulation. Prompt recognition and intensive therapy aimed at controlling cerebral oedema and correcting metabolic imbalance is essential to avoid a high mortality and morbidity. Epidemiological studies suggest that the disorder is triggered by a variety of viruses, possibly acting in combination with either environmental toxins or drugs. Aspirin frequently used during the prodromal illnesses has been incriminated although the evidence is controversial. Family studies suggest that these exogenous factors interact with genetic susceptibility to cause mitochondrial damage and dysfunction.

Wilson disease (hepato lenticular degeneration)

This is a rare and potentially very damaging disease which merits prompt consideration in any child over age six years with unexplained liver disturbance. The pathognomic appearance of copper at the periphery of the cornea (Kayser-Fleischer rings) requires slit lamp examination but is often absent in the young.(The majority of cases have low serum levels of copper and caeruloplasmin. Oral penicillamine facilitates removal of the excess body copper. The disorder is inherited as an autosomal recessive and siblings must be screened for low caeruloplasmin levels.

Chronic aggressive hepatitis

Chronic aggressive or active hepatitis is usually an autoimmune disorder and is relatively more frequent in adolescent girls. The majority have an insidious onset with fever, acneiform rashes, erythema nodosum, colitis, jaundice and hepatomegaly but a significant number have an initial illness resembling infectious hepatitis. Disturbed liver function tests, an elevated ESR and positive antinuclear factor tests favour the diagnosis but it is essential to confirm it by percutaneous liver biopsy. The natural history is one of progressive fibrosis with the development of cirrhosis. Prolonged corticosteroid therapy combined with azathioprine may control this grave development. ＊ (90% 5yr Survival Rate!)

Childhood cirrhosis

Cirrhosis may result from inherited metabolic disorders or from acquired disease of the liver or biliary tract. In the majority of affected children no specific therapy is available and treatment is directed towards combating the resultant malabsorption, bleeding problems and ascites. Liver transplantation is emerging as a realistic procedure: its greatest success, 80% one year survival, has been

Causes and clinical features of cirrhosis in childhood

Causes		Clinical Features
1. Genetic (metabolic/storage) cirrhosis		Portal hypertension
eg. α₁-antitrypsin deficiency		
Wilson disease *Unless Tx early.*		oesophageal varices
galactosaemia		splenomegaly
cystic fibrosis		hypersplenism
		ascites
2. Post-necrotic cirrhosis		Hepatic failure
eg. neonatal hepatitis	biopsy	failure to thrive
chronic aggressive hepatitis		fatigue, anorexia
drugs, toxins, poisons		spider naevi
venous congestion		finger clubbing
		liver palms
3. Biliary cirrhosis		
eg. extrahepatic biliary atresia	regenerating nodules	
intrahepatic biliary hypoplasia	broad bands of fibrosis	
choledochal cyst		

gained in young children. It promises to be a definitive treatment for a range of metabolic disorders, notably α_1-antitrypsin deficiency.

Portal hypertension

This usually presents as intestinal bleeding and splenomegaly, but the spleen may not be palpable immediately after a severe haemorrhage. The majority of cases are due to thrombosis of the portal vein; either idiopathic or secondary to sepsis of the umbilical vein and portal system in infancy. Hepatic cirrhosis and congenital hepatic fibrosis may also cause portal hypertension. The exact cause needs to be established by selective angiography of the coeliac axis and by a liver biopsy. If portal vein thrombosis is diagnosed, the long-term management should be as conservative as possible as splenorenal shunts are technically difficult and seldom successful before the age of ten years. There is a tendency for bleeding from the oesophageal varices to improve with age.

Congenital hepatic fibrosis

Congenital hepatic fibrosis may be either sporadic or familial and is diagnosed by liver biopsy which shows marked portal fibrosis but retention of the normal hepatic lobular architecture. It may be associated with polycystic disease of the kidneys.

Causes of hepatomegaly and clinical signs which may aid diagnosis

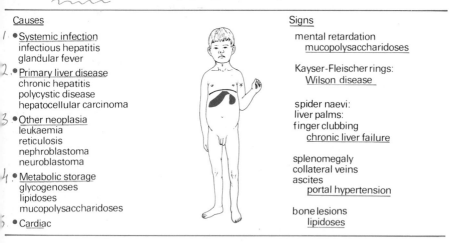

Causes	Signs
• Systemic infection infectious hepatitis glandular fever	mental retardation mucopolysaccharidoses
• Primary liver disease chronic hepatitis polycystic disease hepatocellular carcinoma	Kayser-Fleischer rings: Wilson disease
• Other neoplasia leukaemia reticulosis nephroblastoma neuroblastoma	spider naevi: liver palms: finger clubbing chronic liver failure
• Metabolic storage glycogenoses lipidoses mucopolysaccharidoses	splenomegaly collateral veins ascites portal hypertension
• Cardiac	bone lesions lipidoses

LIVER ENZYME DEFICIENCIES

Glycogen storage diseases

Enzyme deficiencies with their resulting disorders have been recognised for each of the steps in the pathways of glycogen synthesis and degradation. They enter into the differential diagnosis of recurrent hypoglycaemia, hepatomegaly, muscle weakness with cramps, and congestive cardiac failure.

Type I: Glucose-6-phosphatase deficiency is a serious disorder, usually presenting in infancy, and manifest by hepatomegaly, hypoglycaemia and a metabolic acidosis. The enzyme deficiency prevents the normal glycaemic response to intramuscular glucagon and can be confirmed by liver biopsy. Frequent glucose feeds and restriction of galactose and fructose intake are helpful in treatment.

Type III: Debranching enzyme deficiency and type VI: liver phosphorylase deficiency present in a similar although milder fashion and can be diagnosed by measurement of leucocyte enzyme levels.

Type II: Acid maltase deficiency (Pompe disease) results in excessive glycogen deposition in both liver and muscle, with cardiac muscle especially involved. The majority of affected infants present soon after birth with poor feeding, weakness, tachypnoea and cardiac failure. Muscle or leucocyte enzyme analysis confirm the diagnosis but treatment is supportive only and the child will survive only for a matter of months.

Galactosaemia

Galactosaemia is a very rare, recessively inherited disorder but its importance lies in the disastrous consequences of its being overlooked. It results from deficiency of the enzyme, galactose-1-phosphate uridyl transferase, which is essential for galactose metabolism. Affected infants are normal at birth but shortly after the commencement of milk feeds the majority develop jaundice, vomiting, diarrhoea, and fail to thrive. If the disorder remains unrecognised liver disease, cataracts and mental retardation will result. The urine contains galactose and is characteristically Clinitest positive but Clinistix negative, the latter being specific for glucose. Specific enzymatic techniques confirm the diagnosis and establish the necessity of a lactose-free diet.

Hereditary fructose intolerance

This is another rare enzyme deficiency in which prompt recognition can prevent the onset of life-threatening complications. The low activity of aldolase B not only results in the accumulation of fructose-1-phosphate but also causes a secondary inhibition of hepatic pathways responsible for maintaining normoglycaemia. In susceptible children, fructose-containing foods provoke abdominal pain, nausea, vomiting and symptoms of hypoglycaemia. In the longer term hepatomegaly, growth failure and liver failure occur. A detailed dietary history reveals normal health until the introduction of sucrose into the diet, and suspicion may be substantiated by a fructose tolerance test or by liver enzyme analysis. Therapy involves the elimination of all fructose containing items from the diet.

Benign or essential fructosuria. Benign or essential fructosuria is an asymptomatical deficiency of the enzyme fructokinase.

BIBLIOGRAPHY

Apley J 1975 The child with abdominal pains. Blackwell, Oxford
Mowat A P 1979 Liver disorders in childhood. Butterworths, London
Tripp J H, Candy D C A 1985 Manual of paediatric gastroenterology. Churchill Livingstone, Edinburgh
Walker-Smith J A, Hamilton J R, Walker W A 1983 Practical paediatric gastroenterology. Butterworths, London

11

Urinary Tract and Testes

pronephric

mesonephric

metanephric

urogenital sinus

Renal function undergoes a major transition with the onset of extrauterine life and the demands of water conservation and electrolyte homeostasis. Although nephron formation is complete before birth the newborn kidney contains less than 20% of its adult cellular component, and the total renal blood flow is reduced due to higher renal vascular resistance. The glomerular filtration rate at term averages 20 ml per minute per 1.73 m² with adult values only being reached in the second year of life. The functional limitations of the newborn kidney are reflected in higher blood urea and phosphate levels, and a lower plasma bicarbonate concentration.

The higher metabolic rate of the infant in relation to body weight, greater insensible water losses and the inability to control oral intake, increase the susceptibility of young patients to dehydration and metabolic abnormalities. Acute renal failure with acidosis, uraemia and hyperkalaemia can develop very rapidly in the young infant.

RENAL FUNCTION TESTS

Urinalysis
A multiple urine test strip can be employed and it is preferable to examine a fresh morning sample of urine.

Proteinuria
Transient positive readings are common during febrile illnesses or after exercise. Postural or orthostatic proteinuria is suggested by the absence of significant proteinuria on a first morning specimen compared to one tested after the patient has been ambulant. The finding of proteinuria does not necessarily mean that the urine is infected but can signify underlying renal disease.

Haematuria
This may be macroscopic in the case of nephritis or renal tract lesions but is more commonly microscopic. Haematuria may also be a transient finding. Microscopy

of fresh urine should be performed to confirm the presence of red blood cells rather than a false positive test due to free haemoglobin, myoglobin, beeturia or confectionary dyes.

Glycosuria and aminoaciduria
Glycosuria and aminoaciduria may be secondary to elevated serum levels or may be the result of tubular defects.

Urine pH and osmolality
Normal urine pH is between 5 and 7 and is affected by dietary intake. Formal acidification tests may be required if renal tubular acidosis is suspected. A first morning urine sample after fasting overnight provides a useful screening test of renal concentrating ability with normal values being above 800 milliosmoles per kg (specific gravity above 1.020).

Urine microscopy

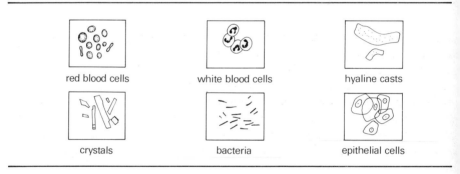

red blood cells	white blood cells	hyaline casts
crystals	bacteria	epithelial cells

Microscopy
This may give useful information especially in the presence of proteinuria or haematuria. Fresh urine should also be used when examining for casts. Red blood cell casts suggest glomerulonephritis. The presence of increased white blood cells, above 5 per high powered field, or motile bacteria suggest urinary tract infection. The latter needs confirmation by urine culture.

Glomerular filtration rate (GFR)
Derived from 24 hour urine volume and measurement of plasma creatinine, this is very liable to error in young children because of difficulty of collection techniques. The approximate GFR can be derived from the plasma creatinine using the equation:

$$\text{GFR}/1.73 \text{ m}^2 \text{ surface area} = 38 \times \text{height (cm)}/\text{plasma creatinine } (\mu\text{mol/l}).$$

The rate of fall in the blood concentration of injected isotope, chromium-51 EDTA or ^{99}Tc-DTPA is used for more precise measurement.

URINARY TRACT MALFORMATIONS

These are relatively common but most are functionally insignificant. A small proportion are fatal and may have important genetic implications. The increased use of ultrasound in pregnancy has resulted in renal malformations being diagnosed more frequently *in utero*. The role of intervention to drain obstructed urinary systems prior to delivery is being evaluated.

Renal agenesis

This results in oligohydramnios and compression of the fetus, Potter syndrome. Other urinary tract malformations such as polycystic kidneys or obstructive lesions may also cause oligohydramnios. The degree of the associated pulmonary hypoplasia is critical to early survival.

[handwritten: post Urethral Valves]

Potter syndrome

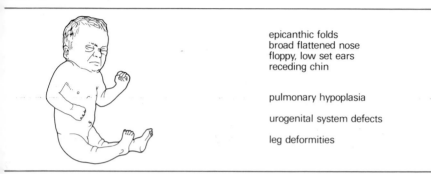

epicanthic folds
broad flattened nose
floppy, low set ears
receding chin

pulmonary hypoplasia

urogenital system defects

leg deformities

Unilateral renal hypoplasia and dysplasia

This may be an incidental finding but a large multicystic dysplastic kidney may present as an abdominal mass in a newborn infant. Differentiation from hydronephrosis is important. The function of the apparently normal contralateral kidney must be carefully assessed as part of the evaluation.

Polycystic kidneys

Infantile polycystic disease results in grossly enlarged spongy kidneys and cystic changes in the liver and other viscera. The bilateral kidney enlargement is conspicuous at birth or in early infancy. There are several varieties each with an autosomal recessive inheritance. The adult form, with autosomal dominant inheritance, can also present in early life although most survive to be young adults and are therefore capable of transmitting the abnormal gene.

Obstructive malformations

These produce unilateral or bilateral hydronephrosis

Pelviureteric junction (PUJ) obstruction. PUJ obstruction is the commonest cause of hydronephrosis and may be produced by intrinsic stenosis, functional obstruction or compression from an aberrant artery or bands.

Horseshoe kidneys. Horseshoe kidneys produce a characteristic IVU picture — the upper poles are further from the midline than the lower poles. Hydronephrosis due to PUJ obstruction may occur. Treatment for PUJ obstruction is by pyeloplasty.

Ureteric duplication. The bifid ureter is more common than complete duplication. Usually there is a strong family history of this abnormality.

Renal tract abnormalities liable to obstruction

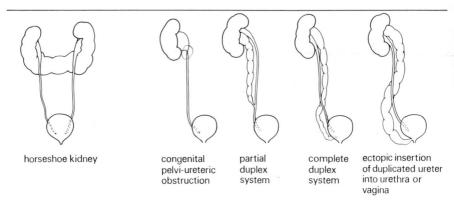

horseshoe kidney

congenital
pelvi-ureteric
obstruction

partial
duplex
system

complete
duplex
system

ectopic insertion
of duplicated ureter
into urethra or
vagina

When the ureters enter the bladder separately the ureter draining the upper renal moiety is situated in a lower position or maybe ectopic. Since it has a longer intravesical course it is liable to become obstructed resulting in hydronephrosis of the upper pole. The ureter draining the lower moiety has a short intravesical course and is therefore prone to vesico-ureteric reflux resulting in chronic pyelonephritis of the lower pole.

Posterior urethral valves. Posterior urethral valves are the commonest cause of lower urinary obstruction in the male child. The diagnosis may be made on antenatal ultrasound or postnatally on routine examination of a healthy neonate who has a distended bladder with a poor urinary stream. Infants may present with a urinary infection or overflow incontinence.

Urethral valves

reflux into dilated
ureter

catheter

dilated posterior
urethra

valves

The kidneys show secondary bilateral hydronephrosis due to obstruction and/or vesico-ureteric reflux. Diagnosis is by MCUG and treatment is by ablation of valves via endoscopy. Temporary diversion is rarely necessary. The reflux should resolve spontaneously after treatment of the obstruction.

Bladder exstrophy. This results from failure of midline fusion of the infra-umbilical midline structures. Males are affected more commonly than females.

Clinically, the bladder mucosa is present as a small contracted circular plaque in the low abdomen, the umbilicus is abnormally low, the penis up-turned and epispadic, the pubic unfused and the lower limbs therefore apparently externally rotated. In girls the genital tract is normal although vaginal stenosis may need surgery in early adult life. Bladder and especially bladder neck reconstruction is extremely difficult and many children are treated by urinary diversion.

Urachal remnants may persist producing blind tracts or cysts in the lower abdominal wall. Complete patency between the bladder and umbilicus is exceptionally rare.

Prune belly syndrome. This occurs almost exclusively in males and is a triad of deficiency of abdominal muscles, complex genito-urinary malformation and bilateral undescended testes. Pulmonary hypoplasia may prove fatal in the newborn period but other less affected children can survive with appropriate therapy.

URINARY TRACT INFECTIONS

This is a common and important paediatric problem because it may be associated with renal damage leading to hypertension and end-stage renal disease. Although 1–2% of schoolgirls and 0.2% of boys have asymptomatic bacteriuria it is now generally accepted that it is the preschool child who is most at risk of developing renal scars.

The most important populations to screen for bacteriuria are newborns and children less than four years of age with unexplained fever. A delay of even a few days in introducing therapy for pyelonephritis will increase the risk of renal damage in these young patients.

In the newborn prolonged jaundice, excessive weight loss or a septicaemic episode may be secondary to urinary tract infection. The young child may also present with relatively non-specific symptoms; poor weight gain, irritability, fever, vomiting and diarrhoea. Urinalysis must be combined with careful urine collection by clean catch or supervised use of a urine bag. Suprapubic aspiration can be used as part of a 'septic screen' of a newborn or to clarify equivocal results in infants.

Organisms derived from bowel flora are the commonest infecting agents. Some individuals are more prone to urinary tract infections that others and this may be associated with abnormal gram negative colonisation of the introitus and peri-urethral areas. Studies showing increased adherence to uroepithelial cells by pyelonephritogenic bacteria may allow improved preventitive measures in the future.

Management

Management of an acute infection combines copious fluids, mild analgesia if required and antibacterial therapy; septicaemia or acute pyelonephritis merits intravenous ampicillin or gentamicin. Oral therapy for less severe cases includes cotrimoxazole or trimethoprim, amoxycillin, nalidixic acid, nitrofurantoin and other agents according to bacteriological sensitivity. A ten-day course of chemotherapy is usually sufficient and a sterile urine culture should be obtained following treatment.

All proven urinary tract infections require radiological evaluation. This has usually been an IVU but an abdominal ultrasound by an experienced paediatric radiologist may well substitute. The important examination particularly in a child less than four years of age is a micturating cystourethrogram (MCUG) to rule out vesicoureteric reflux with which renal scarring and damage may be associated. Reflux can be a familial problem and it may be justified to screen other family members especially if less invasive radionuclide methods are available.

X-ray abnormalities detected in children with bacteriuria (after Smellie and Normand). A classification of vesicoureteric reflux

Grades of vesico-ureteric reflux during micturating cystogram:

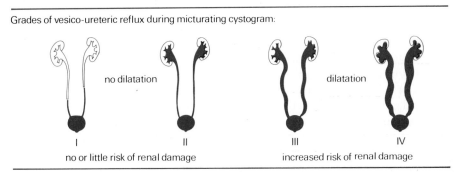

no dilatation   dilatation

I   II   III   IV

no or little risk of renal damage   increased risk of renal damage

The presence of vesicoureteric reflux warrants continuous prophylaxis with antimicrobial agents such as trimethoprim (2 mg/kg/single dose) or nitrofurantoin (2 mg/kg/twice daily). Previously many of these children were subjected to surgery for reimplantation of the ureters, but since reflux will cease spontaneously in a large number of children maintained on prophylactic therapy alone surgery is now generally restricted to cases of urinary obstruction, or to children with 'breakthrough' urinary infections while on prophylaxis.

Drugs commonly used in the treatment of urinary tract infection

Drug	Dose	Comments
Cotrimoxazole or trimethoprim	2 mg/kg trimethoprin twice daily	Useful in prophylaxis Good compliance. Side effects — rashes, vomiting
Amoxycillin	125 mg three times a day	Less useful in prophylaxis. Side effects — rashes, diarrhoea
Nitrofurantoin	2 mg/kg three times a day	Useful in prophylaxis. Side effects — nausea, vomiting
Nalidixic acid	15 mg/kg three times a day	Useful in boys with proteus infection. Side effects — rashes
Gentamycin	1 mg/kg three times a day	Parenteral use only. Side effects — nephrotoxic, ototoxic

It is important to emphasise general preventive measures in all children with urinary tract infection. These include a regular bowel habit, adequate fluids, proper voiding techniques and double micturition, good hygiene and the avoidance of irritants such as bubble baths and nylon underwear.

Older children may complain of an urethral syndrome with frequency and dysuria and no bacteriological confirmation of urine infection. Viral infections may play a role but acute vulvitis or balanitis may be associated with poor hygiene, perineal candidiasis or contact sensitivity to nylon pants.

Screening

Extensive surveys have attempted to monitor the impact of detection, investigation and treatment of asymptomatic bacteriuria in schoolgirls aged 5 to 12 years. The results suggest that such screening is not worthwhile and that kidney damage associated with infection generally occurs before five years. Screening the preschool child is time consuming and the yield of treatable abnormalities is small.

HAEMATURIA

Haematuria may occur as an isolated symptom or may be accompanied by signs of a systemic disorder, for example Henoch Schönlein purpura, acute glomerulonephritis; or by renal colic, due for example to clot, calculus, obstructive malformation; or a loin mass, for example Wilms' tumour or hydronephrosis. Red cell casts and significant proteinuria establish glomerular lesions while pyuria and bacteriuria point to infection. An abdominal ultrasound or IVU is indicated if renal tract pathology is suspected. Cystoscopy is seldom required unless the blood staining is prominent at the start or finish of the stream. Renal biopsy is reserved for children whose haematuria is persistent, and accompanied by significant proteinuria or impaired renal function.

Long-term prognosis of recurrent haematuria (Miller et al 1985)

Recurrent or persistent haematuria

Recurrent macroscopic haematuria exacerbated by upper respiratory tract infections suggests IgA nephropathy or Berger disease. Some healthy children with persistent microscopic haematuria and similar findings in other family members fall into the category of benign familial haematuria. A positive family history of nephritis in association with sensorineural nerve deafness suggests Alport syndrome which is X-linked, and boys with this condition tend to be affected more severely than girls.

Longer term follow of patients with recurrent haematuria suggests that there may be more morbidity and mortality than previously suspected.

Acute haemorrhagic cystitis. This may occur with viral infection, notably adenovirus 11, or as a complication of cyclophosphamide therapy.

ACUTE NEPHRITIC SYNDROME

Post-streptococcal glomerulonephritis

Acute glomerulonephritis occurs predominantly in schoolchildren. Although it characteristically occurs 7 to 14 days after a group A β-haemolytic streptococcal throat infection, an increasing percentage appear to have another, possibly viral explanation. In areas of the world with poor hygiene, glomerulonephritis following streptococcal skin infection with pyoderma is relatively common. Only certain serotypes of streptococcus are responsible and the detection of streptococcal antigen in the glomerular mesangium supports the concept of acute soluble complex injury. Reduced serum complement levels also indicate an immunological pathogenesis.

Many affected children are asymptomatic. Typical complaints include malaise, headache, and vague loin discomfort but it may be the smoky urine which at first causes alarm. Oedema tends to collect around the orbits and on the backs of the hands and feet. Urine microscopy shows gross haematuria with granular and red cell casts. Proteinuria is also present. In the majority of cases oliguria is only mild but severe fluid retention can occasionally produce acute hypertension, with encephalopathy and seizures, or heart failure.

Typical clinical course of acute nephritis

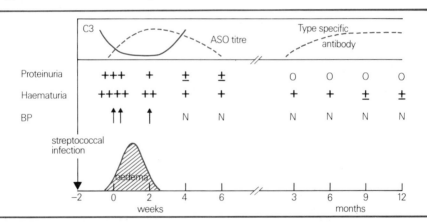

Management. The confirmation of post-streptococcal glomerulonephritis establishes an excellent prognosis in most instances, and therefore all cases should have an antistreptolysin titre determination as well as a throat swab. The remainder of the family should also have throat swabs.

Treatment includes eradication of streptococcal infection with a ten-day course of phenoxymethyl penicillin. Hospital admission is required if there is any suggestion of oliguria, fluid overload or hypertension. The reduced GFR should be assessed by a plasma creatinine estimation and serial progress monitored by daily weight and fluid balance. Oliguria requires salt restriction and water intake balanced against insensible loss, 400 ml per m² surface area per day, plus the previous day's urine output. More aggressive management with diuretics and hypotensive drugs may be needed to control hypertension. Acute peritoneal dialysis is necessary to treat severe fluid overload, hyperkalaemia and a deteriorating clinical state.

The normal course is for the GFR to return to normal in 10 to 14 days. If oliguria persists or progresses, a renal biopsy is justified to define the nature of the glomerular lesion. Rapidly progressive glomerulonephritis with scarring and deteriorating renal function is fortunately rare in the young.

The long-term prognosis of post-streptococcal glomerulonephritis is assumed to be excellent, 92 to 98% achieving resolution. There is still some caution about the eventual status of the non-streptococcal group.

Henoch Schönlein purpura

Although approximately 70% of children with Henoch Schönlein purpura have haematuria and or proteinuria, the glomerulonephritis is usually asymptomatic and non-progressive with an eventual mortality of less than 1 to 3%. This serious complication is, however, responsible for 5% of children entering renal dialysis programmes. Children presenting with an acute nephritic syndrome or rapidly progressing to a nephrotic syndrome have an ominous future. Normal renal function two years after the initial insult is unlikely to deteriorate but there are exceptions. Renal histology is some guide to prognosis, the glomerular lesions varying from minimal change to focal or diffuse mesangial proliferation with crescents, and in the most advanced stages, sclerosis. There is no specific therapy for this nephritis and management is symptomatic. Children with urinary abnormalities after Henoch Schönlein purpura should continue to have urine examinations and blood pressure measurements at periodic intervals in order to detect the late development of hypertension and renal impairment.

H : A,P　(arthritis, Purpura)

Clinical features of Henoch Schönlein purpura　　S : A , R.　(abd. pain　Renal involvement

| Localised oedema
face, hands, feet, scrotum

Arthritis
flitting, large joints

Abdominal pain
melaena
haematemesis
haemorrhage with oedema
of gut wall | | Nephritis
microscopic haematuria
proteinuria
mild focal glomerulonephritis

Maculopapular-purpura rash
buttocks and extensor surface of
legs and arms |

IgA - mild from
IgS } - severe
IgA } complic

NEPHROTIC SYNDROME

The nephrotic syndrome occurs when there is gross urinary protein loss resulting in hypoalbuminaemia and oedema. It is uncommon, with an incidence of 2 per 100 000 children and a peak incidence between 1 and 5 years. Males are more commonly affected than females, 2.5:1. The cause is unknown. Approximately 85% of caucasian children with nephrotic syndrome have the so-called 'minimal change' type.

Peri-orbital or dependent oedema and abdominal ascites are usually noticed first. There may also be abdominal pain, vomiting and diarrhoea. Hypovolaemia and circulatory collapse is a danger in the early phase of the illness since fluid shifts from the intravascular to the extracellular space, and it may be exacerbated by the vomiting and diarrhoea. A careful review of pulse, blood pressure and haematocrit must be maintained until the situation stabilises. Intravenous plasma replacement may be necessary. These children are also susceptible to infection, particularly pneumococcal peritonitis and urinary tract infection. Fever in the presence of ascites justifies a diagnostic ascitic fluid tap for microscopy and culture. Risk of Thrombosis. (Cerebral / Renal Vein).

Pathology. The term minimal change nephrotic syndrome is derived from light microscopy appearance. Electron microscopy shows fusion of the epithelial cell foot processes, a non-specific consequence of proteinuria. Although the pathogenesis of the renal insult leading to proteinuria is uncertain, it is thought to be a combination of structural changes to the glomerular basement membrane and reduced electrostatic inter-reaction between circulating polyanions and fixed negative charge on the glomerular capillary wall. Renal biopsy is not required if the clinical picture matches minimal change nephrotic syndrome and there is a definite response to corticosteroids. Other pathological conditions such as focal segmental glomerulosclerosis and membrano-proliferative glomerulonephritis carry a more guarded prognosis.

Management. Diuretics should be used with care as they promote hyponatraemia and may further reduce the intravascular volume. Salt poor albumin infusion temporarily restores the circulating volume but is required in only a minority of children. Rest is normally guided by the patient's behaviour, and moderate fluid restriction is necessary only while the child is oedematous. Prophylactic penicillin should be given during the oedematous phase. The recovery is monitored by daily weights and proteinuria. Ninety per cent of children with minimal change disease will respond to corticosteroids within eight weeks.

Frequent relapses may be controlled by alternate-day prednisolone, but if corticosteroid toxicity occurs there may be a case for a brief course of cyclophosphamide. Concern about the long-term gonadal effects of cytotoxic therapy restricts its usage.

A scheme for the management of the childhood nephrotic syndrome

Congenital nephrotic syndrome   *↑ αFP antenatally*

Congenital nephrotic syndrome is very rare and either presents at birth with placental oedema or develops in the first year. It may be familial with autosomal recessive inheritance, and is more common in Scandinavia. Dialysis and transplantation can now be offered to children with this previously fatal condition.

Microcystic dil. of Prox Tubule ..--> Fanconi Synd (Cortex)   ->R.F.

Systemic causes of nephrotic syndrome

These include infections (e.g. malaria), poisons (e.g. mercurials), allergies (e.g. bee sting), and collagen vascular disorders (e.g. SLE).

ACUTE RENAL FAILURE

Acute renal failure is an uncommon but important problem in which the kidneys are no longer able to maintain biochemical homeostasis. Oliguria, less than 200 to 250 ml per m² surface area per day, is usually present. The possible causes fall into three main groups; pre-renal, renal, and post-renal.

Classification of acute renal failure

Pre-renal	Renal	Post-renal
Hypovolaemia e.g. burns and acute haemorrhage	Acute tubular nephropathy e.g. ischaemia, nephrotoxins	Obstructive lesions
Circulatory failure e.g. septicaemia, heart failure	Acute interstitial nephropathy e.g. septicaemia, urinary infection	
	Acute glomerulonephritis Haemolytic-uraemic syndrome Renal vein thrombosis	

—Post. Urethral Valves
—Bilat Obst — PU.
— Urethrocoele
—Neurogenic Bladder
—Stone

Management

In practical terms the priorities are to distinguish pre-renal from established renal failure, and to exclude obstruction and pre-existing renal disease (acute on chronic renal failure). The presenting illness, gastroenteritis or septicaemic shock, may be very suggestive of circulatory failure and a pre-renal cause, but if oliguria has developed there is a risk that tubular nephropathy has already occurred. The examination of urine and plasma makes the distinction, as normal kidneys will concentrate urinary urea and reabsorb sodium. Proteinuria, cells and casts also suggest a renal lesion.

Investigations which determine the cause of oliguria

Measurement	Pre-renal	Renal
Urine osmolality (mos/kg)	Above 500	Less than 400
Urine: plasma osmolar ratio	Above 1.3	Less than 1.1
Urinary sodium (mmol/l)	Under 10	Above 20
Urinary urea (mmol/l)	Above 250	Under 100

Pre-renal failure demands urgent vascular volume expansion and careful monitoring of fluid and electrolyte replacement. *Renal failure* may respond to intravenous, high-dosage frusemide but preparations should be made for peritoneal or haemodialysis, especially if the picture is complicated by hypertension, pulmonary oedema or worsening biochemistry. Gentamicin and other drugs with a primarily renal excretion should be used with caution. *Potentially reversible obstruction* must not be overlooked and high dose IVU with tomography, micturating cystourethrograms, ultrasound, and radioisotopic procedures play a role.

Acute renal failure of childhood has in general a good outlook if dealt with expertly. However the survival is less good for acute renal failure complicating other life-threatening conditions such as severe infection or following surgery for complex disease.

Manifestations and management of acute renal failure

DIALYSIS –

	Complication	Therapy	
water overload	hyponatraemia	fluid restriction, twice daily weight	D
sodium overload	hypertension, oedema	salt restriction	I
potassium overload	cardiac arrhythmias	cation exchange resin dietary restriction	A
metabolic acidosis		cautious administration of sodium bicarbonate	L
nitrogen retention ↑		high calorie intake balanced 1st class protein	Y
hypercatabolic metabolism ↑			S
burns, sepsis			I
			S

pre-renal →
renal →
post-renal →

Haemolytic uraemic syndrome (HUS)

This triad of acute renal failure, haemolytic anaemia with fragmented erythrocytes, and thrombocytopenia is a relatively common cause of acute renal failure in infants and children. Small outbreaks occasionally occur in the U.K.. There are endemic foci in other parts of the world such as South America. Typically an episode of vomiting and diarrhoea is followed by pallor, haematuria and oliguria as acute renal failure supervenes. Seizures may reflect hypertension or direct central nervous system involvement. Other organs such as the gut, liver and heart can also be affected.

The epidemic form of HUS has been associated with a variety of bacterial and viral agents with current interest focused on intestinal infection with verotoxin producing *Escherichia coli*. While the pathophysiological mechanisms in HUS are still unclear it is suggested that an initial toxic insult to vascular endothelial cells may disturb the balance between prostacyclin production in endothelial cells and thromboxane synthesis by platelets.

The epidemic form of HUS generally has a good prognosis with supportive treatment alone, but sporadic cases in older children with no clear prodromal illness often result in residual renal impairment.

CHRONIC RENAL FAILURE

The incidence of chronic renal failure in children is much less than in the adult population but the effects on growth and development can be profound. Symptoms do not usually develop until 60 to 80% of renal function is lost. There may be an insidious onset with growth failure, anorexia and nocturia, or an acute on chronic crisis may be precipitated by superimposed infection. Urinary tract infection or salt wasting can cause a rapid deterioration in renal function, while extra-renal infection with increased catabolic demands and vomiting may cause an acute decline in GFR.

Frequency of different causes of chronic paediatric renal disease. (European Dialysis and Transplant Association)

	%
Chronic glomerulonephritis e.g. focal glomerulosclerosis	32.3
Pyelonephritis and urinary tract malformation	21.9
Hereditary — familial, e.g. Alport syndrome	16.1
Renal hypoplasia/dysplasia	12.1
Other diagnoses e.g. Henoch Schönlein purpura	12.5
uncertain	5.1

These children should be supervised by a paediatric nephrology unit which can provide the optimal care consisting of specialist dietary advice, surgical liaison and psychosocial preparation if dialysis and transplantation become imminent. Growth impairment in chronic renal failure is a multi-factorial problem but aggressive feeding regimens with supplements in older children, and nasogastric or gastrostomy feeding in the first two years of life may help to prevent the short stature which has been a feature of such children.

Manifestations and management of chronic renal failure

Effect	Cause	Therapy
growth failure	poor caloric intake deranged biochemistry —acidosis anaemia salt and fluid loss	calorie and vitamin B, C supplements balanced first class protein, sodium bicarbonate and salt supplements in certain patients, early dialysis
renal osteodystrophy	phosphate retention defective Vit D metabolism secondary hyperparathyroidism	dietary phosphate restriction calcium carbonate phosphate binders Vit D supplements
anaemia	nutritional reduced erythropoeitin blood loss	blood transfusion as indicated iron supplements only if iron-deficient folic acid
hypertension	sodium retention renal disease/renin release	sodium restriction, diuretics antihypertensives nephrectomy

Children develop end stage renal disease requiring dialysis and transplantation at approximately 4–6 per million of the child population. Dialysis is seen only as an interim measure before transplantation which offers the best overall form of rehabilitation with growth potential. Haemodialysis can be technically difficult in the smaller child because of problems with vascular access. Continuous ambulatory peritoneal dialysis (CAPD) provides opportunities for more children of all sizes to be treated at home with generally freer diets and improved well being. Dialysis and transplantation are now feasible at any age but such patients place considerable demands on family and treatment resources which can only be met by a full integrated team approach that can decide the best treatment options for each individual.

RENAL TUBULAR DISORDERS

It is essential to consider these disorders when urinalysis reveals glycosuria, aminoaciduria or an impaired ability to concentrate or acidify urine.

Renal tubular disorders; a schematic representation of the renal tubule indicating defects, associated conditions and clinical manifestations

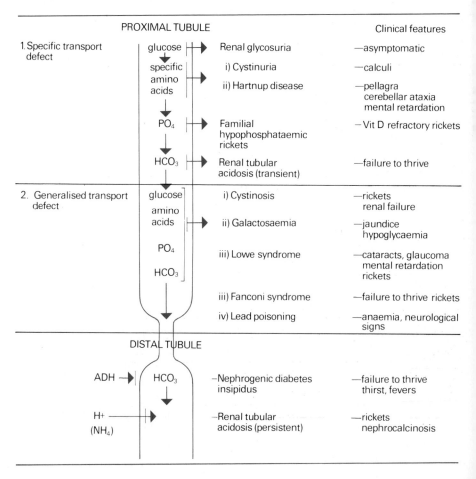

THE TESTES

The testes develop as intra-abdominal structures, entering the inguinal canal during the seventh month of fetal life. At birth the testes are usually in the scrotum but in about 10% of children they are undescended at birth and it is not uncommon for descent to be completed during the first two weeks of life. Descent is unlikely to take place after one year of age. The endocrine control of testicular descent is complex, involving gonadotrophins, androgens and Müllerian inhibitory factor.

Undescended testes

Testes which fail to reach the scrotum may be classified into the following categories:

Incompletely descended testes (20%). Incompletely descended testes lie along the path of descent but fail to reach the scrotum. They may be intra-abdominal or within the canal and hence impalpable. An emergent or high scrotal testis is easily palpable. These testes often appear grossly abnormal at operation, being small, soft and with a disassociated epididymis. Most are accompanied by a large hernial sac. Spermatogenesis is poor and is probably not significantly altered by operation. Orchidopexy may be difficult as the vessels are usually short. Sometimes no testicular tissue can be found and is either the result of intrauterine torsion or true agenesis. In the latter case abdominal ultrasound should be performed to determine whether there is associated renal agenesis.

Maldescent and undescent of the testes

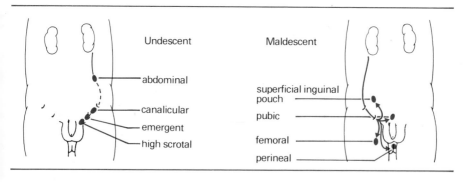

Ectopic or maldescended testes (80%). Ectopic or maldescended testes pass through the inguinal canal and emerge from the superficial inguinal ring, thereafter following an abnormal course. Ectopic sites include superficial, inguinal perineal, femoral and pubic. All ectopic testes are easily palpable. The testis is usually normal in appearance and a hernial sac is only occasionally present. Orchidopexy is easy because of adequate cord length. Spermatogenesis is almost normal with or without operation. The main indication for orchidopexy is to achieve optimal gonadal function. This is temperature dependent, the temperature of the scrotum being 1°C less than the intra-abdominal temperature. Previously orchidopexy was performed late in childhood but now most paediatric

Features which distinguish maldescent and undescent of the testes

	Maldescent	Undescent
Frequency of occurrence	80% of cases	20% of cases
Presence of hernia	Some cases	100% of cases
Prognosis for fertility	Good	Poor
Technique of orchidopexy	Inguinal approach	Abdominal approach
Likelihood of getting testis into scrotum	Easy in all cases	Unpredictable
Normality of testis naked eye and histology	Normal	Abnormal
Risk of torsion	Increased	Slightly increased
Risk of malignancy (*Both* sides in unilateral presentation)	Slightly increased	Increased

surgeons operate at the age of 2 to 3 years. The other indications for orchidopexy are cosmetic, psychological, and to reduce the risks of torsion, trauma and unrecognised malignancy. Testicular malignancy in the fourth decade of life is known to occur more frequently in individuals born with their testes outside the scrotum. Orchidopexy does not diminish the incidence of malignancy but does bring a previous impalpable testis into a palpable position.

Torsion of the testis
Approximately 20% occur in the perinatal period and present as a discoloured scrotum. Unfortunately the diagnosis is often delayed and orchidectomy inevitable. However the opposite testis must be fixed in a stable position.

The majority of torsions occur around puberty and present acutely as abdominal pain radiating to the testis or as intermittent testicular pain. There may be associated anomalies; a clapper bell testis due to high attachment of the tunica vaginalis or a long meso-orchium. The twist usually occurs in the spermatic cord. The undescended testis is also at risk of torsion. Urgent surgery is indicated when torsion is suspected.

Torsion of the hydatid of Morgagni
This is very common and can usually be distinguished from torsion of the testis because the pain is less severe, and as a consequence the history is usually longer than six hours. Sometimes it is possible to feel the torted hydatid and to demonstrate it by transillumination.

Varicoceles
Varicoceles occur infrequently in children. They do not usually need treatment during childhood.

Inguinal hernias and hydroceles
During its descent into the scrotum the testis is accompanied by a pouch of peritoneum, the processus vaginalis. The processus begins to close at birth and is normally obliterated during the first year of life. Both inguinal herniae and hydroceles are due to persistent patency of the processus. Where the processus remains very narrow, it allows peritoneal fluid to enter its cavity creating a hydrocele. If the hydrocele is present at birth and does not vary in size, it is

called a non-communicating hydrocele and will usually resolve within 4 to 6 months of birth. Beyond this age it is more common for the hydrocele to vary in size, a communicating hydrocele, and spontaneous closure is unlikely. In these children ligation of the patent processus is performed at the internal ring. In an older child sudden development of a hydrocele without a history of trauma may be a feature of a testicular tumour.

Where the processus remains sufficiently wide in part or all of its course, the bowel may enter the cavity resulting in an inguinal or scrotal hernia. Spontaneous resolution does not occur and an operation is essential. In children there is no underlying muscular weakness and therefore excision of the sac, a herniotomy, is all that is necessary. The younger the child the more urgent the operative procedure. Irreducibility is more common in young babies and it not only puts them at risk of bowel ischaemia but also of testicular necrosis.

Inguinal hernia and hydrocele

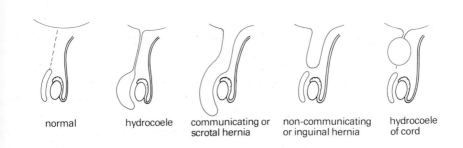

| normal | hydrocoele | communicating or scrotal hernia | non-communicating or inguinal hernia | hydrocoele of cord |

The child with a hernia may present with a history of swelling which comes and goes and the only clinical evidence of the hernial sac may be thickening of the spermatic cord on the affected side. Almost as commonly however, the swelling appears suddenly and is apparently irreducible, thus requiring emergency admission. If the history is of less than 12 hours and there is no reddening of the skin over the hernia, Gallows traction is applied to the legs and the child sedated with diamorphine. In 99% of children undisturbed sleep will result in the hernia reducing spontaneously or as a result of easy manipulation. Following such an episode the child should be kept in hospital and a herniotomy performed within days as the oedema subsides. If the hernia does not reduce with conservative means, or if the bowel within the hernial sac is clearly strangulated, emergency operation is essential. This can be one of the most difficult operations in paediatric practice. All infants noted to have a hernia should be referred to a surgeon promptly for elective surgery.

THE PREPUCE

The prepuce is closely adherent to the glans penis during the first year of life and any attempt at retraction must be avoided until spontaneous separation occurs. This is usually in the second year but may be delayed until four years of age. Ammoniacal dermatitis of the prepuce is common, and often confused with balanitis. Because of this, circumcision should never be performed until a child is out of nappies.

Phimosis

Phimosis refers to stenosis of the preputial orifice. It may be congenital but more often results from recurrent balanitis or traumatic retraction of the foreskin. It leads to ballooning and a poor stream during urination, as well as further attacks of balanitis. Treatment is by circumcision.

Paraphimosis

This can only occur in a child with a moderate phimosis, a preputial aperture slightly less than the size of the coronal sulcus. Following forcible retraction the foreskin is trapped in the retracted position. Treatment is by reduction under anaesthesia, with or without a dorsal slit, followed six weeks later by circumcision.

Hypospadias

The urethra opening on to the ventral aspect of the penis, at a point proximal to a normal site, is one of the commonest congenital abnormalities of the male genitalia, occurring in 1 in 350. The severity varies from a glandular orifice to scrotal and perineal types. There may also be a ventral curvature or chordee of the penis distal to the abnormal urethral meatus which becomes more conspicuous during erection. Failure of fusion of the ventral part of the foreskin results in a redundant dorsal hood. Surgical repair is indicated if the boy is incapable of a socially acceptable urinary stream while standing, or where the deformity may interfere with normal sexual intercourse. It is absolutely essential to conserve the foreskin so that it may be used in these corrective procedures.

BIBLIOGRAPHY

Edleman C Jr 1978 Pediatric kidney disease. Little Brown & Co, Boston Massachusetts
Fine R N, Gruskin A B 1984 End stage renal disease in childhood. W B Saunders Company, Philadelphia, London
The Pediatric Clinics of North America 1982 Volume 29 No. 4 W B Saunders Company, Philadelphia, London
International Study of Kidney Disease in Children 1978 The nephrotic syndrome in children. Prediction of histopathology from clinical and laboratory characteristics at the time of diagnosis. Kidney International 13:159
Levin M, Barratt T M 1984 Haemolytic uraemic syndrome Archives of Disease in Childhood 59: 397–400
Smellie J M, Ransley P G et al. 1985 Development of new renal scars: a collaborative study. British Medical Journal 290: 1957–1960
Miller P F W, Speirs N I et al. 1985 Long term prognosis of recurrent haematuria Archives of Disease in Childhood 60: 420–425

12
Blood

The interpretation of haemoglobin concentrations and white blood counts during infancy and childhood demands some knowledge of the physiological adjustments occurring during this period. The polycythaemia present at birth is followed by a progressive fall in haemoglobin concentration, reaching its minimum at two to three months. This fall is paralleled by relative erythroid hypoplasia in the marrow; however the haemoglobin concentration of healthy infants seldom falls below 10 g/100 ml.

During the fourth and fifth months, iron deficiency contributes to the anaemia and may be corrected by oral iron supplements. Folate deficiency may also occur particularly in infants born before term. Premature infants are also liable to develop anaemia during the first four months of life simply because the blood volume, in line with body size, increases rapidly at a time when the bone marrow is relatively hypoplastic.

The white cell count, which is high at birth, rapidly falls to normal adult

Age-related changes in haemoglobin concentration

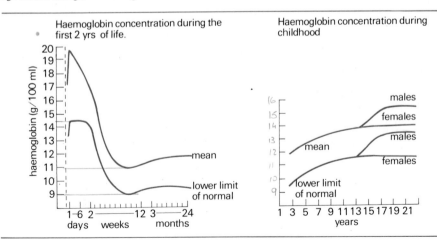

Haemoglobin concentration during the first 2 yrs of life.

Haemoglobin concentration during childhood

Age-related changes in white-cell count

	neutr.(%)	lymphoc. (%)
cord	60	30
1 day	70	25
1 wk	45	40
6 mths	30	60
1 yr	50	60
4 yrs	40	50
8 yrs	50	40
12 yrs	55	40

evels. During the first four years of life lymphocytes predominate rather than neutrophils.

IRON DEFICIENCY ANAEMIA

Anaemia in children may be suggested by tiredness, lethargy or pallor, but it is often only discovered during investigation for other conditions, particularly infection and poor weight gain. Overt gastrointestinal bleeding is rare in childhood. Although it is important to exclude serious underlying problems, the majority of childhood anaemia is due to dietary iron deficiency.

Three-quarters of the total body iron of a newborn infant is found in circulating haemoglobin. In the full-term infant this reserve is adequate to meet

Causes of anaemia

	Neonatal	Infancy	Childhood
Haemorrhage	Feto-Maternal Twin-to-twin Placental Subaponeurotic Cephalhaematoma	Hiatus hernia	Hiatus hernia Meckel diverticulum Epistaxis
Haemolytic	Rhesus incompatibility ABO incompatibility Spherocytosis G6PD deficiency	Sickle cell Thalassaemia Spherocytosis	Sickle cell Thalassaemia Spherocytosis
Infection	Intra-uterine (CMV, rubella) Septicaemia Urinary tract	Urinary tract	Chronic infection Chronic disease
Bleeding disorders	Haemorrhagic disease of the newborn	Haemophilia Christmas disease	Haemophilia Christmas disease
Deficiency		Physiological Prematurity Iron Folate Bone marrow depression	Iron Folate Bone marrow depression

Iron balance in infancy

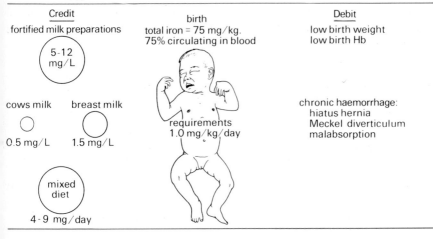

Credit	birth	Debit
fortified milk preparations 5-12 mg/L	total iron = 75 mg/kg. 75% circulating in blood	low birth weight low birth Hb
cows milk 0.5 mg/L breast milk 1.5 mg/L	requirements 1.0 mg/kg/day	chronic haemorrhage: hiatus hernia Meckel diverticulum malabsorption
mixed diet 4-9 mg/day		

requirements for the first four to six months but probably lasts only six weeks in the premature. The dietary requirements of a normal infant for elemental iron are 1 mg/kg/day. Although breast milk has a relatively low iron content, it is probably unnecessary to give iron supplements, particularly if mixed feeding is introduced at four to six months. It might even be contraindicated because recent research has demonstrated that the iron binding globulin of breast milk, lacto-ferrin, has bacteriocidal properties and that this effect is reduced if the protein becomes iron saturated.

In any community between 10 and 60 per cent of children may be iron deficient, depending on dietary and social habits. The higher figures occur in children of immigrant populations or those who live in impoverished inner city areas. A hypochromic microcytic blood film is usually sufficient evidence to justify a trial of oral iron therapy. The history may provide clues to alternative diagnoses, for example recurrent vomiting indicating reflux oesophagitis or pica suggesting lead poisoning. Children who fail to respond to an adequate course of iron warrant more detailed investigation including serum iron and iron binding capacity, radiological studies of the gastrointestinal tract, and renal and thyroid

Serum iron and iron bending capacity in the investigations of anaemia

Fe(µg)

0 100 200 300 400 500

normal 1 yr old
iron deficiency
infection
haemolytic anaemia

0   20   40   60   80   100
µmol/L

□ iron binding capacity
■ serum iron
■□ total iron binding capacity

function tests. Intestinal malabsorption may present with iron deficient anaemia, and there may be associated folate deficiency. There is some evidence that severe iron deficiency may itself impair the integrity and function of the intestinal mucosa. Iron treatment should be continued for three months to replenish iron stores as well as correct haemoglobin concentrations.

Iron preparations

Ferrous gluconate (Ferlucon) elixir	250 mg/5 ml dose contains 30 mg of elemental iron
Ferrous fumerate (Fersamal) syrup	140 mg/5 ml dose contains 45 mg of elemental iron
Ferrous sulphate (BPC) mixture	60 mg/5 ml dose contains 12 mg of elemental iron
Ferrous gluconate tablets	300 mg contains 36 mg of elemental iron
Ferrous sulphate tablets	200 mg contains 60 mg of elemental iron

APLASTIC ANAEMIA

A pancytopenia necessitates marrow examination which may show either reduced cellularity without infiltration, aplastic anaemia, or invasion by malignant cells. Aplastic anaemia may be inherited or acquired.

Fanconi anaemia
An autosomal recessive condition, Fanconi anaemia is the most common of the inherited types, and presents in boys at four to seven years of age and in girls between six and ten years of age. Bruising and purpura are the usual presenting complaints with anaemia appearing more insidiously. Associated features include abnormal pigmentation, short stature, skeletal and renal malformations and there may be chromosomal breakages. The condition is progressive but the deterioration may be delayed with androgens and corticosteroids. Most children with Fanconi anaemia die within a few years of diagnosis and some develop acute leukaemia. Bone marrow transplantation from a compatible sibling or donor offers the main hope of therapy.

Acquired aplastic anaemia
This may occur at any age. Although some cases follow the ingestion of certain drugs such as chloramphenicol, the majority have no obvious provoking factor. Aplastic anaemia may occur following hepatitis B infection. If the bone marrow is moderately cellular at diagnosis there is a greater chance that spontaneous remission may occur. The majority have pancytopenia, respond poorly to corticosteroids and androgens, and are at risk of dying of infection. Compatible bone marrow transplantation is now the treatment of choice. Transplantation is more successful in those patients who have had the least blood transfusions and it is important therefore to explore the availability of suitable donors early in the course of the illness.

HAEMOLYTIC ANAEMIAS

Haemolytic anaemias may be congenital or acquired. Some of the acquired group produce problems in the first days of life and are due to maternal antibodies haemolysing the infant's cells.

The pathogenesis of haemolytic anaemias

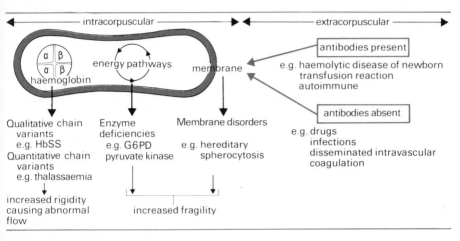

Hereditary haemolytic anaemias

The majority of haemolytic anaemias encountered in infancy and childhood are due to disorders of the red cells. They are characterised by anaemia, an increased reticulocyte count, an unconjugated hyperbilirubinaemia and skeletal changes secondary to compensatory marrow hyperplasia.

Hereditary spherocytosis. This is an autosomal dominant condition with a high new mutation rate in which the red cell membrane is abnormally permeable to sodium. The resulting spherocytes are not diagnostic of hereditary sphero-cytosis as they are found in a wide variety of autoimmune haemolytic anaemias. The disorder may present as neonatal jaundice and has been confused with ABO incompatibility. In later childhood it produces anaemia, chronic malaise and sple-nomegaly. The continuous high rate of bilirubin excretion leads to pigmented gall stones so that, eventually, gall bladder disease is common. The haemoglobin concentration generally runs in the range of 9 to 11 g/100 ml, but may drop during an infection because of an increased rate of haemolysis and also because there may be an associated hypoplastic crisis. Jaundice may also become conspic-uous in these episodes. The diagnosis is confirmed by demonstrating the increased osmotic fragility. Splenectomy is indicated in all symptomatic cases but is usually delayed until after the age of four years because of the risk of over-whelming septicaemia in young splenectomised children. Continuous prophy-lactic antibiotics and pneumococcal vaccine are recommended to prevent this hazard. Following splenectomy the red cell survival is returned to normal although spherocytosis persists.

Hereditary red cell enzyme deficiencies

Two important pathways are essential for the normal function of the mature red cell. The hexose-monophosphate pathway provides a supply of reduced nicotin-amide adenine-dinucleotide phosphate ($NADPH_2$) which is essential for protection against oxidative damage. The glycolytic or Emden-Meyerhof pathway provides the majority of energy for the cell. Deficiency of many of the enzymes in these two pathways has been described but the most important deficiencies are those of glucose-6-phosphate dehydrogenase (G6PD) and pyruvate kinase.

Metabolic pathways of the red blood cell

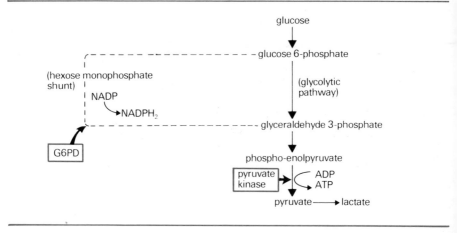

Glucose-6-phosphate dehydrogenase deficiency. There are many variants of this enzyme, each having a different geographical distribution. The form seen in black Americans results in haemolysis when the person is exposed to anti-malarial and other drugs. The Mediterranean and oriental variants often present in the newborn period with jaundice due to excess haemolysis and they may require an exchange transfusion. These conditions are also 'drug sensitive'. Inges-tion of Fava beans is a well recognised hazard in affected Mediterranean peoples. Patients with glucose-6-phosphate dehydrogenase deficiency should be given a list of drugs to avoid. The condition is inherited by the X-linked.

Pyruvate kinase deficiency. This is considerably less common and affects mainly North European populations. It causes neonatal jaundice, anaemia and splenomegaly. Splenectomy is occasionally of benefit. *

An abbreviated list of drugs to be avoided by patients with glucose-6-phosphate dehydrogenase deficiency. A typical drug induced crisis in such a patient

The developmental changes in the haemoglobins of intra- and extrauterine life

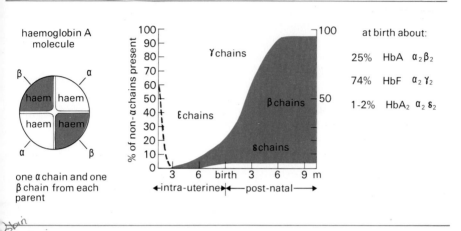

Haemoglobin A molecule — one α chain and one β chain from each parent. At birth about: 25% HbA $\alpha_2\beta_2$, 74% HbF $\alpha_2\gamma_2$, 1-2% HbA₂ $\alpha_2\delta_2$.

Disorders of haemoglobin synthesis

These fall into two main categories: those in which there is an aminoacid substitution in the globin portion of the molecule, the(1) haemoglobinopathies; and those in which there is relative failure of globin chain synthesis, the(2) thalassaemia syndromes. It is unusual for these conditions to present in the newborn period when fetal haemoglobin is the predominant haemoglobin type.

Sickle cell anaemia. Sickle cell anaemia is by far the most common of the haemoglobinopathies; 15% of all black people carry the gene that causes valine to replace glutamine in the sixth position of the beta chain. The homozygous condition is referred to as sickle cell anaemia or disease, and the heterozygote as sickle cell trait. The disease is a serious condition with a number of important complications in addition to the chronic anaemia. Painful swelling of the hands and feet is a common early presentation. The splenomegaly of the younger child becomes less prominent as repeated infarctions produce an 'autosplenectomy'. *Rare >10*

Features of sickle cell disease   *Hb: 6-8g /dl : Reticulocytes 10-20%.*

Crises		Clinical features
Thromboses: painful		pallor; icterus
rare - haemolytic		
aplastic *- Due Parvovirus*		haemic murmur; hepatomegaly
cold, hepatic *(Sequestration: RBC*		splenomegaly (after 8 yrs of age only 10%)
Dehydration, megaloblastic *trapping!)*		chronic leg ulcers
infection *(muscular Exertion)*		
Ischaemia Acute infarction:		renal involvement:
abdominal		haematuria
pulmonary		defective urine concentration
neurological		
hands and feet syndrome		infections:
aseptic necrosis—femoral		pneumococcal septicaemia
and humeral heads		salmonella osteomyelitis *

Priapism -prolonged erection.

4. Child - good health c̄ Crises
Older - Chr ill health. - R.F, Bone Necrosis, osteomyelitis (
leg ulcers

BLOOD 193

Normal and abnormal haemoglobins in later childhood

normal			abnormal		
different polypeptide chains in various haemoglobins			HbS	α_2 β_2^s	sickle cell disease
	% after age 3 yrs		HbAS	α_2 β β^s	sickle cell trait
HbA	α_2 β_2	(98-99%)			
HbF	α_2 γ_2	(0-2%)	Hb Barts	γ_4	thalassaemia
HbA₂	α_2 δ_2	(1-3%)	HbH	β_4	

Crises are usually precipitated by infection and may be complicated by dehydration, poor tissue perfusion, hypoxia and acidosis. The anaemia is sometimes exacerbated by temporary marrow failure secondary to parvovirus infection. Treatment is largely symptomatic with antibiotics, warmth and adequate fluids. In developed countries the prognosis for a normal life is moderately good. The heterozygote is asymptomatic except under conditions of low oxygen tension as might occur at high altitude or under general anaesthesia.

Thalassaemia syndromes are most common among Asian and Mediterranean races, and are subdivided into alpha and beta thalassaemia depending on the chain affected by the synthetic failure. Beta thalassaemia is the more common, the homozygous state resulting in a severe haemolytic anaemia with hypochromic microcytic cells. The compensatory bone marrow hyperplasia produces a characteristic overgrowth of the facial and skull bones, as well as fragile limb bones. Although death may be delayed by repeated transfusion, this resource is unavailable to the majority of the world's affected children. Repeated transfusion introduces the hazard of chronic iron overload and tissue damage. Continuous nocturnal desferrioxamine subcutaneous infusion is moderately effective in

Features of thalassaemia major

anaemia
growth failure

skull bossing
maxillary overgrowth

hepatosplenomegaly

brittle long bones

repeated transfusions

haemosiderosis
cardiomyopathy
cirrhosis
skin pigmentation
endocrine failure
— Due to Iron Overload !

world distribution of thalassaemia

reducing the positive iron balance. Bone marrow exchange is being explored as a definitive therapy but currently the risks outweigh the benefits.

In the first trimester fetal diagnosis for haemoglobinopathies is now available based on the techniques of trophoblast biopsy and restriction endonuclease analysis of fetal DNA.

The heterozygous beta thalassaemia produces a mild anaemia which may be confused with iron deficiency. Haemoglobin electrophoresis permits identification of these abnormal haemoglobin types.

Classification of bleeding disorders

Presentation		Mechanism	Diagnosis
Injury provoked skin and mucosal bleeding		defective blood vessels	hereditary haemorrhagic telangiectasia allergic or post-infectious vasculitis Vit C deficiency—scurvy
		thrombocytopenia	immune
		platelet function defect	drug induced thrombasthenia
Spontaneous and injury provoked deep haematomas haemarthrosis haematuria		coagulation disorder	haemophilia A, B Von Willebrand's disease Vit K deficiency liver disease

BLEEDING DISORDERS

A variety of disorders may lead to excessive bleeding in childhood. A past history may be important in distinguishing congenital from acquired problems. Previous surgery, including dental extractions, without undue bleeding provides good evidence against an inherited disorder. Tonsillectomy is notorious for putting a considerable strain on coagulation systems and may uncover mild haemophilia. A family history is often helpful in diagnosing sex-linked recessive disorders such as haemophilia or Christmas disease, but may be absent in up to a third of new cases. Von Willebrand disease and hereditary telangiectasia have a dominant pattern of inheritance. The character of the bleeding problem together with four basic tests of coagulation should make it possible to decide from which group of disorders a patient is suffering. These tests also serve as screening procedures in cases of suspected child abuse or before liver or jejunal biopsy.

Key investigations in the evaluation of a bleeding disorder

- Full blood count including platelet count (normal 150–400 × 10⁹/l; bleeding occurs when below 40 × 10⁹/l).
- Ivy's bleeding time (normal less than six minutes). An abnormal result with normal platelet count is suggestive of a qualitative platelet abnormality.
- Prothrombin time. A test of the extrinsic pathway: Factors II (prothrombin), V, VII and X together with fibrinogen. (Normal = control ±20%).
- Partial thromboplastin time. A test of the intrinsic pathway: Factors, V, VIII, X, XI, XII and XIII together with prothrombin and fibrinogen. (Normal = control ±20%).

Normal results in these four tests exclude all deficiencies other than factor XIII, (fibrin stabilising factor) deficiency.

Inherited deficiencies of each of the coagulation factors have been described; they are all rare with the exceptions of haemophilia A and B, and von Willebrand disease.

Haemophilia

Haemophilia A occurs in approximately 1 in 14 000 males and is six times more common than haemophilia B, otherwise known as Christmas disease. Haemophilia A is due to the synthesis of abnormal factor VIII with resulting reduced biological activity. It is transmitted as a sex-linked recessive, and carrier females are asymptomatic but may be detected because of an excess of immunoreactive factor VIII over that which is biologically active. The severity of haemophilia is linked to the degree of deficiency of factor VIII; concentrations of factor VIII less than 1% of normal causes severe problems, 1 to 5 per cent causes moderate problems, and 5 to 20 per cent only mild symptoms. Spontaneous bleeding into joints and muscles with resulting orthopaedic problems is the main hazard.

It is essential to treat all bleeding incidents promptly by replacing the missing factor. Until relatively recently, this necessitated the use of fresh frozen plasma, but currently the availability of cryoprecipitate concentrates and purified dried human factor VIII have enabled the use of small volumes and therefore simplified treatment. Many families have now been trained to treat bleeding episodes at home. In general, the aim of replacement is to increase the factor VIII level to a biologically effective concentration of 10 to 20 per cent. Activity up to 50% of normal may be necessary to combat severe trauma or surgery. Physiotherapy has a vital role in maintaining the strength of muscles which might otherwise become weakened during periods of immobilisation and therefore increase joint susceptibility to further damage.

It is recognised that repeated factor VIII administration carries risks of transfusion hepatitis and chronic liver disease. AIDS is an additional threat but

Coagulation pathways. Characteristic laboratory results in immune thrombocytopenia (ITP), Van Willebrand disease, haemophilia, and vitamin K deficiency

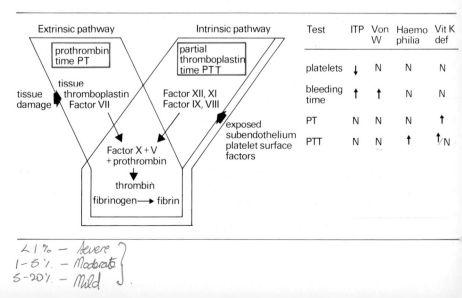

Test	ITP	Von W	Haemophilia	Vit K def
platelets	↓	N	N	N
bleeding time	↑	↑	N	N
PT	N	N	N	↑
PTT	N	N	↑	↑/N

Extrinsic pathway — prothrombin time PT — tissue damage — tissue thromboplastin Factor VII — Factor X + V + prothrombin — thrombin — fibrinogen → fibrin

Intrinsic pathway — partial thromboplastin time PTT — Factor XII, XI Factor IX, VIII — exposed subendothelium platelet surface factors

<1% — severe
1–5% — Moderate
5–20% — Mild

heat treatment is capable of excluding this agent from pooled factor VIII.

Von Willebrand disease

Von Willebrand disease is an autosomal dominant disorder characterised by prolonged bleeding time, low factor VIII and reduced platelet adhesiveness. Treatment is as for haemophilia. Aspirin should not be given.

Thrombocytopenia   E leukaemia, Aplastic Anaemia.

Immune thrombocytopenic purpura. This is the most common of the thrombocytopenias and is thought to have an immunological basis as it often follows one to two weeks after a viral infection. There is a clear relationship with rubella. Platelet bound IgG antibodies are detectable in a significant proportion of cases. Problems usually develop when the platelet counts fall below $40 \times 10^9/l$, and is the severe cases the count may be below $5 \times 10^9/l$. The common presenting features are petechiae and superficial bruising but mucosal bleeding may also occur. Rarely haemorrhage occurs into the brain or viscera. As the differential diagnosis includes acute leukaemia and aplastic anaemia, it is justifiable to perform a marrow examination immediately to demonstrate the normal or increased number of megakaryocytes which are characteristic of idiopathic thrombocytopenia.

In children, 85% have an acute self-limiting course and the majority have recovered spontaneously by six months. In those who have only mild symptoms no treatment is necessary, but where there is a risk of severe generalised bleeding or bleeding into a solid organ, a short course of corticosteroids may help by producing a temporary elevation of the platelet count. Intravenous human immunoglobulin infusions are also effective in elevating the platelet count. Long courses of corticosteroids should be avoided and refractory cases should be considered for splenectomy; if this fails immunosuppression with azathioprine may be successful.

Drug-induced thrombocytopenia is unusual in childhood but is becoming increasingly recognised following the use of cotrimoxazole. Thrombocytopenia may occur in the neonatal period as a complication of rhesus disease, intrauterine infection or due to maternal drug ingestion. It may also occur transiently in the infant of a mother with idiopathic thrombocytopenia. There is also a group of rare hereditary thrombocytopenias.

Wiscott-Aldrich syndrome. This is a sex-linked familial disorder in which boys present with early thrombocytopenia, eczema and susceptibility to infection. It is generally fatal in early childhood but is now amenable to bone marrow transplantation.

Disseminated intravascular coagulation (DIC)

Severe disturbances such as septicaemia, shock and acidosis may promote simultaneous activation of both the coagulant and the fibrinolytic pathways, with a resulting consumption of platelets, fibrinogen, factors V and VIII but without the formation of insoluble fibrin. Soluble complexes of fibrin monomers circulate as fibrin degradation products and their detection is a further indication of consumptive coagulopathy. DIC should be suspected in a gravely ill child with both shock and generalised bleeding. Every attempt should be made to determine and treat the underlying cause. In the neonatal period this may be asphyxia, profound hypothermia, infection or severe rhesus disease. In infancy it may complicate hypertonic dehydration and produce renal vein thrombosis, manifest by oliguria, haematuria and bilateral renal masses.

BIBLIOGRAPHY

Biggs R 1978 The treatment of haemophilia A and B and von Willebrand's disease. Blackwell, Oxford
Oski F A, Jaffé E R, Mieschet P A 1975 Current problems in paediatric hematology. Grune & Stratton, New York
Miller D R 1984 Blood diseases in infancy and childhood. Blackwell Scientific Publications, Oxford
Weatherall D J, Clegg J B 1972 The thalassaemia syndromes, 2nd edn. Blackwell, Oxford
Willoughby M L N 1977 Paediatric haematology. Churchill Livingstone, Edinburgh

13
Malignancy

Malignancies are now second only to accidents in the mortality tables of children aged 1 to 15 years. Childhood malignancies fall into two main categories: those which are found more commonly and almost exclusively in children; and those which are manifestations of tumours found in all age groups. The former group which includes nephroblastomas, neuroblastomas and retinoblastomas evolves from malignant transformation of developing tissues. Genetic influences are probably greater than environmental factors and the spectrum of susceptible organs is quite different to that seen in adults where bronchus, gastrointestinal tract and breast predominate. It has long been recognised that complete cure is possible in nephroblastoma, and the carefully monitored introduction of more aggressive modes of therapy has demonstrated that an increasing number of malignancies are amenable to cure. This progress is the result of better understanding of the natural history of tumours and the introduction of expert multidisciplinary management schedules. These schedules are often very intensive and require specialised supportive care that is usually available only in paediatric oncology centres. Intensive treatment brings rewards in terms of survival but imposes a great strain on families.

Malignancy as a cause of mortality

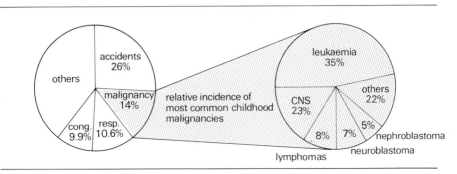

LEUKAEMIA

Leukaemia is the most common malignant disease in childhood with an annual incidence of 3.5 per 100 000 under the age of 15 years. Acute lymphoblastic leukaemia accounts for 86%, acute myeloblastic leukaemia for 13% and chronic myeloid leukaemia for 1%. Acute leukaemias are characterised by the presence of blast cells in the peripheral blood, as distinct from chronic leukaemias where excessive numbers of normal looking leucocytes are present.

Age distribution of acute leukaemia

The aetiological basis of leukaemia remains a mystery. A familial incidence is very rare. It is a relatively common cause of death in children with Down syndrome as the incidence is 10 to 18 times that in normal children. It is unlikely that a single cause of leukaemia will be found, and the role of background radiation and viral infections has yet to be clarified.

Clinical manifestations

A minority, 15%, of children with acute leukaemia present rapidly over a few days; the majority, 85%, develop symptoms more insidiously over weeks and

Clinical features of acute leukaemia

fatigue and pallor	80%		hepatomegaly	60%
anorexia	45%		splenomegaly	70%
fever	55%		abdominal pain	20%
skin or mucosal bleeding	30%		lymphadenopathy	25%
Infections:			bone pain	25%
sore throats	20%		CNS signs	5%
other	20%			

months. Common initial complaints include pallor, fever, recurrent infections, malaise and abnormal bruising. Childhood leuakaemia is notorious for its varied presentations, and it must be considered in the diagnosis of any unusual illness especially if accompanied by hepatosplenomegaly, lymphadenopathy or bone tenderness.

Clinical suspicion must not be conveyed to parents until laboratory investigation has provided complete confirmation. Doctors and nurses must also be sensitive to the sometimes irrational fears of leukaemia that arise when parents have failed to grasp the meaning of relatively innocent diagnoses such as iron deficiency anaemia and infectious mononucleosis. Idiopathic thrombocytopenia may alarm doctors until the characteristic bone marrow appearance has been revealed!

Careful examination of peripheral blood and a bone marrow aspirate is generally sufficient to confirm or refute the diagnosis of acute leukaemia. Blast cells are usually apparent and account for between 1% and nearly 100% of the white cell count. The total white cell count is typically in the range 20 to 50 $\times$ 10^9/l but can be lower than 10×10^9/l. In subleukaemic leukaemia peripheral blood blast cells may be undetectable. By contrast the total white cell count may be in excess of 100×10^9/l, a presentation which indicates a poor prognosis. A normochromic normocytic anaemia and a thrombocytopenia are invariable. Bone marrow examination is essential to the diagnosis, and provides an important parameter by which to judge subsequent remission. Immunological techniques enable classification of the lymphoblasts so that three broad classes of leukaemia are now recognised; T-ALL, B-ALL and non-T, non-B ALL. The latter class includes common ALL the most frequent variety in childhood, 75%, and Null-ALL, 11%, most often seen in the very young child or in adult life.

Leukaemia: complications of the disease and its treatment

1. Systemic
   malnutrition
   growth failure
   hair loss
2. Gastrointestinal
   mucosal
   atrophy/ulceration
   hepatic impairment
3. Respiratory
   pneumonia
4. Cardiac
   cardiomyopathy

5. Haematological
   marrow failure
   coagulation disorders
6. Endocrine
   hypothalamic/pituitary
   deficiency
   testicular relapse
   impaired fertility
7. Metabolic
   hyperuricaemia
8. Skeletal
   bone pain
   pathological fractures

9. Neurological
   meningeal relapse
   cerebral infiltration
   radiation encephalopathy
   peripheral neuropathy
10. Infective
   varicella, measles
   septicaemia
   opportunistic e.g.
   pneumocystis carinii
11. Secondary malignancy

Management

As soon as the diagnosis has been made with certainty both parents are seen together so that the nature of the disease, its treatment and prognosis may be discussed in detail. This initial talk has usually to be repeated because of the distress of the first conversation. While the ultimate aim is one of curing the disease, this has to be balanced against the ability of the child and family to tolerate all components of management.

In the U.K. specific treatment plans have evolved as the result of controlled studies under the auspices of the Medical Research Council. Chemotherapy lasts two to three years and aims at as complete eradication of malignant cells as is possible. This eradication must be directed not only at the bone marrow but also at the central nervous system, and current programmes include cranial irradiation and intrathecal methotrexate. In judging the effectiveness of therapy it is a useful concept to consider the total leukaemia cell load, which may be 10^{11} to 10^{12} cells,

The tumour cell mass

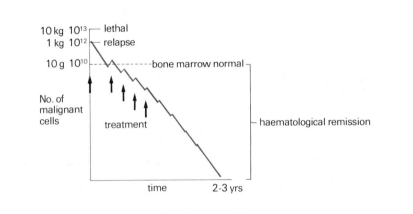

or more than a kilogram of malignancy at the time of diagnosis. Each course of treatment is thought to produce a 'two log kill', equivalent to reducing the tumour mass from 1 kg to 10 g. Apparent remission with a normal marrow examination is compatible with the persistence of 10 g of malignant cells in the body. This model of total tumour mass is also applicable to disseminated solid tumours. Chemotherapeutic agents are selected on the basis of selective toxicity towards tumour cells, speed of effect, and according to their impact on the phases of cellular divison.

Treatment of acute leukaemia

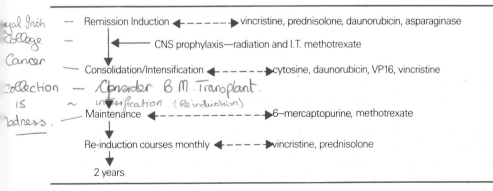

Supportive Tx

Haematology
Biochemistry
Immunosuppression
Nutrition
General Morale.

Drugs used in acute lymphoblastic leukaemia

Drug	Mode of administration	Side effects
Vincristine	i.v.	Neuropathy, bone marrow suppression (mild)
Prednisolone	oral	Cushingoid effects
Daunorubicin	i.v.	Cardiomyopathy, bone marrow suppression
Asparaginase	i.v/i.m.	Allergic reactions
Mercaptopurine	oral	Skin rashes, bone marrow suppression
Methotrexate	oral/i.v.	Mouth ulcers, bone marrow suppression

Immunosuppressed children are susceptible to infection and up to 15% die from this cause without any evidence of marrow relapse. Live vaccines must be avoided during the treatment phase. Chickenpox and measles are particular hazards and protection must be offered to at-risk children with appropriate immunoglobulin. Acyclovir provides specific therapy for herpes virus infections.

Current treatment regimens have resulted in the survival of 40 to 60 per cent of children for more than four years and it is hoped that survival for this length of time indicates cure. The question of stopping potentially toxic therapy after a sufficiently prolonged remission is important as unnecessary immunosuppression has a mortality risk of its own. *>60% survive 5yrs (85% of those → adult life cured.*

Chemotherapy still provides the best chance of success for children with good prognosis leukaemia but any child who relapses on treatment is unlikely to survive for more than two years. Bone marrow transplantation has been introduced as a potentially curative treatment in childhood leukaemia. At the moment it considered for those presenting with a high initial white blood cell count and for those in their first relapse on treatment. Transplants may be homologous, from an HLA compatible donor such as a sibling. The alternative is an autologous transplant which involves removing bone marrow from the child when in remission, purging it of any malignant cells using a panel of monoclonal antibodies, and then reinfusing the treated marrow after total body irradiation combined with cytotoxic therapy. Cyclosporin reduces the incidence of graft versus host reactions. An approximate 50 per cent success rate has been achieved in patients with AML but results are less satisfactory with ALL.

Survival rates in acute leukaemia

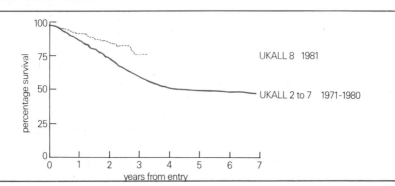

Nephroblastoma: clinical features and investigations

Presentation:

fever
poor appetite
vomiting

abdominal mass
(lateral, superficial, nodular)

abdominal pain

haematuria

Investigation:

urinalysis
blood count
chest X-ray
IVP
bone marrow
skeletal survey

ultrasound
CT and NMR scans
chromosomes

distortion of
Lt. pelvicalyceal
system

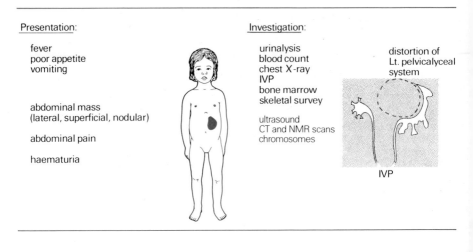

IVP

NEPHROBLASTOMA (WILMS TUMOUR)

A nephroblastoma originates from embryonal kidney and is made up of tissues in various stages of differentiation. The incidence is approximately 1 in 10 000 live births (i.e. 70 new cases each year in the U.K.). Sixty per cent present before the age of three years, and it is marginally more common in boys than girls. The left kidney is affected more frequently than the right, and 10% of tumours are bilateral.

The resulting abdominal mass is usually asymptomatic and often comes to light through accidental palpation. It is important to investigate all cases of haematuria with this diagnosis in mind. The IVP is sometimes, but not always, diagnostic of nephroblastoma, showing the intrarenal origin of the tumour and the resulting distortion of the pelvicalyceal system. It is also necessary to determine whether the contralateral kidney is normal. Forty per cent of tumours have metastasised by the time of diagnosis but secondaries amenable to surgery or irradiation do not necessarily prevent complete cure. Nephrectomy is no longer regarded as an emergency but should be performed promptly. The involved kidney together with ureter, lymph nodes and adjacent infiltrated tissues is removed and formal staging is decided upon. Vincristine is administered at the time of surgery and further treatment protocols are decided after clinical and histological staging, the latter incorporating the degree of tumour differentiation as well as invasion. The long-term results in children with stage I and II tumours are excellent and they may be placed more at risk by inappropriate chemotherapy. Triple chemotherapy using vincristine, adriamycin and actinomycin, combined with radiotherapy to the site of the tumour is now used only for stages III, IV and those of unfavourable histology which alone account for 50% of deaths. It is unusual for a child to relapse if maintained disease-free for two years after presentation.

In some children nephroblastoma is associated with deletions in chromosome 13, and other features such as aniridia and body hemihypertrophy.

Neuroblastoma: clinical features and investigations

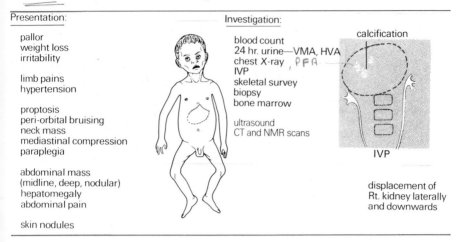

Presentation:

pallor
weight loss
irritability

limb pains
hypertension

proptosis
peri-orbital bruising
neck mass
mediastinal compression
paraplegia

abdominal mass
(midline, deep, nodular)
hepatomegaly
abdominal pain

skin nodules

Investigation:

blood count
24 hr. urine—VMA, HVA
chest X-ray , PFA
IVP
skeletal survey
biopsy
bone marrow

ultrasound
CT and NMR scans

calcification

IVP

displacement of
Rt. kidney laterally
and downwards

NEUROBLASTOMA

A neuroblastoma originates from tissues of neural crest origin namely the adrenal medulla and sympathetic nervous system. Although they are usually highly malignant, there is an interesting spectrum of disease and histological examination of infant deaths show that localised, 'in situ' tumours may occur 14 to 40 times as frequently as those which are symptomatic. There is also a gradation between the rapidly proliferating neuroblastoma and the benign ganglioneuroma. Cases have been reported in which neuroblastomas have spontaneously matured into ganglioneuromas. *— Commonest malignancy in Infancy!!*

These tumours occur most commonly in the first years of life with an incidence of approximately 1 in 8000 live births, so that there are about 80 new cases each year in the U.K.

The clinical manifestations are varied depending on the site of the primary tumours and the extent of metastases. The latter are commonly responsible for the symptoms. Sixty-five to 75 per cent of cases are abdominal, most arising in the adrenal medulla but some in the retroperitoneal sympathetic ganglia. The remainder arise in sympathetic ganglia in the neck, thorax and pelvis, and the extra-abdominal sites appear to have a better prognosis.

Those tumours which are abdominal in origin usually produce a mass which crosses the mid-line and which may be difficult to distinguish from the liver. The liver may well be involved in metastases. It is therefore important to exclude primary liver pathology such as a hepatoblastoma. Features useful in confirming the presence of a neuroblastoma include the diffuse, speckled calcification sometimes seen on a plain abdominal x-ray, and elevated levels of catecholamine degradation products in the urine. Raised levels of homovanyllic acid (HVA) and especially vanilmandelic acid (VMA) are present in over 90% of affected children. The high frequency of metastases makes a careful systemic review and skeletal survey important. Bone metastases are more common than pulmonary.

Surgery is directed towards complete resection where possible but not at the expense of causing severe mutilation. Postoperative irradiation is invariably

[handwritten annotations at top: Prognosis — Good: <1 yr. Neck, Post Med. — Ganglioneuroma / Ganglioneuroblastoma. — Bad: >2 yrs. — Abd. — Del. of Short arm of Chrom 1, Long arm ChR.]

indicated but in immediate proximity to the spine and kidneys it introduces problems of subsequent scoliosis and radiation nephritis. A case for chemotherapy has not been fully established but combined treatment with vincristine and cyclophosphamide are frequently used.

Unfortunately the prognosis for children with this tumour has not shown any significant improvement over the last 20 years. The prognosis is influenced by the site of the tumour and by the age of the child. The figures are more favourable in children under the age of two years and an interesting group of infants show spontaneous recovery in spite of metastases to subcutaneous tissue, liver and bone marrow. A recent advance has been the use of autologous bone marrow transplantation after purging the marrow with appropriate monoclonal antibodies and total body irradiation. Monoclonal antibodies may also have a role in targeting cytotoxic drugs.

Survival rates for nephroblastoma (staged) and neuroblastoma by age of presentation

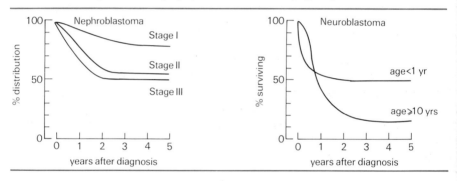

HISTIOCYSTOSIS X

Histiocytosis X is a term used to describe a spectrum of disease in which there is an abnormal proliferation of histiocytes. Histiocytes occur throughout the body as circulating monocytes, cutaneous Langerhans cells, Kupffer cells, bone osteoclasts, microglial cells and alveolar macrophages. Traditionally histiocytosis X has been regarded as a malignant disease but there is a high incidence of spontaneous remission and there are histological features unlike genuine malignancy. It therefore seems increasingly probable that the disease has an immunological basis. Most patients have a deficiency of circulating suppressor lymphocytes and therefore an increased helper: suppressor ratio.

The clinical presentation is likely to fall into one of three categories. It is a rare disease, only 30 to 40 cases presenting each year in the U.K.

Eosinophilic granuloma of bone

This is the most benign end of the spectrum and consists of isolated lesions of bone occurring most commonly in the skull, ribs, clavicles and vertebrae. They present with pain, swelling, a lump and occasionally spinal cord signs. The typical radiographic appearance is of a well-demarcated lytic lesion but a full skeletal survey and a biopsy are necessary to confirm the diagnosis. Accessible lesions are treated by currettage at the time of biopsy or by local injection of methyl prednisolone. Inaccessible and threatening lesions may be treated by radio-therapy. Only 5% become multi-focal.

Hand-Schuller-Christian disease

This is a more disseminated variety commonly presenting as a persistent ear discharge but there may also be a seborrhoeic-like rash, bone lesions of the skull and mastoid, exophthalmos, diabetes insipidus and hepatosplenomegaly.

Letterer-Siwe disease

Letterer-Siwe disease is at the most severe end of the spectrum and behaves as a highly malignant and generalised disorder. It typically presents in infancy as failure to thrive, fever, a haemorrhagic seborrhoeic rash, lymphadenopathy and hepatosplenomegaly. There may be pancytopenia and the ESR is elevated. The diagnosis is largely based on clinical appearance but should be confirmed by biopsy of either the enlarged glands or the skin rash.

Because spontaneous remission occurs at the more benign end of the disease spectrum it is not always necessary to treat eosinophilic granuloma or Hand-Schuller-Christian disease. Hypothalamic dysfunction may require endocrine evaluation and treatment with, for example, growth hormone and DDAVP. Complex cytotoxic regimens including prednisolone, vinblastine and CP 16 are currently used in Letterer-Siwe disease. The prognosis depends not only upon the extent of the disease but also the degree of impaired function within the involved organs. The child may recover from overt histiocytic infiltration only to be severely disabled by pulmonary and hepatic fibrosis combined with severe growth failure.

OTHER MALIGNANCIES

Rhabdomyosarcoma

This is a rare but highly malignant tumour originating from striated muscle and occurring most frequently in the first two years of life. It may present as a swelling around the orbit or nasopharynx, in the bladder, vagina or uterus and occasionally in the limbs. It can be responsible for a haemorrhagic vaginal discharge. In the past therapy involved disfiguring radical surgery. Currently the aim is to reduce the size of the tumour with chemotherapy using vincristine, actinomycin, adriamycin and cyclophosphamide combined with radiotherapy. The resulting tumour is then amenable to less radical surgery.

Non-Hodgkin lymphoma

This highly malignant disorder used to be termed lymphosarcoma. Malignant cells, usually derived from T-lymphocytes, proliferate in lymph glands, bone marrow and not infrequently the central nervous system. Mediastinal involve-ment may lead to superior vena-caval obstruction. The lymphoma may also present within abdominal lymph nodes, producing intestinal obstruction and intussusception. Malignant cells in this site more commonly derive from B-lymphocytes. Treatment is intensive incorporating multiple chemotherapy, surgery and radiotherapy.

Hodgkin disease

This is rare in children but there is some evidence that genetic factors play a part in its aetiology, there being a significant association with certain HLA types. It is also four times more common in boys than girls. The presenting features include lymphadenopathy, with or without systemic symptoms such as fever, sweating and weight loss. The staging and treatment programmes which have proved so successful in adult practice are being increasingly applied in the childhood disease but splenectomy is less commonly practised because of the risk of septicaemia. Radiotherapy is most effective for localised disease, particularly that in cervical lymph glands. Chemotherapy used in systemic disease includes chlorambucil, vincristine, procarbazine and prednisolone.

Retinoblastoma   *40% AD. (60% New Mutations)   Chr. 13*

This is a very rare but important tumour of the eye with frequency of approximately one in 30 000 live births. There is a strong familial incidence particularly if the condition is bilateral. The spread is either into the orbit or along the optic nerve, and intracranial extensions are the usual cause of death. The diagnosis must be suspected whenever a white pupillary reflex replaces the normal red one and must be rapidly followed by an adequate opthalmological examination. Treatment may involve enucleation of the eye together with radiotherapy and chemotherapy.   *25% Bilat.*   *Clinical   leucocoria.*

(if ≥ 1/2 Retina affected)   *Strabismus.*
Coloboma - ?
Painful Red eye

BIBLIOGRAPHY

Altman A J 1985 Pediatric oncology in Pediatric Clinics of North America 32:3. W. B. Saunders, Philadelphia
Broadbent V, Pritchard J 1985 Histiocytosis X — current controversies. Archives of Disease in Childhood 60: 605–607
Chessels J 1981 Acute leukaemia in childhood. In: Hull D (ed) Recent advances in paediatrics — 6. Churchill Livingstone, Edinburgh
Schweisguth O 1982 Solid tumours in children. John Wiley & Sons, New York

14
Growth

Accurate measurements of height, weight and head circumference plotted on record charts provide an invaluable illustration of growth and development. Growth reflects not only general health but also the nutritional and emotional environment of a child, and disordered growth may be the only obvious manifestation of disease or deprivation.

HEAD GROWTH

At birth the head circumference, 32 to 37 cm, is three-quarters of its adult value, 52 to 57 cm, and the majority of post-natal growth occurs in infancy. The anterior fontanelle which normally measures approximately 2.5 by 2.5 cm at birth, may no longer be palpable by six months but often remains patent until 18 months.

Head circumference chart (after Nellhaus)

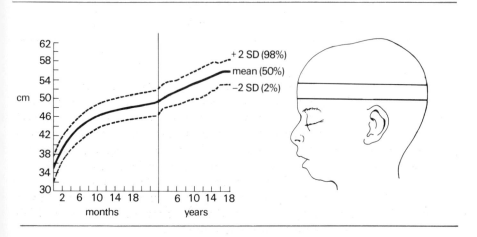

Microcephaly
Microcephaly is commonly associated with brain hypoplasia or previous brain damage.

Macrocephaly
Macrocephaly refers to a large head from whatever cause. With hydrocephalus the increased volume is due to accumulation of CSF within the ventricular system. In megalencephaly the brain itself is larger than usual and this is responsible for the large head. Megalencephaly is commonly benign and often familial but is occasionally associated with mental handicap.

Hydrocephalus
Hydrocephalus must be considered when serial head circumference measurements deviate away from a normal growth curve and where there are signs of raised intracranial pressure. This condition more than any other emphasises the need for accurate measurement and careful plotting on an appropriate chart.

Asymmetrical skulls
Asymmetrical skulls are caused by inequality of growth rates at the coronal, sagittal and lambdoid sutures. The inequality may be an innocent postural effect as is commonly the case in mild plagiocephaly or may be due to premature fusion of the sutures, craniosynostosis.

Asymmetrical skulls and craniosynostosis

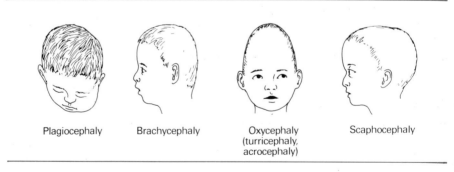

Plagiocephaly   Brachycephaly   Oxycephaly
(turricephaly,
acrocephaly)   Scaphocephaly

Premature craniosynostosis
Premature craniosynostosis occurs as an isolated congenital deformity, as a component of certain inherited syndromes, and secondary to metabolic disorders such as hypophosphatasia and idiopathic hypercalcaemia. It has also been reported after excessive thyroxine replacement therapy. Localised forms of craniosynostosis produce characteristic skull shapes and in some there are potentially damaging pressure effects upon the brain, eyes, and cranial nerves. Infants suspected of having this condition require prompt referral to a neurosurgical centre experienced in assessing and treating these problems. Craniectomy or reconstruction of the sutures is usually performed in the first few months of life, and may have to be followed by cosmetic procedures.

Growth charts (after Tanner and Whitehouse)

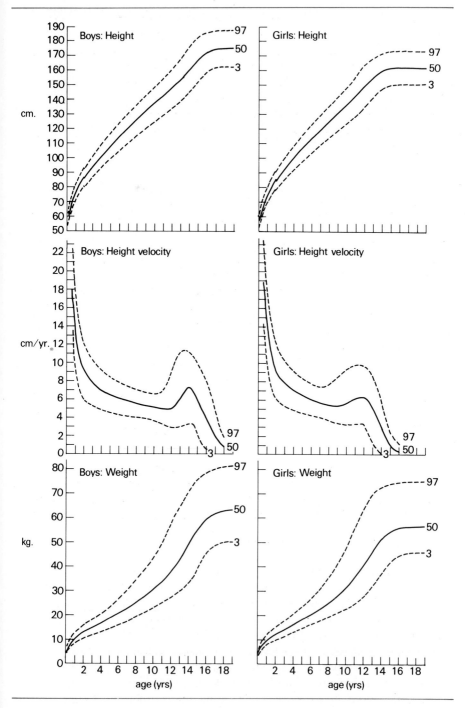

HEIGHT AND WEIGHT

Height increase or velocity is rapid in infancy and then progressively slows until the pubertal growth spurt. Birth length is doubled by approximately four years and trebled by 13 years. Puberty causes acceleration of the height velocity from a mean of 5 to 6 cm per year to a brief peak of approximately 10 cm per year. Linear growth ceases when the long bone epiphyses fuse, an event closely related to sexual maturity and adrenal androgen release.

Body weight is the most sensitive index of nutritional status and general health. On average half the adult weight is reached by 9 to 11 years.

SHORT STATURE

Short stature, defined as a height below the third centile, occurs in many healthy children but each case should be carefully evaluated and particular attention must be paid to those who are severely short with a height less than minus three standard deviations, those whose parental heights suggest that they should be above the third centile, and those in whom serial measurements show progressive deviation from the normal. The investigation of these children must take into account the multiple genetic and environmental factors which influence growth.

Genetic and environmental causes of short stature

Familial short stature. Adult height is subject to polygenic inheritance and has therefore a normal distribution. In assessing a problem of short stature it is useful to plot the parents' height centiles on the child's growth chart. In calculating the mid-parental height for a boy add 12 cm to his mother's height; for a girl subtract 12 cm from her father's height. It must be remembered that parental short stature may have resulted from inherited disease, for example skeletal dysplasia, or from still relevant environmental influences.

Familial growth delay. A separate group of genes regulates the tempo of growth and there may be a familial pattern of delayed puberty with retarded skeletal maturation but eventually normal adult height. This variant is commoner in boys and can cause considerable distress in adolescent years. Recognition of the

Causes of short stature (after Lacey and Parkin)

Newcastle Community Study: 98 ten-year-old children below 3rd height centile

82 normal short

16 organic short

6 chromosomal abnormalities
1 cystic fibrosis
1 chronic renal failure
1 Fallot tetralogy
1 juvenile rheumatoid
1 Hurler syndrome
4 mental handicap

1 growth hormone deficiency

Longitudinal growth assessment

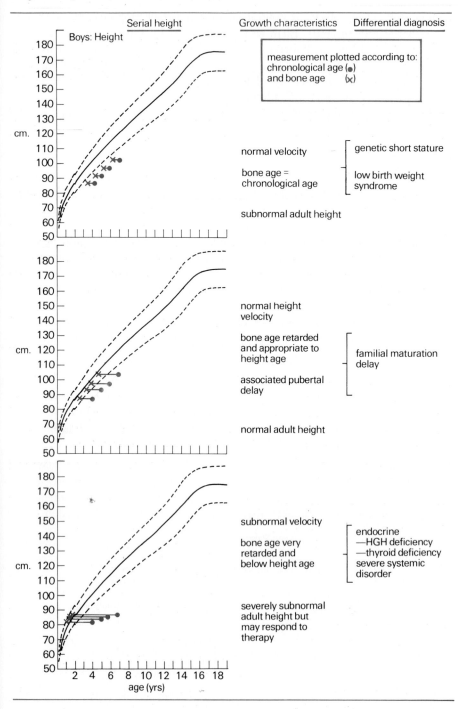

Serial height   Growth characteristics   Differential diagnosis

Boys: Height

measurement plotted according to:
chronological age (●)
and bone age (x)

normal velocity

bone age =
chronological age

subnormal adult height

genetic short stature

low birth weight
syndrome

normal height
velocity

bone age retarded
and appropriate to
height age

associated pubertal
delay

normal adult height

familial maturation
delay

subnormal velocity

bone age very
retarded and
below height age

severely subnormal
adult height but
may respond to
therapy

endocrine
—HGH deficiency
—thyroid deficiency
severe systemic
disorder

age (yrs)

problem and sympathetic explanation provides a considerable boost to their morale and it is rarely justified to artificially accelerate puberty with exogenous androgen treatment.

Low birth weight conditions. The majority of pre-term and small-for-gestational age infants achieve normal adult size. A minority have permanently restricted growth. They are a heterogenous group consisting of infants exposed to external influences such as congenital infection or maternal drugs, or having intrinsic disorders, for example chromosomal anomalies. A number of syndromes include low birth weight and subsequent growth restriction. Russell-Silver syndrome combines these features with a triangular facies, small mandible and body asymmetry.

Social deprivation. Short stature is most prevalent in the lower social classes and reflects the superimposition of a disordered environment on genetic potential. It is not easy to define the latter as successive generations have usually been exposed to the same adverse factors. Growth hormone release is depressed in emotionally deprived children but rapidly reverts to normal when they are provided with love and reasonable care. These disturbed children may also show bizarre, compulsive eating behaviour, to the extent that they develop distended abdomens and bouts of vomiting.

Nutritional starvation produces a different response with exaggerated growth hormone secretion but a block at the hepatic level where there is diminished synthesis of the somatomedins, growth factors which mediate in the peripheral anabolic effects of growth hormone.

Systemic causes

Those sufficient to restrict growth are usually severe and can be diagnosed by careful history and examination. Exceptions are chronic renal disease and malabsorption. Coeliac disease is a particular problem in that it may mimic hypopituitarism producing subnormal height velocity, delayed bone age and suppressed growth hormone responses. A jejunal biopsy may therefore be necessary in doubtful cases.

Endocrine causes of short stature

Growth hormone deficiency. This is relatively uncommon but has provided a major stimulus to basic research in this field, and its therapy has resulted in the establishment of specialised growth clinics. In the majority of affected children it is an isolated deficiency and an underlying fault cannot be defined. Ten to 15 per cent have a familial basis. Multiple pituitary hormone failure suggests secondary hypopituitarism produced by inflammatory, traumatic or neoplastic disorders in the suprasellar region.

Growth hormone deficiency must be confirmed by serial accurate height measurements and by a subnormal response to provocation tests such as an oral clonidine test or insulin-induced hypoglycaemia. The hypothalamic growth hormone releasing factor, GRF, has now been extracted and synthetic analogues show promise as diagnostic and therapeutic agents. Until recently the established therapy was human pituitary derived growth hormone but this is now being replaced by biosynthetic human growth hormone. Early recognition and initiation of treatment in children with proven deficiency can give the promise of satisfactory adult height.

Craniopharyngioma. This is a rare but important condition to exclude whenever there is a possibility of secondary hypopituitarism. The tumour is composed of expanding cystic remnants of Rathke's pouch, a dorsal protrusion of the embryonic stomatodoeum, and its strategic location results in life threatening pressure effects. Headache and defective vision are more common initial complaints than short stature, but visual field assessment and a lateral skull X-ray are essential in the assessment of short children.

Pressure effects and clinical features of craniopharyngioma

III ventricle—hydrocephalus

post. pituitary
–diabetes insipidus

optic chiasma–
–asymmetrical
bitemporal
hemianopia

ant. pituitary–
–growth failure

headache 80%:   defective vision 65%

X-ray -expanded sella with calcification

Juvenile hypothyroidism results in progressive growth failure and is characterised by severe retardation of skeletal development. It is readily confirmed by performing thyroid function tests and responds well to thyroxine replacement.

Adrenal insufficiency, hypoparathyroidism and pubertal disorders account for a small number of children with short stature. Corticosteroid therapy at a dosage in excess of prednisone 5 mg per day or its equivalent interferes with linear growth. Alternate day single dose corticosteroid regimens permit more normal growth.

Investigation of short stature
In the majority of children the history will reveal a genetic or social basis for their problem and detailed investigation is therefore inappropriate. Those lacking such an explanation, having definitely abnormal growth, or having additional signs or symptoms, require accurate measurement or anthropometry. In addition to an accurate measurement of height, which provides the basis for longitudinal growth assessment, there must be some comparison of trunk versus leg length to allow recognition of disproportionate short stature. Pubertal staging, optic fundi and visual field assessment are essential parts of the physical examination. Laboratory investigations are guided by the clinical findings but in general are limited to total blood count, plasma electrolytes, creatinine, calcium, phosphorus, alkaline phosphatase and thyroid function. Turner syndrome is not rare and hence there is a case for chromosomal analysis in short girls. Random measurements of basal

growth hormone levels are misleading and a more formal provocation is required. A commonly used out-patient procedure is the exercise test in which the serum growth hormone level is measured 20 minutes after finishing 10 minutes of strenuous exercise. Radiographs of the left wrist and hand for bone age determination and a skull X-ray for pituitary fossa examination complete the initial assessment.

It is unnecessary to subject children to more formal assessment of growth hormone secretion, such as insulin-induced hypoglycaemia, until they have had at least six months of longitudinal growth assessment. Exact height measurement at three monthly intervals enables the height velocity to be determined. A subnormal velocity confirms the case for further detailed investigation. The combination of serial height measurements and bone age determinations is not only a useful tool in the diagnosis of short stature, but provides a parameter by which therapy may be judged.

Disproportionate short stature

Calculation of the ratio of upper and lower body segment lengths will reveal cases of disproportionate short stature. Skeletal disorders account for the majority of this group and may be classified into those where abnormality originates in the skeleton, or has a systemic metabolic basis, for example mucopolysaccharidoses. They may also be divided into those with short limbs or short trunks, the latter usually having kyphoscoliosis. Exact diagnosis, confirmed by radiological and metabolic studies, is essential for genetic counselling.

Achondroplasia

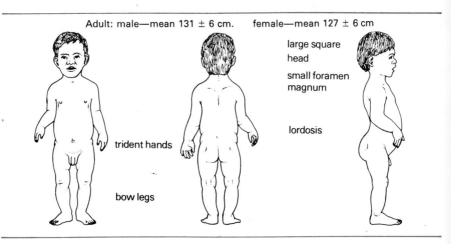

Adult: male—mean 131 ± 6 cm.   female—mean 127 ± 6 cm

large square head

small foramen magnum

lordosis

trident hands

bow legs

EXCESSIVE HEIGHT

The great majority of tall children come from tall families and accept their stature as normal. An unusually tall child may have an underlying disorder but these are usually readily excluded. Occasionally, girls apparently destined to have an adult height above 5 feet 10 inches (178 cm) are brought for advice and possible medical intervention. Prediction of final height is not easy as it is influenced by the time of menarche and the rate of skeletal maturation as well as by the linear growth rate in childhood. Tables are available for predicting adult height but they are liable to errors of approximately 5 cm either way. Exogenous oestrogen therapy has been used to promote accelerated skeletal maturation and a premature cessation of linear growth in girls but the benefits are often marginal, and there is concern about the risks of interfering with the humoral mechanism of puberty and of increasing the incidence of reproductive tract neoplasia. The orthopaedic approach to this problem, epiphyseal stapling, retains its place in a very small group of children with asymmetrical growth. Irradiation of the growing epiphyses has rightly been abandoned because of the high risk of inducing osteosarcomata.

Pathological causes of excessive height

Endocrine disorders	Other disorders
Pituitary — eosinophilic adenoma	Cerebral gigantism (Soto syndrome)
Thyrotoxicosis	Marfan syndrome
Precocious puberty (early stages)	Homocystinuria

BIBLIOGRAPHY

Beighton P 1978 Inherited disorders of the skeleton. Churchill Livingstone, Edinburgh.
Brook C G D 1982 Growth assessment in childhood and adolescence. Blackwell Scientific Publications, Oxford
Lacey K A, Parkin J M 1974 Causes of short stature. A community study of children in Newcastle-upon-Tyne. Lancet i: 42–45.
Marshall W A 1977 Human growth and its disorders. Academic Press, London.
Nellhaus G 1968 Head circumference from birth to eighteen years. Pediatrics 41: 106–114.
Tanner J M, Whitehouse R H, Takaishi M 1965 Standards from birth to maturity for height, weight, height velocity and weight velocity; British children. Archives of Disease of Childhood 41: 613–635

15
Endocrine

TSH
ACTH
FSH, LH
HGH
prolactin

Although the fetus is totally dependent on a maternally regulated environment, fetal endocrine systems differentiate and commence autonomous activity in the first trimester. The placenta is relatively impermeable to peptide hormones so that most fetal hypothalamic-pituitary-endocrine gland circuits evolve independently of any direct interference from maternal hormone levels. The adrenal cortex is an exception in that the placenta actively participates in steroid metabolism and this is reflected in the major transition from fetal to adult cortex activity with birth.

Trophic hormones are first detectable in the anterior pituitary between five and eight weeks' gestation, and serum levels of thyroid stimulating hormone (TSH) and the gonadotrophins (LH and FSH) reach adult levels by 16 to 20 weeks. This early surge of trophic hormone activity may relate to endocrine gland development prior to the establishment of sensitive feedback mechanisms.

The endocrine factors which control human fetal growth have yet to be defined. Anencephalic infants with absent growth hormone have relatively little reduction in body weight although there are delays in skeletal and lung maturation. The mean birth weight of hypothyroid infants is greater than normal. These apparent anomalies may be resolved by greater knowledge of the role in fetal growth of the new generation of growth promoting peptide hormones, somatomedins, epidermal growth factor, fibroblast growth factor and nerve growth factor.

Delivery and the demands of an independent existence result in major endocrine adjustments. In the case of TSH and thyroid hormone release the change is abrupt, but for other systems such as the gut and pancreas the transition occurs progressively with the introduction of oral feeds.

PUBERTY

Puberty is a series of physical and physiological changes which convert the child to an adult capable of reproduction. The physical events include a growth spurt,

The normal age range of puberty, girls (after Marshall and Tanner)

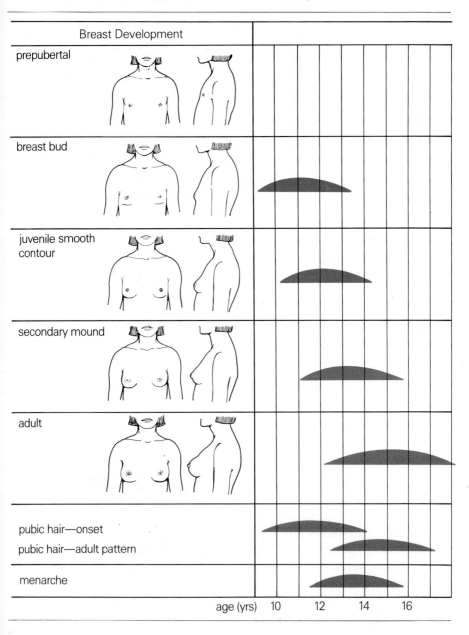

alteration of body proportion and the development of sexual organs and secondary sexual characteristics. There is great variability in the onset and order of these events. Ninety-five per cent of girls commence puberty between 9 and 13 years with breast formation (80%) or pubic hair growth (20%) as a first event. Menarche occurs at a mean age of 13.5 years and is closely correlated with skeletal maturity so that it is suspicious to find a girl still amenorrhoeic with a bone

The normal age range of puberty, boys (after Marshall and Tanner)

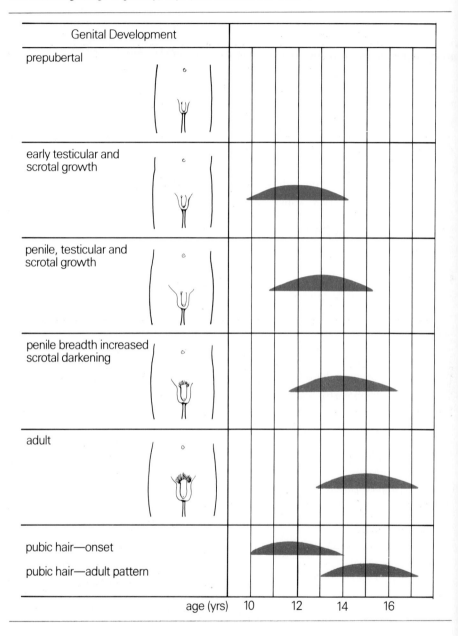

age of over 15 years. Boys have a later puberty with onset for 95% being between 9.5 and 13.5 years, the first sign being enlargement of the testes, rapidly followed by growth of the penis and pubic hair. It is not unusual to find infantile genitalia in a boy aged 15 years if there is delayed skeletal maturation. A standardised scheme for recording genital, breast and pubic hair maturation has been described by Tanner.

Physiology of puberty

The newborn infant is capable of releasing high levels of gonadotrophins, testosterone and oestradiol but this transient hormonal activity is subsequently inhibited by a very sensitive gonadohypothalamic feedback mechanism. Puberty follows the elevation of the threshold for this feedback inhibition but the mechanisms responsible for this readjustment are not known. The pineal gland may be partly responsible for hypothalamic suppression of gonadotrophin release as tumours which destroy this gland or its connections sometimes result in precocious puberty. Longitudinal studies show that from the age of 6 years nocturnal pulses of LH release gradually increase in frequency and amplitude. Ovarian ultrasound examination also reveals increasing follicular activity from mid-childhood. The onset of puberty is not an abrupt event but is preceded by several years of endocrine adjustment. Adrenarche describes the increase in adrenal androgen release which commences between 6 and 8 years of age. Gonadarche and adrenarche are closely parallel events but the exact link between the two remains a mystery. Adrenal androgens, particularly in girls, are responsible for sexual hair growth and skeletal maturation.

Precocious puberty

Precocious puberty is termed 'true' or intracranial when it is controlled by the hypothalamic-pituitary axis, and 'false' when an extracranial or exogenous source of hormone is responsible.

Early puberty is relatively common in girls and there may be a family history. Detailed assessment is unnecessary unless puberty commences before the age of six years or menses before eight years, or if puberty pursues an abnormal sequence of events with virilisation or is accompanied by other problems such as neurological symptoms, hypertension or abnormal growth. Of girls commencing puberty early, 90% have no demonstrable abnormality. Precocious puberty in boys (defined as having an onset earlier than nine years) is more frequently pathological (60% of cases) and requires careful evaluation.

Causes of precocious puberty

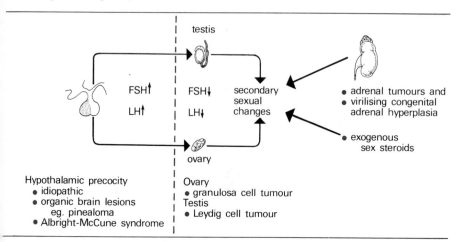

testis

FSH↑   FSH↓   secondary
LH↑   LH↓   sexual
                changes

ovary

- adrenal tumours and
- virilising congenital
  adrenal hyperplasia

- exogenous
  sex steroids

Hypothalamic precocity
- idiopathic
- organic brain lesions
    eg. pinealoma
- Albright-McCune syndrome

Ovary
- granulosa cell tumour
Testis
- Leydig cell tumour

The Albright-McCune syndrome. This consists of unilateral pigmentation, cystic bone lesions and precocious puberty. It is far commoner in girls. The basic endocrine derangement involves autonomy of normally pituitary dependent glands.

Premature thelarche. This is an isolated transient phase of breast development in girls and is not uncommon during infancy and childhood. There are no other signs of puberty and recognition of this innocent occurrence should obviate further investigation.

Premature pubarche. This refers to isolated development of pubic and axillary hair and is again more common in girls. There may be slight advance in the bone age and a marginal increase in plasma adrenal androgens but other signs of sexual development are absent.

Gynaecomastia in adolescent boys. This is common and may be uni- or bilateral. It is usually transient and does not indicate underlying endocrine problems unless there is other evidence of testicular failure. Very occasionally it can be sufficiently prominent to merit a cosmetic reduction procedure.

Delayed puberty
Delayed puberty may indicate a gonadal failure with elevated gonadotrophin levels, or a disorder of the hypothalamic-pituitary axis in which case they are reduced. Ovarian dysgenesis is a component of Turner syndrome, XO karyotype, but it can also occur independently. In males, various degrees of testicular failure occur in Klinfelter syndrome, XXY karyotype. Gonadal failure may also follow irradiation or exposure to cytotoxic therapy.

The testicular feminisation syndrome. This syndrome is suggested by amenorrhoea and absent pubic hair in a girl with normal breast development. In this familial disorder genetic males with testes develop as phenotypic females because of end-organ resistance to testosterone.

Normal sexual differentiation

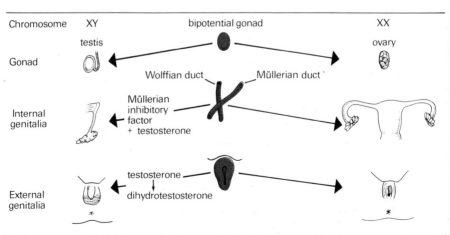

Haematocolpos. Increasing abdominal distention and monthly discomfort without bleeding calls for examination of the vulva, as an imperforate hymen may produce retention of menstrual products.

DISORDERS OF SEXUAL DIFFERENTIATION

The bipotential gonadal and genital tissues of the early fetus require the Y chromosome in order to undergo male differentiation. Female differentiation represents the basic organisational direction and will occur independantly of functioning gonads. Girls with Turner syndrome may have fibrous streaks instead of ovaries but have otherwise normal internal and external genitalia. There are many potential faults in the more complex pathway leading to maleness and these manifest as varying degrees of cryptorchidism, micropenis and hypospadias.

Parents expect the sexual identity of their offspring to be immediately obvious. Ambiguity of the external genitalia at the time of birth causes great distress and sensitive explanation is vital. Complete diagnostic evaluation requires special expertise as it has to consider the long term functional role of the individual as well as the precise gender. A genetic male with functioning testes but feminised external genitalia is better reared as a girl.

A classification of ambiguous genitalia

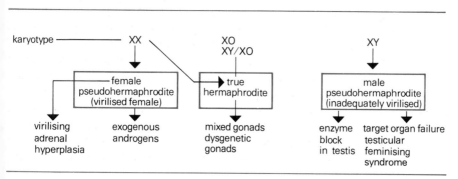

The majority of intersex problems represent female or male pseudohermaphroditism rather than true hermaphroditism. The recognition of virilising congenital adrenal hyperplasia must be a priority in order to avert a salt-losing crisis. The exact nature of other types may necessitate pelvic scans, laparotomy and gonad biopsy. After assigning the appropriate gender, management may involve reconstructive surgery, hormonal substitution and possibly removal of gonads. The latter is particularly indicated in gonadal dysgenesis because of the risk of neoplastic transformation. Reconstructive surgery to the external genitalia should be completed before 18 months of age if possible because of the psychological implications.

ADRENAL GLANDS

During intrauterine development the adrenal cortex is considerably enlarged due to a thick inner fetal zone. This zone, which accounts for 80% of the cortex at full term, involutes rapidly after birth leaving the outer adult zone to synthesise essential mineralocorticoids and glucocorticoids. The fetal cortex acts in a mutually dependent relationship with the placenta to synthesise oestriol and dehydroepiandrosterone. The measurement of these steroids in the maternal serum or urine provides an index of feto-placental health. The increasing development of the adult zone at term may be a factor in initiating the onset of labour; anencephalic infants with secondary adrenal hypoplasia but without poly-hydramnios tend to have prolonged gestation.

Congenital adrenal hyperplasia

This group of inherited, autosomal recessive disorders is caused by the absence of essential enzymes in the pathway of cortisol and aldosterone synthesis. The resulting interruption of the adrenohypothalamic feedback stimulates excessive corticotrophin (ACTH) release and overactivity of the biosynthetic steps prior to the block, with an accumulation of androgenic steroids. The commonest variety is 21-hydroxylase deficiency, approximately 1 in 5000 live births. Affected female infants are virilised at birth with clitoral hypertrophy and variable fusion of the labia minora. The most masculinised girls may be confused for males with hypospadias and cryptorchidism. Prompt recognition of this problem is less easy in males and they may not be diagnosed prior to an adrenal crisis in the second week of life. The crisis, often preceded by vomiting and poor weight gain, is biochemically characterised by low serum sodium and high potassium. Grossly elevated serum ACTH and 17-hydroxyprogesterone levels suggest the 21-hydroxylase deficiency. This may be confirmed by elevated concentrations of urinary pregnanetriol and 17-oxosteroids. A salt-losing crisis demands urgent therapy with intravenous saline, glucose and hydrocortisone. Long-term management must aim to suppress the hyperplastic adrenal glands and provide replacement hydrocortisone and a salt-retaining steroid, fludrocortisone. The correct replacement is that which permits normal linear growth and maintains serum 17-hydroxyprogesterone and adrenal androgens within acceptable limits. Surgical correction of the masculinised female perineum is commenced in the first year.

Congenital adrenal hyperplasia

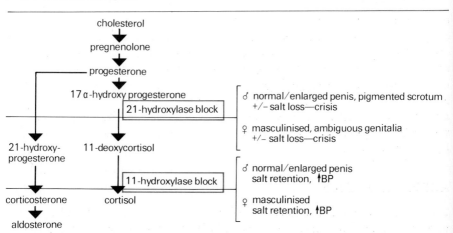

Adult men and women are capable of normal fertility but should remain on hydrocortisone and fludrocortisone. Among the rarer forms of congenital adrenal hyperplasia, 11-beta-hydroxylase deficiency results in virilisation and salt retention with hypertension. Affected children may present with excessive growth, but the advanced bone age considerably limits their final adult stature.

Cushing syndrome

This disorder is due to sustained high circulating cortisol levels of either exogenous or endogenous origin. Iatrogenic disease is now less common with the introduction of effective alternatives to systemic corticosteroid therapy in for example asthma. Endogenous Cushing syndrome is fortunately rare in childhood but is likely to be due to a potentially malignant adrenocortical tumour. It should be considered when acne and masculinisation accompany the usual signs of cortisol excess. Distinction must be made between these potentially malignant unilateral tumours and the rarer problem of bilateral adrenal hyperplasia due to pituitary microadenomata. An IVP will probably show kidney displacement in the former. ACTH levels are suppressed by the tumour and elevated urinary steroid metabolites fail to diminish during a dexamethasone load. Adrenal tumours require unilateral adrenalectomy and additional radiotherapy if there is histological evidence of capsule invasion. In acquired bilateral adrenal hyperplasia, management is directed against the pituitary adenomata using high voltage radiation or trans-sphenoidal microsurgery.

Cushing syndrome

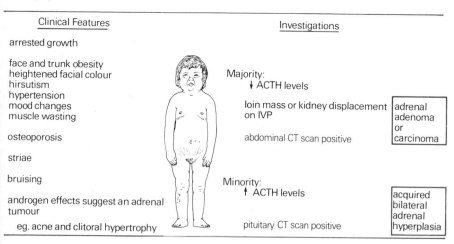

Clinical Features	Investigations	
arrested growth		
face and trunk obesity	Majority:	
heightened facial colour	$\downarrow$ ACTH levels	
hirsutism		
hypertension		
mood changes	loin mass or kidney displacement	adrenal adenoma or carcinoma
muscle wasting	on IVP	
osteoporosis	abdominal CT scan positive	
striae		
bruising	Minority:	
	$\uparrow$ ACTH levels	acquired bilateral adrenal hyperplasia
androgen effects suggest an adrenal tumour		
eg. acne and clitoral hypertrophy	pituitary CT scan positive	

Adrenal cortical failure (Addison disease)

This uncommon disorder has an autoimmune basis and may occur in association with diabetes mellitus, thyroiditis and hypoparathyroidism. Children either present with an insidious onset of weakness, weight loss and increased pigmentation or become acutely ill following a brief episode of diarrhoea and vomiting. An adrenal crisis demands urgent therapy with intravenous glucose and saline together with hydrocortisone. Long-term replacement consists of hydrocortisone (15–20 mg/m² surface area/day) and fludrocortisone (0.1 to 0.2 mg daily). With all patients on corticosteroid replacement therapy, the child must be provided with a steroid warning card and the parents advised of the necessity of increasing the dosage during times of illness.

THYROID

The thyroid originates from a ventral extension of the endoderm foregut which migrates caudad to lie at the level of the upper trachea. Developmental failures may be classified as hypoplasia or maldescent. Hypoplasia varies from absence of detectable thyroid and early severe hypothyroidism, to lesser degrees which remain asymptomatic until later childhood. An ectopic gland may account for a lingual mass or produce at thyroglossal cyst. A sinus may occur along the line of descent.

Physiology

The fetal thyroid contains colloid and iodoproteins by ten weeks gestation; plasma TSH is detectable at this stage and there is evidence for early activity of the pituitary-thyroid axis. The fetal thyroid preferentially releases 'reverse T3', a molecule which differs from tri-iodothyronine by the location of a single iodine atom. Reverse T3 is thought to be inactive and its place in physiology has not been established. There is minimal transplacental passage of maternal thyroxine to the fetus.

Following birth there is a surge of TSH release later paralleled by increased thyroxine (T4) and tri-iodothyronine (T3). TSH levels return to the normal adult range by one week but T4 and especially T3 show a slower decline to adult values. The definition of normal neonatal thyroid function is essential for the development of screening programmes to detect congenital hypothyroidism.

Hypothyroidism

Congenital hypothyroidism. Congenital hypothyroidism is relatively common, 1 in 4000 live births. Central nervous system development appears critically

Ectopic sites of the thyroid gland. Neonatal thyroid function

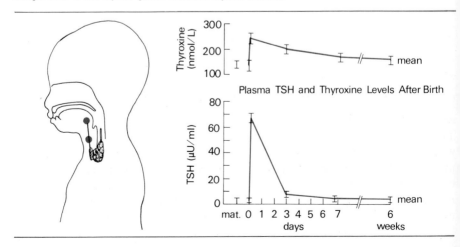

Plasma TSH and Thyroxine Levels After Birth

Congenital hypothyroidism

coarse facies

dry skin

hoarse cry

hypotonia

umbilical hernia

constipation

prolonged jaundice

TSH ↟↟
thyroxine ↓

dependent on thyroxine from late pregnancy through the first months of infancy. In some infants brain development may be irreversibly damaged before birth, in others brain damage may be avoided by early detection and adequate treatment. It is important that affected infants are identified as soon as possible after birth. Available data suggests that screening programmes can protect over 80% of affected infants from significant neurological sequelae.

Goitrous hypothyroidism. A hypothyroid infant with a goitre has probably been exposed to maternal goitrogens such as antithyroid drugs, iodine-containing preparations, phenylbutazone or PAS. The goitre may cause life threatening tracheal compression. Inborn errors of thyroxine biosynthesis account for familial goitrous hypothyroidism but these conditions seldom present in the newborn.

Juvenile hypothyroidism. Hypothyroidism occurring in later childhood presents with growth failure and abnormal skeletal delay. It is most commonly due to autoimmune thyroiditis. The neonatal screening programmes have permitted much earlier recognition of structural thyroid deficiencies. As thyroxine levels are adequate in the early critical phase of brain development, there is no intellectual impairment.

Thyroxine is the standard therapy for hypothyroidism. Infants require a relatively higher dose, 5 μg per kg per day, diminishing to 2 to 3 μg per kg in later childhood. The dose is monitored by checking height and bone age increments as well as biochemical parameters. Therapy must be life long.

Hyperthyroidism

Neonatal hyperthyroidism. This is an uncommon disorder but must be anticipated in all infants of mothers with a history of thyrotoxicosis. Maternal thyroid stimulating immunoglobulins may traverse the placenta to overstimulate the fetal thyroid producing irritability, fever, diarrhoea and poor weight gain. Although transient the condition is potentially fatal and may require antithyroid therapy or propanolol.

Juvenile hyperthyroidism. This is uncommon but the features are similar to those seen in adults with the addition of excessive growth and occasional abnormal choreiform movements. The diagnosis is confirmed by elevated plasma thyroxine levels. Medical management using carbimazole is the treatment of choice. An initial two year course may result in spontaneous remission in 25 to 75% of cases, and a further course should be completed before considering surgical management. Radioactive iodine is to be avoided in childhood.

Autoimmune thyroiditis
Goitres due to autoimmune thyroiditis are less rare than previously considered. The majority are asymptomatic but there may be signs of mild hyperthyroidism or progressive hypothyroidism. A positive thyroid antibody test confirms the diagnosis. Therapy with replacement thyroxine is indicated for significantly enlarged goitres or biochemical hypothyroidism. Goitrogen consumption and familial goitrous hypothyroidism enter the differential diagnosis.

Isolated thyroid nodules
These must be carefully investigated by isotope scans and biopsy to exclude carcinoma.

PARATHYROID GLANDS

Hypoparathyroidism
Transient hypoparathyroidism is a common neonatal event and the resulting hypocalcaemia may cause convulsions or apnoeic episodes. Permanent hypoparathyroidism is rare and has to be distinguished from conditions in which there is organ unresponsiveness to circulating parathyroid hormone, the pseudohypoparathyroidism syndromes.

Features of hypoparathyroidism

Acute Hypocalcaemia	Chronic Hypocalcaemia
Convulsions	Convulsions
	calcification of basal ganglia
Neuromuscular excitability	headache, vomiting (raised intracranial pressure)
Chvostek sign	photophobia
Trousseau sign	cataracts
carpopedal spasm	poor dentition
	chronic diarrhoea
	Investigation: serum calcium ↓ serum phosphorus ↑ alk. phos.—normal

True hypoparathyroidism. True hypoparathyroidism is confirmed by demonstrating undetectable plasma PTH levels, and increased urinary phosphate or cyclic AMP excretion during an infusion of parathyroid hormone.

Pseudohypoparathyroidism syndromes. These syndromes are refractory to parathyroid administration and the children may show the other features; short stature, round facies, short metacarpals, ectopic calcification and mental retardation.

Pseudopseudohypoparathyroidism. This is part of the group of X-linked disorders in which the typical physical abnormalities are not accompanied by biochemical derangement.

Classification of hypoparathyroidism

Transient neonatal	Prematurity, cerebral injury Maternal diabetes Maternal hyperparathyroidism

Permanent life-long	Isolated hypoplasia
	Di George syndrome. Thymus aplasia, defective
	  immunity, candidiasis, cardiac lesions
	Autoimmune — associated diabetes mellitus,
	  Addison disease, chronic hepatitis, etc.
	Post-thyroidectomy

Pseudohypoparathyroidism syndromes

Treatment of hypoparathyroidism. Acute symptomatic hypocalcaemia requires urgent correction with intravenous calcium, 0.1 mmol elemental calcium per kg bodyweight per hour. Ten per cent calcium gluconate should be diluted to 2% for use and the infusion must be carefully monitored.

Permanent hypoparathyroidism and pseudohypoparathyroidism are treated with supraphysiological doses of vitamin D or related compounds which act by promoting intestinal calcium absorption and by mobilising bone calcium. The dose of vitamin D is adjusted to maintain the plasma calcium level in the low normal range (2.15 to 2.40 mmol/l). Chronic overdosage carries the risk of nephrocalcinosis and renal failure.

DIABETES

Diabetes mellitus is the disorder which results from insulin deficiency. In most juvenile diabetics, this is due to irreversible islet beta cell damage. Diabetes is rare in infancy but the incidence rises so that by age 16 years, 2 per 1000 are affected. Children account for only 4 to 6% of the total diabetic population but the life-long implications of the disease emphasise their importance.

Aetiology

The failure of islet beta cells appears to reflect both genetic and environmental factors. HLA-DR3 and DR4 are linked to increased incidence and are present in 95% of type 1 or insulin dependent diabetics. The HLA system is carried on chromosome 6 and is linked with determinants of immune function. There is growing evidence of auto-immune beta cell damage, paralleled by circulating islet cell antibiodies for months or even years before clinical diabetes becomes manifest. It is however unclear how environmental influence converts inherited susceptibility into overt disease. Viral involvement is favoured by seasonal peaks of presentation, case clustering and the occasional isolation of Coxsackie B virus from newly recognised but fatal diabetes. We are no nearer defining a specific group of viral pathogens against which immunisation might be developed. Other still speculative evidence favours early dietary exposure as an environment trigger.

Clinical features

The symptoms are characteristic and the diagnosis is seldom in doubt if hyperglycaemia, glycosuria and ketonuria are detected. Young diabetics always require prompt diagnosis and therapy, but the correct diagnosis may be confused by a coincidental febrile illness and the hyperventilation mistakenly interpreted as being due to pneumonia. Diabetes may be confirmed by a single blood glucose estimation and glucose tolerance tests are rarely necessary. Early diagnosis saves lives and allows an organised introduction to the principles of diabetic management; often as an out-patient. Ketoacidosis obviously necessitates urgent admission.

Features and duration of symptoms in childhood diabetes

Clinical Features

Early:	Late:	
polyuria	vomiting	
(secondary nocturnal	abdominal pain	Duration of symptoms before diagnosis
enuresis)	hyperventilation	
thirst	(metabolic acidosis)	0-2 wks 20%
lethargy	shock	
weight loss	coma	2-6 wks 52%
anorexia		
(increased appetite		6 wks plus 28%
unusual)		
constipation		

Diabetic ketoacidosis

The basic principles of treatment consist of insulin therapy, fluid and electrolyte replacement and the correction of provoking factors. Low dose insulin regimens are favoured as these provide for more predictable control of blood sugar and largely avoid hypoglycaemia and hypokalaemia. Although metabolic acidosis may be prominent it is unnecessary to administer sodium bicarbonate unless there is severe circulatory failure.

Long-term management

It is not possible to return diabetics to a physiologically normal state with current methods of insulin administration. Management must be a compromise aimed at the following objectives; a happy child leading a full life and equipped for a normal adult role; normal growth; education and motivation to maintain the best possible diabetic control. Current clinical and experimental studies support the belief that optimal control reduces the long-term risk of microvascular disease. In practice good control means freedom from symptoms and satisfactory blood glucose profiles confirmed by regular glycosylated haemoglobin levels. This can only be achieved at the expense of occasional hypoglycaemic episodes. The essentials of management are diet, appropriate insulin and education in the techniques and understanding of diabetes.

A scheme for the management of diabetic ketoacidosis

---

1. **Initial management**
   Assess circulatory status
   Weigh
   Insert I.V. line and send samples to laboratory
   Stop oral intake and insert nasogastric tube
   Attach ECG monitor

2. **Identify provoking factors**. e.g. infection

3. **Treat shock**
   i.v. N saline or plasma

4. **Fluid and electrolyte management**   **Insulin management**
   Calculate total fluid requirement
   (deficit + maintenance + losses)
   Replace ⅓ 0–4 hr
           ⅓ 4–12 hr
           ⅓ 12–24 hr

   • Extracellular replacement: i.v. short-acting insulin
     i.v. N saline + KCl until blood glucose initial dose 0.25 u/kg
     < 14 mmol/l   continue 0.10 u/kg/hr
                                              using infusion pump until blood glucose
                                              < 14 mmol/l

   • Intracellular replacement: reduce insulin to 0.05 u/kg/hr
     i.v. 0.2 N saline in 5% glucose + KCl   (adjust according to blood glucose)

   • Graded re-introduction of oral fluids 2- start 8-hourly short-acting insulin
     hourly milk/sugar drinks   0.5–2.0 u/kg/day

   • Regular diet   establish on medium-acting insulin

Diet. The modern diabetes diet emphasises good nutrition based on a normal proportion of appropriate carbohydrates, particularly those high in fibre. This approach has replaced the restricted carbohydrate intake which placed too great a reliance on fat-based calories. Dieticians assist the family in adjusting their previous diet and provide a meal and snack structure based on readily recognised 10 g portions.

Insulin. Most children require a twice daily insulin injection regimen based on combinations of short and medium duration insulins. Modern highly purified pork or human insulins avoid antibody generation and the resulting injection site fat atrophy. Dosage has to be individually tailored and based on blood glucose profiles.

Injections are the focal points of the diabetic day and correct techniques must be stressed. Modern disposable syringes (0.5 ml = 50 units) have simplified the injection so that most older children can perform their own. Injection problems include pain from too shallow needle insertion and fat hypertrophy due to inadequate spacing of injections.

Monitoring. Regular capillary blood glucose measurement is now part of the modern diabetic way of life. The problem is to devise a compromise between the child's variable lifestyle and worthwhile data collection. There are often short and

A selection of insulins

Type		Species	Approximate time of action (hour)		
			Onset	Peak	Duration
Short-acting (neutral insulin)	Actrapid Velosulin Humulin S	Pig/Human[1] Pig/Human[1] Human[2]	$\frac{1}{2}$	1–3	6–8
Medium-acting (isophane insulin)	Protaphane Insulatard Humulin I	Human[1] Pig/Human[1] Human[2]	1–1$\frac{1}{2}$	2–12	18–24
Medium-acting (insulin zinc suspension)	Monotard Humulin Zn	Pig/Human[1] Human[2]	2–3	6–14	22–24

Human[1] = modified pig (emp)
Human[2] = biosynthetic (c & b)

medium term problems in achieving good control but hopefully the child and family will grasp the longer term objectives of understanding and achieving good diabetes control.

Problems in diabetic control
Poor control and so-called brittle diabetes with recurrent ketoacidosis and hypo-glycaemia may arise several causes.

Hypoglycaemia. Parents have a great fear of insulin reactions and this naturally leads to caution in attaining normoglycaemia especially in the evening tests. All diabetic children must have immediate access to glucose tablets or drinks. Families should be provided with glucagon injection for emergency management of hypoglycaemia.

The dawn phenomenon. This refers to the common finding of refractory hyperglycaemia in the early part of the day. It results from waning insulin action after the previous evening's injection exacerbated by circadian rhythms of growth hormone and cortisol release.

Behaviour. Parents require advice on how to cope with injection trauma, dietary delinquency, fake tests and pseudo-hypoglycaemia. Clinic visits must not

Factors which influence diabetic control

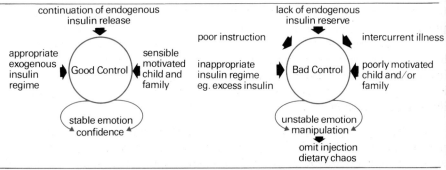

be regarded as times of judgement. Adolescents may become introspective and depressed about the future so that poor control and carelessness may be a symptom of their distress.

Diabetes and growth
Children with diabetes can look forward to a normal adult stature, although comparison between identical twins discordant for diabetes shows some loss of final height. Modest pubertal delay is more frequent; marked delay especially in girls is an indication for excluding co-existent auto-immune hypothyroidism.

Long-term complications
The challenge of preventing microvascular disease in this generation of diabetic children is highlighted by life table analysis of earlier cohorts showing a mortality rate 2 to 6 times in excess of age matched non-diabetic controls. The bulk of this excess mortality is due to renal failure and myocardial infarction. Approximately 25 to 40% die in renal failure, the incidence peaking after approximately 15 years of diabetes. Persistent proteinuria is a late feature predicting established renal failure within 4 to 5 years. Current efforts are being directed at recognising the sub-population at risk of developing nephropathy while they are potentially amenable to strict metabolic control. Early pointers include elevated glomerular filtration rate, increased kidney volume and raised albumin excretion.

Diabetic eye disease is the commonest cause of blindness in young and middle-aged people in the developed world. However, it is seldom detectable by conventional examination before diabetes has been established 10 to 15 years. Subcapsular snowstorm cataracts occasionally develop in childhood.

The introduction of intensified insulin management programmes based on either multiple injections or subcutaneous infusion pumps offers the potential for delaying the evolution of microvascular disease. Short-term studies in selected groups of patients have provided ground for optimism but it remains to be seen whether an impact can be made on a wider spectrum of young diabetics.

HYPOGLYCAEMIA

Hypoglycaemia is rare after the newborn period but must be considered in the assessment of non-febrile seizures, particularly those occurring early in the morning and after prolonged fasts. A blood glucose of less than 2.2 mmol/l is diagnostic and the urine should also be tested for ketones, a helpful step in distinguishing the two main categories of disorders which cause recurrent hypoglycaemia: substrate deficiency and hyperinsulinism. In children in whom there is no obvious explanation, a carefully monitored period of starvation with serial determinations of plasma glucose, insulin, cortisol, growth hormone, beta-hydroxybutyrate and lactic acid is the most useful investigation.

Substrate deficiency

Ketotic hypoglycaemia. This is the commonest cause of hypoglycaemia after the first year. Affected children are usually small, slim and more susceptible to attacks during coincidental illness. Nocturnal fits associated with vomiting and unconsciousness develop and ketonuria is prominent. Monitored starvation results in a more pronounced hypoglycaemia and ketonaemia than normal, but insulin levels are very low. Limited gluconeogenic reserves probably account for this disorder. Hypoglycaemia can be avoided by regular bedtime snacks and additional glucose drinks during illness. The problem resolves spontaneously in later childhood.

Causes of hypoglycaemia in infancy and childhood

Substrate deficiency (ketones usually present)	Hyperinsulinism (ketones absent)
• ketotic hypoglycaemia	• pancreatic
• hepatic enzyme deficiencies	nesidioblastosis
glycogen storage diseases	insulinoma
galactosaemia	• mesenchymal tumours
hereditary fructose intolerance	• prediabetes mellitus
• exogenous hepatotoxins and poisons	
Reye syndrome	
alcohol, aspirin	
unripe Akee fruit	
• endogenous hepatotoxins	
tyrosinosis	
maple syrup urine disease	
• endocrine deficiencies	
pituitary, adrenal	

Hyperinsulinism

Nesidioblastosis is a rare problem of young infants in which developmental disorganisation of the islet cells and inappropriate insulin release results in refractory hypoglycaemia. The latter may be partially controlled using continuous infusions of glucose, and diazoxide. The most successful long-term therapy is a 75 to 80% resection of the pancreas.

Insulinomas account for most cases of hyperinsulinism in older infants and children, and again extensive resection of the pancreas is indicated.

BIBLIOGRAPHY

Aynsley-Green A 1984 Paediatric endocrinology in clinical practice. MTP Press, Lancaster
Brook C G D 1981 Clinical paediatric endocrinology. Blackwell Scientific Publications, Oxford
Craig O 1981 Childhood diabetes and its management 2nd edn. Butterworths, London

16
Skin

Man consists mainly of water and it is his skin which stops him from drying out. In addition, the skin protects the body from physical, chemical and biological insult. The superficial layer of the epidermis, stratum corneum, with its compact horny cells provides an effective barrier to the passage of substances in either direction. The dermis, with its high collagen content, gives skin its ability to stretch and mould. Its numerous blood vessels and sweat glands are important in the control of body temperature.

The epidermis develops in the third week of fetal life, and is initially composed of two layers, an outer periderm and an inner basal layer. The periderm is equipped with absorptive microvilli and actively transfers substances between amniotic fluid and fetal tissues. It is normally shed long before term, but occasionally it persists as a horny cocoon, creating the so-called 'collodion baby'. The basal or germinative layer gives rise to the definitive multi-layered epidermis, and this differentiation is largely complete when keratinisation establishes the stratum corneum in the sixth month of fetal life. An extremely premature infant has thin, poorly keratinised epidermis, and is therefore vulnerable to excessive skin water losses after birth.

The sebaceous glands are active from mid gestation, and their secretion, together with the residue of the periderm, accounts for the vernix caseosa. The vernix provides a greasy coating to the newborn skin and may have bactericidal properties. Term infants are able to sweat within two to five days after birth, but there may be a delay of two to three weeks in the premature. Sebum and sweat retention are common in the newborn.

Milia

These are minute sebaceous material cysts which give rise to yellowish-white specks over the nose and face. Although they may be very conspicuous in the first days of life, they disappear spontaneously after three to four weeks.

Miliaria

This is possibly the most frequent skin eruption in the first weeks of life, and reflects sweat gland immaturity and the tendency to overheat babies. It arises as crops of papules or papulo-vesicles over the face, trunk and napkin area. It generally resolves rapidly with appropriate clothing and ventilation, but may occasionally become secondarily infected.

RASHES OF EARLY INFANCY

Infantile seborrhoeic dermatitis

Seborrhoeic dermatitis is a distinctive erythematous and scaly, non-eczematous eruption of unknown cause. It usually starts during the second or third month of life as cradle cap or napkin dermatitis which spreads rapidly, sometimes giving psoriasis-like lesions over much of the body. The child is never ill and is not

Seborrhoeic dermatitis

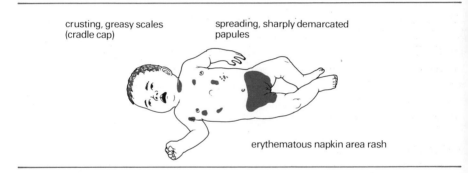

crusting, greasy scales (cradle cap)

spreading, sharply demarcated papules

erythematous napkin area rash

distressed by it. In its mildest form, just one or two lesions may be present in the flexures giving rise to an erroneous diagnosis of atopic eczema. Very mild corticosteroid and antiseptic combinations such as 1% hydrocortisone and 3% clioquinol will usually clear it.

Axilla

Napkin rashes

Rashes in the napkin area are very common and not always indicative of poor

Napkin area rashes

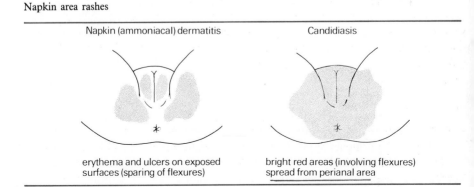

Napkin (ammoniacal) dermatitis

Candidiasis

erythema and ulcers on exposed surfaces (sparing of flexures)

bright red areas (involving flexures) spread from perianal area mothering. The main causes are napkin dermatitis, candidiasis and seborrhoeic dermatitis.

Napkin dermatitis. Napkin dermatitis is caused by prolonged contact with wet napkins. Bacterial conversion of the urine to ammonia creates an alkaline irritant. Simple measures are usually effective; frequent napkin changes, careful washing at each change and the application of a protective cream such as zinc and castor oil ointment. The napkin should be rinsed thoroughly after washing and used with disposable napkin liners.

Candidiasis. Candidiasis is commonly superimposed on a napkin rash and warrants treatment with nystatin ointment.

ATOPIC ECZEMA

Atopic eczema affects 3% of children and usually has its onset between two and eighteen months of age. There is often a family history of other atopic disorders, hay fever or asthma. Itching is very prominent and scratching frequently results in secondary infection. It has a fluctuating course with approximately 50% resolving by eighteen months and few continue to have a problem beyond childhood. Although skin prick tests for specific allergens are often positive, they provide little guide to clinical management as multiple factors are usually involved. There is some preliminary evidence that breast feeding and total avoidance of cow's milk protein in the first few months of life may reduce the incidence of atopic problems in genetically susceptible infants.

Management

Atopic eczema is a very taxing illness for child and family. Disturbed nights, irritability and the often alarming appearance add to the burden. The parents have an active role in management and need careful sympathetic instruction.

Atopic eczema

The skin is often dry because of an associated ichthyosis; the avoidance of all soap and the use of emulsifying ointment in its place helps to correct this. Corticosteroid ointments applied once or twice daily benefit the affected areas but should be used sparingly and the potency kept to the minimum necessary to control the disease. One per cent hydrocortisone cream or ointment, or betamethasone cream diluted to 1 in 10 with cetomacrogol cream, are usually adequate for all but the most stubborn patches. Secondary infection may be treated with a topical antibiotic, for example chlortetracycline or neomycin combined with a corticosteroid. If the child is pyrexial, or deeper spread of infection occurs, a systemic antibiotic should be given. The control of scratching and the provision of undisturbed nights are valuable assets. Antihistamines, for example trimeprazine tartrate or promethazine, used as night sedation are well tolerated and valuable if given as a short course during exacerbation. Other useful measures include using cotton underclothes rather than wool, avoiding heat, and light bandaging of the limbs at night. The hands must never be tied to prevent scratching. There is no contraindication to immunisation against diphtheria, whooping cough, tetanus and poliomyelitis, but these should be given when the eczema is in a less acute phase. Primary infection with herpes simplex virus may give a very severe reaction known as Kaposi's varicelliform eruption.

INFECTIONS AND INFESTATIONS

Bacterial

Impetigo. This is a highly contagious superficial skin infection which passes rapidly through a vesicular phase and usually presents with typical golden brown crusts. Topical therapy with the application of 3% chlortetracycline cream is adequate for limited infections. More extensive lesions require a systemic antibiotic, for example erythromycin. Refractory or atypical cases raise the possibility of an underlying cause such as scabies, scalp pediculosis or an immune deficiency.

Bacterial skin infection

Scalded skin syndrome

Impetigo

golden crusts

staphylococcus

streptococcus

Bullous impetigo of the newborn. This may have serious complications, for example osteomyelitis and pneumonia, and the mortality is high. Systemic antibiotics are required, for example flucloxacillin.

Toxic epidermal necrolysis (Lyell's disease, Ritter's disease or staphylococcal scalded skin syndrome). Toxic epidermal necrolysis results from epidermal cleavage due to toxins of staphylococcus phage type 71. Typically, young infants and children develop acute inflammation and soreness which evolves into a generalised exfoliation, the scalded skin syndrome. Even ordinary handling can result in skin loss and extreme care is necessary in the nursing of these children.

Viral

Primary herpes simplex. Primary herpes simplex infection is usually asymptomatic but it can produce a gingivostomatitis in young children. It presents with fever, irritability, and difficulty in swallowing. The latter is caused by extensive shallow ulcers of the buccal, gingival and pharyngeal mucosae. Occasionally there may be a vulvovaginitis or a keratoconjunctivitis.

Herpetic encephalitis is a rare but grave complication. Gingivostomatitis requires careful nursing to ensure an adequate fluid intake. Idoxuridine paint may accelerate healing if it can be successfully applied to the ulcerated mucosa.

Herpes zoster. This is not uncommon in children and usually settles without leaving post herpetic neuralgia. Povidone-iodine paint will reduce infectivity and the likelihood of secondary infection.

Viral warts. Viral warts affect most children at some time during childhood. They are harmless and self limiting, and treatment is only indicated if there is discomfort. This is most likely on the pressure bearing areas of the soles. The application of a salicylic acid based wart paint is usually all that is required.

Molluscum contagiosum. This is more likely to affect covered areas of the body. The individual lesions can be cleared by pricking the centre with a sharpened stick dipped in liquid phenol.

Fungal skin infection

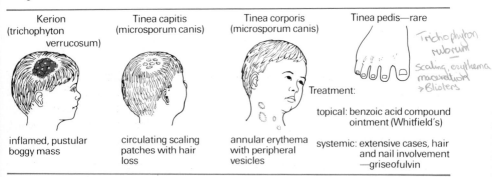

Kerion (trichophyton verrucosum)	Tinea capitis (microsporum canis)	Tinea corporis (microsporum canis)	Tinea pedis—rare
inflamed, pustular boggy mass	circulating scaling patches with hair loss	annular erythema with peripheral vesicles	Treatment: topical: benzoic acid compound ointment (Whitfield's) systemic: extensive cases, hair and nail involvement —griseofulvin

Fungal infection

Fungal infections due to the usual human dermatophytes are uncommon in childhood; a diagnosis of athlete's foot is nearly always wrong. Susceptibility to animal ringworm, especially *Microsporum canis* from cats and dogs, is quite high and scalp involvement is unique to children.

Infestations

Scabies is due to a mite which is spread by close family contact and invades the horny layer of the skin where it lays its eggs. The burrows are generally over hands, wrists, elbows, feet and genitalia but can occur on the face of babies. Infestation provokes an intense itch and a secondary erythematous papular rash. The mite may be identified using a low power lens and a needle. The whole family should be treated by a single application of benzyl benzoate emulsion to all the skin surfaces below the neck. A less irritating alternative is 1% gamma benzene hexachloride.

Skin infestation

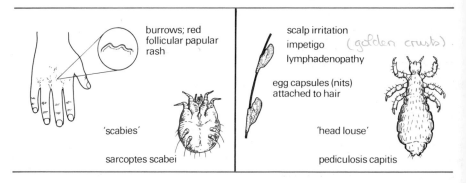

Pediculosis capitis or head lice infestation is common in our schools. It may present as a persistent itch with secondary dermatitis or be found on routine hair examination. The oval nits are easily seen firmly adhering to the hair shaft. The mature lice are less often visible. The application of 0.5% malathion solution is effective against the lice and nits.

CONGENITAL SKIN LESIONS

Birth marks

Strawberry naevus (superficial cavernous angioma). A third of these elevated lesions occur on the face and become conspicuous and grow rapidly in the first month of life. In spite of parental pressure, management must be conservative with the reassuring knowledge that spontaneous disappearance occurs by the age of five or six years.

Capillary naevus (port wine stain). This defect in dermal blood vessels can occur anywhere but is commonest on the upper half of the body. There is no tendency to fade or spread. Usually it is an isolated cosmetic problem, but occasionally there may be meningeal involvement as well, for example in the Sturge-Weber syndrome.

Pigmented naevi. These naevi are rarely evident at birth and start to appear at the age of two years. In childhood they are usually flat or only slightly elevated. Histologically they show junctional activity but malignancy is extremely rare. With maturation the majority lose their junctional elements and become intra-dermal and completely benign. Extensive macular pale brown 'café au lait' spots are a feature of neurofibromatosis.

Ichthyosis

The most frequent form is an autosomal dominant condition characterised by dry finely scaling skin. It may coincide with and complicate atopic dermatitis. Restoration of skin moisture with an emollient cream is the basis of treatment.

Congenital anhidrotic ectodermal dysplasia

This is a rare, sex-linked, recessive condition producing loss of sweat glands, dental hypoplasia, and sparse hair, eyebrows and eyelashes. These children are intolerant of heat.

Epidermolysis bullosa

This condition is a pathological susceptibility to blistering and there are a number of genetic varieties. The severity ranges from blistering with unusual trauma to serious life threatening scarring and deformity, despite careful handling.

Incontinentia pigmenti

This rare condition is almost exclusively restricted to females and is usually obvious at birth. Groups of vesicles evolve through warty papules to bizarre patterns of pigmentation. There is associated eosinophilia, dental and eye abnormalities.

Xeroderma pigmentosum

This autosomal recessive condition is manifest by dry photosensitive skin liable to freckling, keratoses and malignant transformation.

Acrodermatitis enteropathica

This produces progressive mucocutaneous ulceration and is associated with bowel pathology. It responds to treatment with zinc.

OTHER COMMON SKIN DISORDERS

Psoriasis

B-Haemolytic Strep

This commonly presents as an acute guttate rash following an upper respiratory tract infection. An eruption of small discrete red scaling lesions may develop rapidly and cover much of the body. Resolution usually occurs after two months or so, but the existence of the psoriatic tendency has been indicated and the more typical plaques on elbows, knees and scalp may develop at any time. Treatment should be kept to a minimum compatible with asymptomatic control. The application of coal tar and salicylic acid ointment after bathing is a useful measure.

May get Pustular form on One digit only!

Pityriasis rosea   *adults.   ↑ Spring + Autumn   Red-Brown*

This is an acute self limiting eruption giving rise to erythematous scaling macules *2-6 cm* with a central distribution. It may superficially resemble guttate psoriasis but is distinguished by a herald patch, which appears three or four days before the main eruption, and by the frequent presence of itching and fine scaling. A mild corticosteroid ointment may help resolution. *mild.*

Lasts 6-8 wks.

Granuloma annulare

These skin lesions consist of asymptomatic dermal nodules usually on the fingers or toes. It is a harmless condition but resolution may be slow, taking years rather than months.

Alopecia areata

These areas of localised hair loss on the scalp have a characteristic margin of exclamation mark hairs. The alopecia is usually self-limiting and possibly related to periods of school or other stress. Rare cases progress to alopecia totalis. It should be distinguished from habitual hair pulling, trichotillomania, and ringworm of the scalp in which there is an obvious inflammatory element.

Acne

Acne occasionally occurs in a child less than eighteen months old and reflects physiological adjustments in the responsiveness of sebaceous glands to postnatal hormone changes. Its occurrence later in childhood, but before the onset of puberty, requires further investigation in case of underlying adrenal pathology. It is, of course, very common in adolescence but the problem should not be discounted because it may dominate life and give rise to self-imposed isolation. It is linked to the onset of sebaceous gland activity and the production of free fatty acids in follicles which are blocked, with resulting comedones or blackheads, inflammation and pustules. Treatment is directed at removing the keratin plugs, for example with benzoyl peroxide, and suppression of lipolytic bacteria with long-term low dose antibiotics, usually tetracycline 250 mg twice daily.

Erythema nodosum

These tender erythematous nodules occur most frequently over the pretibial region. They appear in crops and may be associated with fever and arthralgia. An underlying problem may be streptococcal infection, tuberculosis, *Mycoplasma pneumoniae*, food or drug sensitivity. In the majority no underlying condition will be found.

BIBLIOGRAPHY

Solomon L M, Esterly N B 1973 Neonatal dermatology. Saunders, Philadelphia.
Solomon L M, Esterly N B, Loeffel E D 1978 Adolescent dermatology. Saunders, Philadelphia.

17
Bone and Joint

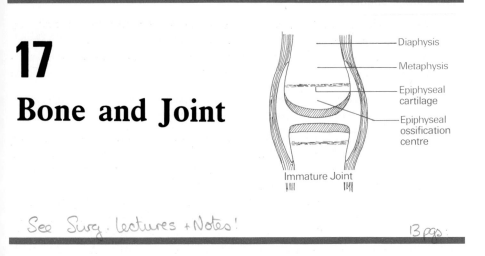

Diaphysis

Metaphysis

Epiphyseal cartilage

Epiphyseal ossification centre

Immature Joint

See Surg. lectures + Notes! *13 pgs.*

Bone tissue can be detected in the eight-week fetus. It arises from precursor mesenchymal cells which either evolve into osteoblasts and osteocytes capable of primary ossification, or into chondroblasts and chondrocytes which give rise to an initial cartilagenous model. Tissue oxygen concentration, mechanical stress and hormonal agents are some of the factors known to dictate the type of bone development. In the limbs there are also complex interactions between skeletal formation and the ectodermal covering. Mineralisation which is essential to bone structure depends on the transplacental passage of calcium, phosphorus and vitamin D or its metabolites. This mineral transfer is maximal in later gestation and the calcium content of the fetus is doubled in the last month. The calcium deficit created by premature delivery increases the requirement for vitamin D in the postnatal period. Following delivery, the skeleton continues its growth, both in length and weight. It also undergoes considerable remodelling, particularly in the first two years when the rate is 10 times that which occurs in adult life. Maturation is accompanied by progressive endochondral ossification with the appearance of epiphyseal centres and the disappearance of the growth cartilages. This maturation is subject to genetic and environmental controls and may be quantified to provide the bone age, a valuable parameter in assessing growth and its disorders.

Polyarthritis in childhood

Infection	Bacterial — pyogenic, tuberculosis
	Viral — rubella, mumps, infectious mononucleosis.
Post-infectious	Rheumatic fever
Allergic	Henoch Schönlein purpura, other allergies
Collagen vascular disease	Rheumatoid arthritis, systemic lupus erythematosis, dermatomyositis
Haematological disease	Leukaemia, haemophilia, sickle cell disease
Gastrointestinal tract disorders	Ulcerative colitis, Crohn disease, dysentery
Trauma and synovitis	

242

ARTHRITIS

A swollen, painful joint requires prompt evaluation as it may be the first sign of severe systemic illness. Young children present with fever, limp or pseudo-paralysis rather than specific joint symptoms. The problem may be localised to a single joint, in which case pyogenic infection must be excluded, or involve several joints, a polyarthritis.

Pyogenic arthritis

In pyogenic arthritis the joint is usually hot, swollen and acutely tender and more than one joint may be involved. Movement of the affected joint is restricted and very painful. The joint must be aspirated and the fluid examined by microscopy and culture, and also blood samples taken for culture at the same time. Osteomyelitis adjacent to a joint may produce a sympathetic effusion but the tenderness will be on the bony metaphysis rather than over the joint. The commonest infecting organism is *Staphylococcus pyogenes*, and flucloxacillin given intravenously is the treatment of choice. Surgical drainage is frequently required if the diagnosis is delayed beyond 48 to 72 hours from the onset of symptoms. During the acute phase of the illness the joint is splinted, but later physiotherapy and mobilisation is essential to prevent joint flexion from developing into a permanent deformity.

Rheumatic fever

See Chapter 9.

Tuberculous arthritis

Tuberculous arthritis is now very rare in Europe but occasionally presents in the spine and the larger synovial joints.

Viral arthritis

Viral arthritis may be confused with rheumatic fever or juvenile chronic polyarthitis.

Henoch Schönlein purpura

This is a diffuse, self-limiting allergic vasculitis. It is common in young children but the precipitating factors have not been fully identified. The clinical picture is readily recognisable; the majority resolving quickly and requiring only analgesics. A minority have more severe gastrointestinal manifestation and may warrant a brief course of corticosteroid therapy. The renal lesion is discussed elsewhere (p. 176).

Allergic polyarthritis

A transient allergic reaction consisting of an urticarial rash and synovitis is not uncommon. It may follow mild upper respiratory tract infections, drug or dietary allergen exposure.

Juvenile chronic arthritis (JCA)

Chronic arthritis is uncommon in childhood and is seldom accompanied by specific laboratory evidence of rheumatoid disease. The diagnosis of JCA must be based on clinical features, and other systemic disorders manifesting arthritis have to be excluded. The aetiology of JCA is unknown although there is growing evidence of genetic susceptibility with links to HLA tissue types and inherited immune deficiencies. The natural history of children with JCA has revealed the following main sub groups.

Features of systemic onset juvenile chronic arthritis

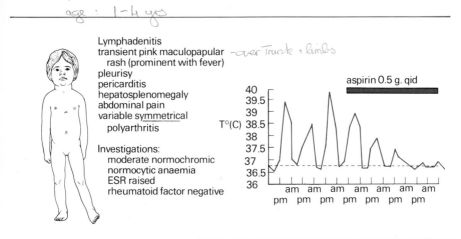

Lymphadenitis
transient pink maculopapular
   rash (prominent with fever)
pleurisy
pericarditis
hepatosplenomegaly
abdominal pain
variable symmetrical
   polyarthritis

Investigations:
   moderate normochromic
   normocytic anaemia
   ESR raised
   rheumatoid factor negative

aspirin 0.5 g. qid

T°(C)

40
39.5
39
38.5
38
37.5
37
36.5
36

am am am am am am am
pm pm pm pm pm pm pm

Systemic onset JCA (20%). Systemic onset JCA usually presents in young children between 1 and 4 years. The systemic symptoms often precede arthritis, and the diagnosis must be considered when there is difficulty establishing the cause of a remitting fever, prominent adenopathy and hepatosplenomegaly. An evanescent macular rash often coincides with the peaks of fever. The majority of patients have a self-limiting illness although there may be a pattern of relapsing and sometimes destructive arthritis.

Polyarticular onset JCA (15%). Polyarticular onset JCA is commoner in girls and affects a wider age range. It presents with symmetrical, painful swelling and stiffness of both large and small joints. These may include the cervical spine and temporo-mandibular joints.

Pauciarticular onset JCA (60%). Pauciarticular onset JCA refers to involvement of four or less joints. Younger children, predominantly girls, commonly have a positive antinuclear factor test and are prone to chronic uveitis. Older boys possessing the tissue type HLA B27 develop lower limb arthritis and may then progress to ankylosing spondylitis of variable severity. They are more vulnerable to acute iritis.

Management. The priorities in therapy are to reduce joint inflammation and to avoid deformity. Physiotherapy, drug and surgical intervention all play a role, and ophthalmic review is essential. As with other chronic and potentially handicapping disorders, affected children benefit from the skills of a specialised team.

Features of pauciarticular onset juvenile chronic arthritis

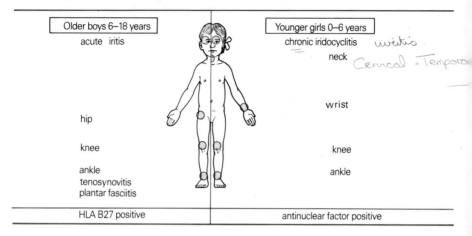

Older boys 6–18 years		Younger girls 0–6 years
acute iritis		chronic iridocyclitis _uveitis_
		neck _Cervical + Temporo_
		wrist
hip		
knee		knee
ankle		ankle
tenosynovitis		
plantar fasciitis		
HLA B27 positive		antinuclear factor positive

Aspirin in a dose of up to 80 mg per kg per day is an effective anti-inflammatory drug but young children are susceptible to salicylate toxicity without recognisable warning signs. Other non-steroidal anti-inflammatory drugs (NSAIDS) such as ibuprofen, naproxen and indomethacin are useful in JCA. Chronic active disease may justify the use of potentially hazardous drugs, for example gold, penicillamine and chloroquine. Corticosteroids are avoided if possible but may be required to control severe systemic problems, for example pericarditis. Exercise, hydrotherapy and joint splints are designed to provide each child with a carefully tailored programme aiming at maximal long-term mobility.

Prognosis differs in the various sub-groups but overall 75 to 80 per cent should have no or only minor disability after 15 years.

OSTEOMYELITIS

Osteomyelitis affects the metaphyses of long bones and is usually haematogenous in origin. The principal exception is that at the proximal femur, as the metaphysis is intracapsular, the infection may spread to the bone by direct inoculation from a primary pyoarthrosis of the hip joint. The growth plate normally acts as a barrier to extension of infection from a primary metaphysal focus to the associated epiphysis. *Staphylococcus pyogenes* accounts for 90%, with *Haemophilus influenzae* and *Streptococcus pyogenes* as less common isolates. Children with sickle cell disease are susceptible to salmonella infections and the site is frequently atypical.

Clinical features. The infected limb is painful and held immobile, pseudo-paralysis. Swelling and occasionally redness may be seen if diagnosis is delayed. Examination of all inexplicably febrile children must include careful palpation of the limbs looking for areas of local swelling and tenderness. The adjacent joint may contain a sterile, sympathetic effusion. Repeated blood culture is the most satisfactory method of determining the responsible organism and therefore establishing its antibiotic sensitivity. X-rays are not of diagnostic help in the first 10 to 14 days. The first radiological signs are subperiosteal new bone formation and

The anatomy of osteomyelitis and is distribution in 93 children, 89 with a single site and four with double sites — in parenthesis (after Mollan and Piggot)

spotty rarefaction. Radionuclide bone scan will almost always demonstrate a zone of high emission at a much earlier stage and has proved to be a most useful tool to confirm diagnosis and localise the pathology.

Management. Prompt, effective parenteral antibiotic therapy is essential for a successful outcome. Neglected cases are liable to develop irreversible bone necrosis, draining sinuses and limb deformity. Appropriate antibiotic regimens include high-dosage, intravenous flucloxacillin or fusidic acid (to cover staphylococcal infection) with ampicillin (to cover gram negative organisms) until there is an unequivocal clinical response and then effective oral therapy for up to six weeks until all the clinical, radiological and haematological parameters indicate healing of the disease. Lack of response in the first 48 hours of therapy is an indication for surgical exploration and drainage.

NORMAL POSTURAL VARIATIONS

These are common problems which arouse much parental anxiety. Reassurance is usually more appropriate than expensive shoe modifications or unnecessary physiotherapy.

In-toe gait. This may originate in the foot (metatarsus varus), in the tibia (tibial torsion), or in the femora (persistent anteversion of the femoral neck).

Causes of in-toe gait

femoral anteversion   tibial torsion   metatarsus varus

These conditions are symmetrical, pain free and are accompanied by normal mobility. They generally resolve in three to four years.

Out-toe gait. Out-toe gait is also common in the first two years of life and may be unilateral. It always corrects spontaneously.

Genu varum (bow legs). Outward curving of the tibia is usually assciated with internal tibial torsion, is not uncommon and always corrects with growth. Severe examples should raise the suspicion of rickets (nutritional in susceptible groups, or the congenital hypophosphataemic form) or Blount disease, a rare developmental abnormality of the proximal tibial epiphysis.

Genu valgum (knock-knees). This is frequent in the 2 to $4\frac{1}{2}$ year age-group and is usually innocent if symmetrical and independent of any other abnormality. Severe and progressive cases raise the possibility of rickets which is most frequently seen among Asian immigrant children. Rickets may be confirmed by the x-ray appearance of the typical frayed metaphyseal changes and by an elevated serum alkaline phosphatase.

Knock knees and flat feet

genu valgum

pes planus

Flat feet. The medial arch of the foot develops within two to three years of walking. It is largely obliterated by a fat pad in younger children. Persistent flat feet may be familial or reflect joint laxity. It is insignificant if the foot is pain free, mobile and develops an arch when standing on tiptoe. Neurological problems and pathological joint laxity are occasional underlying causes. Severe convex flat foot is occasionally due to congenital vertical talus, in which condition early surgical treatment can avoid crippling deformity in later life.

SCOLIOSIS

Scoliosis, a term coined by Galen, refers to a spinal curve in the coronal plane. Scoliosis may be postural or structural. Structural curves are fixed and associated with vertebral rotation which produces, in the thoracic region, rib asymmetry detectable most easily when the child bends forwards. A postural curve will correct with adjustment of posture and is not accompanied by rotation. Such a curve will not evolve to a structural scoliosis.

Structural scoliosis, its anatomy and clinical detection

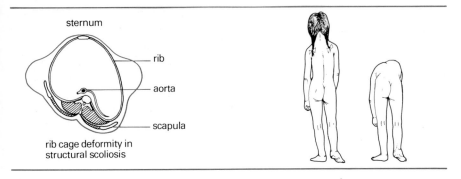

sternum

rib

aorta

scapula

rib cage deformity in
structural scoliosis

Structural scoliosis. This may be idiopathic, either infantile ('early onset') or adolescent ('late onset'), congenital (with hemivertebrae or unsegmented lateral bony tethers) or secondary to other disease, such as osteogenesis imperfecta, Marfan syndrome or neurofibromatosis. Neuromuscular imbalance, as in poliomyelitis, cerebral palsy, or muscular dystrophy, can also result in a severe scoliosis.

Idiopathic adolescent scoliosis. Eighty to 85 per cent of all structural scoliosis falls into this group, affecting mainly girls in the age range 10 to 14 years. Great efforts have been made in the last decade to detect such cases early by programmes of school screening and this has resulted in many early curves being treated successfully by bracing; it is not, however, established that this has reduced the need for surgery. Thus, the value of screening programmes is uncertain and as the late onset curve, even allowed to progress unchecked, is unlikely to produce life-threatening cardio-respiratory compromise from thoracic deformity, the problem is primarily a cosmetic one, albeit severe. The WHO has suggested that screening for cosmetic problems is not a justifiable resource allocation.

Physiotherapy has no place in the treatment of structural scoliosis. Curves of up to 40° or 50°, depending on age of onset, are usually treated by a thoraco-lumbo-sacral orthosis (TLSO) which controls progression in about 70% of cases.

HIP DISORDERS

Congenital dislocation of the hip

Early detection of the lax hip at birth is important as it permits a relatively simple and safe treatment protocol with a high expectancy of a normal hip as the outcome. Delay in diagnosis leads to progressively severe dysplasia of both the femoral head and the acetabulum resulting in the need for more complex management, including the possibility of a long surgical programme.

The precise aetiology is unknown. Wynn-Davies (1970) found a high incidence of both shallow acetabulum and of congenital joint laxity in the first order relatives of CDH patients. There is wide variation in the geographical incidence of the condition. Established, irreducible CDH, in the absence of a neonatal screening and treatment programme is found in about 1.5 per 1000 live births in most European groups. The Lapps and the North American Indians, who swaddle their infants with the hips extended and the legs together, have a much higher incidence; the Island Lake Manitoba Indian community, who still use the cradleboard have a 4% incidence of CDH. It is a rare condition among ethnic groups who carry the infant with its legs astride the mother's pelvis, as in black Africans and the Chinese. It is against this background that it is believed that posturing the hips in subtotal abduction-in-flexion (the 'human' position as opposed to the 'frog' position) is believed to prevent the evolution of the lax neonatal hip into a fully established, irreducible dislocation. Screening for neonatal hip laxity and treatment by splintage is likely, with a well-controlled programme, to reduce the incidence of late-diagnosis CDH.

Neonatal screening. These techniques must be learnt by practical instruction from an experienced clinician. The infant should be well-fed, warm, relaxed and lain on a firm surface. The hips and knees are flexed to 90° with one examining hand to each leg. The thumb should be on the inner side of the babe's knee and the ring and little fingers behind the greater trochanter. Gentle but firm pressure is applied in the line of the femur, so that a lax hip would be dislocated posteriorly. The thighs are then abducted fully with a gentle motion, at the same time lifting the greater trochanter forwards; this motion is less like opening a book and more like opening a surgical 'peel pack'. It is the movement which has to be learned. If a hip is lax, the reduction which occurs as the legs are abducted will be felt as a clunk or jumping sensation. Many normal hips 'crack' or click (like pulled finger joints!) and only experience can teach the distinction between clunks and clicks.

A variant of this test is to steady the pelvis with one hand with the thumb over the pubic symphysis and the fingers of the same hand behind the buttocks, and then with the other hand holding the examined leg as before, attempt to rock the head of the femur backwards and forwards in and out of the socket. This test must be applied in different degrees of abduction until the 'lax arc' is found.

Any doubt about a hip should lead to referral to an orthopaedic surgeon with paediatric experience. Any child whose hip has been suspect should be x-rayed at 3 to 6 months of age.

Infants statistically at risk are relatives of other lax hip children, first born females, babies born by breech delivery (or by LSCS after a breech intrauterine

Ortolani test for congenital dislocation of hip

hips flexed 90°   knees flexed

clunk+

Congenital dislocation of hip: radiology and management

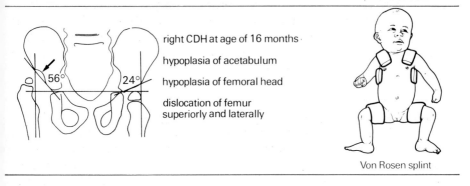

right CDH at age of 16 months

hypoplasia of acetabulum

hypoplasia of femoral head

dislocation of femur
superiorly and laterally

Von Rosen splint

position) and those with³foot deformities orʰsternomastoid 'tumour'.

Management. The infant whose hips remain suspect by the second or third week of life should be splinted and referred for orthopaedic follow-up. The use of an appropriate splint (von Rosen or Craig type), properly applied and adjusted, for a period of about three months will in most cases be all that is required. X-rays must be used to confirm normal hip joint development until independent walking. X-rays are of little use under three months of age. The finding of limited abduction in flexion at the hip is a feature of the established dislocation and is, therefore, not a sign which develops until about three to four months of age. Conversely, the clunk will disappear at about three weeks of age when the hip first becomes irreducible. The lack of a diagnostic clinical or radiological indicator in this three-week to three-month period has led to it being referred to as the 'grey' diagnostic period. Sadly, it is within this period, at about six weeks of age, that most infants have their major post-natal check!

It is unfortunately true that dislocated hips are still missed in spite of the widespread introduction of screening procedures. Suspicion is raised by a child with a shortened leg, or with a gait in which the affected foot is placed flat on the ground while the opposite knee is flexed. It does not generally delay the onset of walking but may well cause frequent falls. Bilateral cases have a symmetrical gait and tend to present even later if missed in the neonatal period. Attempted reduction of the hip involves initial traction followed by more prolonged splintage or in the event of failure, operative intervention. The latter may involve open reduction, femoral osteotomy and acetabular reconstruction.

Transient synovitis   2-12 yrs.
This is the most common cause of limp, with hip and/or knee pain, in young children. It is a unilateral, self-limiting condition of ill-defined aetiology although many follow a mild upper respiratory tract infection. Boys in the age group 2 to 12 years (average six years) are most susceptible. It usually has a sudden onset with limp, and pain of variable severity. Abduction, full extension and internal rotation are restricted and there may be tenderness over the anterior aspect of the hip. There is usually no leucocytosis, and the ESR is normal or only mildly elevated. X-rays are normal. The diagnosis can only be made after exclusion of

Exclude 1. infection - at/near hip jt.
2. Perthes Disease
3. Slipped Upper femoral epiphyses.
4. 1° Neoplasm — Benign
— Malignant.

BONE AND JOINT   251

an infective process at or adjacent to the hip joint, Perthes' disease, slipped upper femoral epiphysis or even a primary neoplasm, benign or malignant.

Transient synovitis seldom lasts for more than a few days or weeks and treatment consists of simple analgesics and bed rest often with simple skin traction. Approximately 6% of cases considered to have transient synovitis subsequently develop features of Perthes' disease.

Perthes disease   4-8yo.

This results from episodes of segmental avascular necrosis of the femoral head. The necrotic bone is gradually replaced by new bone, but recovery can be complicated by residual deformity of the femoral head. It is most common in the four to eight-year age group and the ratio of boys to girls is 5:1. The underlying cause has not been established but it is suspected that the femoral head disorder is part of a more generalised growth disturbance in which skeletal development is retarded.

Limp, with or without pain, is the presenting complaint and hip mobility, especially abduction and internal rotation, is limited. The hip x-ray reflects the natural history of the bone necrosis; initial increase in density followed by fragmentation and reossification. The identification of the femoral head at risk of deformity is central to management; the head at risk is usually treated by 'containment' in the acetabulum either by femoral osteotomy or bracing. The healing phase during which the head requires protection lasts two to four years.

Slipped upper femoral epiphyses   ♀ 10-14 yrs   ♂ : 12-16yo.

This condition, occurring during the adolescent growth spurt (10 to 14 years in girls; 12 to 16 in boys), is a posterior slipping of the epiphysis of the femoral head in relation to its metaphysis, a shearing failure of the growth plate resulting. The slip may be acute after minimal trauma (massive trauma is required to displace a normal proximal femoral epiphysis) or gradual. Atypically early presentation should lead to the search for an underlying endocrine disease, the commonest being hypothyroidism.

The condition is bilateral, but not necessarily synchronous, in about 25% of cases. Obese children with delayed secondary sexual development, or tall thin boys, appear to be especially susceptible. Pain in the hip, the thigh or the knee associated with limp in this age group demands urgent referral for investigation. Slipped upper femoral epiphysis is a true emergency, as massive further slipping may supervene without warning at any time.

Treatment is by pin fixation in situ for mild slips and by either open reduction and fixation or femoral osteotomy for major slips. Manipulation should never be attempted, it either fails to improve the position or, if it produces a reduction, avascular necrosis of the femoral head is then highly likely.

KNEE DISORDERS

The knee is a common source of complaint among adolescents. In assessing the cause of knee pain, the hip must also be examined as hip pain is often referred to the knee.

Osgood Schlatter syndrome

Osgood Schlatter syndrome is a painful, tender swelling of the tibial tubercle due to repeated minor avulsion trauma at the site of insertion of the patellar tendon — a traction apophysitis. It is an example of an overuse syndrome and is caused by excess physical exertion before skeletal maturity. Most cases will resolve with a total embargo on sport, swimming, physical education, cycling, etc. for up to six months. Return to these activities should then be graduated and moderated if a recurrence is to be avoided. Resistant cases usually resolve after a period of rest for 6 to 8 weeks in a plaster cylinder cast.

Chondromalacia patellae

Chondromalacia patella indicates softening of the articular cartilage of the patellae usually as the result of indirect trauma, for example unaccustomed games activity. The retropatellar pain is worse on rising from prolonged sitting or on stairs, and is accompanied by crepitus. Avoidance of repetitive knee bending and physical recreation is usually adequate advice. Occasional cases have patellar misalignment worthy of surgery.

TALIPES (CLUBFOOT)

Talipes equinovarus

The fixed clubfoot is one of the most complex deformities facing orthopaedic surgeons as it represents disruption of complicated interrelationships between bone, ligament and muscle. The incidence is 1.2 per 1000 live births, rising by 20-fold where there is an affected first degree relative. Males are more at risk by a ratio of 3:1, and 50% of cases are bilateral. All cases must be examined carefully to exclude an underlying neurological problem

Treatment is largely determined by the rigidity of the deformity and by the secondary changes. In the earliest stages, gradual manipulative correction is combined with strapping. Over a period of six to eight weeks this results in correction of approximately 60% of cases. If the hind foot remains in an equinus position operation is required to release the responsible soft tissue shortening. Manipulation and strapping are continued until the foot will evert and dorsiflex beyond the neutral position. In the final stages, Denis Browne's bootee splints,

[handwritten margin notes: ⊕ XRay ? 3/12 ? operal]

Talipes

Talipes —   equinovarus   calcaneovalgus

in which open-ended boots are attached to a crossbar, are worn at night. The whole course of treatment may continue until at least five years of age. A true correction must be obtained by three months of age and if this goal has not been reached, then surgical soft tissue release is usually undertaken without delay. Failure to achieve early true correction may result in th need for corrective bone surgery later in childhood.

Talipes calcaneovalgus

In this deformity the foot is dorsiflexed and everted but the underlying structural abnormality is less profound and the foot is more amenable to simple manipulation.

GENETIC BONE AND JOINT DISORDERS

Marfan disease (autosomal dominant)

This disease consists of arachnodactyly, hypermobile joints, ocular abnormalities, and a high arched palate. There are commonly associated deformities of the spine and chest. The prognosis is determined by associated cardiovascular problems such as dilated aortic root, dissecting aortic aneurism and billowing mitral valve incompetence.

Cleido-cranial dysostosis (autosomal dominant)

The features include absence of part or all of the clavicle, and delayed ossification of the skull with persistent open skull sutures. Affected children also tend to be short.

Diaphyseal aclasis, multiple cartilagenous exostoses (autosomal dominant)

This disorder of the growth plate results in multiple cartilage capped osteomas arising at the ends of long bones. The multiple bony swellings make their appearance in infancy and increase in number and size during growth. They may cause pain, deformity and growth impairment. A proportion of patients, probably less than 5%, are liable to malignant sarcoma transformation in adult life.

Osteogenesis imperfecta (autosomal dominant, occasionally recessive)

In this condition there is an underlying failure in collagen metabolism resulting in multiple fractures of fragile bones, lax joints and thin skin. Blue sclerae, scoliosis, hypoplastic teeth and progressive deafness are also features. The congenital form may be of such severity that the fetus dies *in utero* or shortly after birth. The later onset variety is compatible with a reasonable prognosis and may present in adolescence as 'osteoporosis'.

Osteopetrosis or marble bone disease (autosomal recessive or autosomal dominant)

The recessive form is more severe causing bone marrow failure and early death. The dominant or less severe form presents in childhood as facial paralysis, bone fractures and osteomyelitis. Bone marrow transplantation has had limited success in reintroducing normal osteoblast and osteoclast function.

BONE TUMOURS AND ALLIED DISORDERS

Features suggestive of a bone tumour include pain, swelling or a limp. Fortunately the majority of underlying lesions are benign; atypical osteomyelitis, incomplete fracture of normal bone, a simple cyst or an osteoid osteoma.

Simple bone cysts (unicameral cysts)

These are most frequently see in the metaphyseal regions of long bones and are discovered usually only when they fracture and cause pain. The x-ray features are characteristic. They fill in spontaneously and disappear shortly after skeletal maturity. The fractures heal readily but the cyst often remains. Treatment is usually by washout of the cyst using two wide-bore needles inserted under anaesthetic and x-ray control, followed by the instillation of triamcinolone acetate.

Osteoid osteoma

This may present with intermittent and often nocturnal pain, classically responding to aspirin. X-rays show extensive periosteal thickening with a focus of dense new bone surrounding a centrally placed radiolucent nidus. The majority are so painful that surgical removal of the nidus is required. These lesions concentrate bone-seeking radionuclides such as technetium-99 m compounds and this can be exploited to locate them at surgery by the use of sterilisible miniature gamma ray detectors. Recurrence is virtually unknown after successful removal of the nidus tissue.

Ewing tumour and osteosarcoma

These are the two most common malignant primary bone tumours in childhood. The former has to be distinguished from secondary neuroblastoma which commonly metastasises to bone. Radiology can normally distinguish Ewing tumour, which produces characteristic periosteal new bone formation, from osteosarcoma where there is more prominent bone destruction and infiltration. The introduction of combined local radiotherapy, or ablative surgery with chemotherapy, has brought a note of optimism to these previously dismal conditions. Osteosarcoma is less responsive to chemotherapy but recent programmes combining high dosage methotrexate, folinic acid 'rescue', adriamycin and early radical amputation demonstrates remarkably improved results up to the present time. It is however emerging that adjuvant chemotherapy may only delay metastasis and some long-term studies are showing a late reduction in survival figures. A period of chemotherapy prior to surgical ablation, followed by a cyclical adjuvant regimen is a recent promising protocol.

BIBLIOGRAPHY

Ansell B M 1980 Rheumatic disorders in childhood. Butterworths, London
Asher C 1975 Postural variations in childhood. Butterworths, London
Blockey, N J 1976 Children's orthopaedics — practical problems. Butterworths, London
Craft A W 1985 Arthritis in children. British Journal of Hospital Medicine 33: 188–194
Fixsen J A 1977 Borderline orthopaedic abnormalities in children. Hospital Update 3: 185–191
Lloyd-Roberts G C 1971 Orthopaedics in infancy and childhood. Butterworths, London
Mollan R A B, Piggot J 1977 Acute osteomyelitis in children. Journal of Bone and Joint Surgery 59B:2
Wynne-Davies R 1970 Acetabular dysplasia and joint laxity. Journal of Bone and Joint Surgery 52B:704

18
Brain, Nerve, Muscle

All who are concerned with the safe passage of children from conception to adulthood, have as a prime goal the preservation of normal brain development. Potential hazards have effects which are largely determined by the degree of differentiation of the nervous system. In the first trimester genetic and environmental influences may disrupt embryogenesis and produce malformations which either abort or reach term as gross anomalies, for example anencephaly and spina bifida. In later fetal life and during infancy insults are more likely to produce focal, irreversible pathology in differentiated tissue, lesions which may well be the basis of cerebral palsy.

In addition to interference with structural differentiation, the brain is also susceptible to problems during its various growth spurts. In the human fetus maximal neuronal proliferation occurs in the mid-trimester and is relatively protected from maternal malnutrition and placental dysfunction, but is vulnerable to viral infection, radiation, drugs and excessive alcohol. Glial multiplication and myelination occurs over a more extended period from the third antenatal trimester through the first two years of life and is therefore exposed to the effects of intra- and extrauterine malnutrition, perinatal asphyxia and inborn errors of metabolism. We are only on the threshold of understanding how these hazards may influence the subtler components of growth, dendritic proliferation and synaptic connectivity.

INTRA-CRANIAL INFECTION

Acute infection of the meninges may be viral (aseptic meningitis), or bacterial (acute purulent meningitis) in origin. Meningitis may also be due to tuberculosis and rarer pathogens such as fungi and protozoa. Leukaemic cell infiltration can cause a sterile meningitis.

Acute purulent meningitis
Purulent meningitis is relatively common in childhood especially in preschool years, 35% of childhood cases occurring in the first and 80% in the first five years

Bacterial meningitis: clinical features and common causative organisms

fever
irritability, drowsiness
vomiting, diarrhoea

bulging   high pitched cry   limited extension of knee
fontanelle   and hip (Kernig sign)
(infants)

otitis media does not   arched back
exclude meningitis   neck stiffness

Neonate:

E coli and other gram -ve organisms
group B haemolytic streptococcus

Infant and child:

H. influenzae
N. meningitidis
pneumococcus

of life. In the U.K. one in 500 children suffer from purulent meningitis between the age of one month and ten years. It is essential to make an early diagnosis as delay increases the risk of death or neurological complications.

The characteristic features of meningeal irritation, neck stiffness and Kernig sign are often absent in children under 18 months of age. Such young infants are more likely to present with a fever, poor feeding, vomiting and drowsiness. Some in this age group have a convulsion as the first sign of illness. An infant who has a fever with convulsion almost invariably warrants a lumbar puncture. The development of complicating meningitis may be the reason why a child with an otitis media or other upper respiratory tract infection fails to respond to an antibiotic and becomes increasingly drowsy. On the other hand children with an upper respiratory tract infection, cervical lymphadenitis or pneumonia may show meningismus, that is they have the signs of meningeal irritation in the absence of intracranial disease.

Treatment. For children older than three months an intravenous high dosage cefotaxime regime, 200 mg/kg/day is appropriate until the microorganism and its antibiotic sensitivies have been identified. *Haemophilus influenzae* infection requires the cefotaxime to be continued for at least 10 days. *Neisseria meningitidis* and *Diplococcus pneumoniae* are usually very sensitive to parenteral benzylpenicillin, 250 000 units/kg/day.

[handwritten margin notes: Brudzinski's sign (flex 2nd h during K.S) Opisthotonus (1 Ext of head + S]

[handwritten: STEROIDS !]
[handwritten: Antiepileptic.]

Lumbar puncture

*[handwritten:
Causes of Meningism
1 meningitis, encephalitis
2. Acute otitis media.
3. Severe tonsillitis
4. Cervical lymphadenitis
5. Pneumonia.
6. Retropharyngeal abscess]*

blood glucose
blood culture

LP needle with
introducer

CSF avoid cooling (N. meningitidis is fragile)

microscopy—gram stain, culture (tuberculosis needs Zeil Nielson
                                    or immunofluorescent stain)
chemistry—protein and glucose

Cerebrospinal fluid findings in meningitis

	Normal*	Acute purulent meningitis	Aseptic (viral) meningitis	Tuberculous meningitis
appearance	clear	cloudy	usually clear	opalescent
cells/mm^3	0–5 lymphocytes	10–100 000 polymorphs	15–2000 lymphocytes	250–500 lymphocytes
glucose mmol/l	2.8–4.4 (CSF >60% blood)	low (CSF <60% blood)	normal (CSF >60% blood)	very low (CSF <60% blood)
protein g/l	0.15–0.35	0.5–5.0	0.2–1.25	0.45–5.00

* in the postnatal period normal CSF contains a higher cell and protein content.

Children with meningococcal infections often have a widespread purpuric rash and are liable to develop septicaemic shock. Purpura in a febrile child suggests major infection and must always be regarded seriously, for treatment should be commenced as soon as possible. Other children in the family are also vulnerable and should be provided with prophylaxis, rifampicin 20 mg/kg/day for four days. Chronic nasal carriage of *N. meningitidis* is relatively common but difficult to eradicate.

Complications. Meningitis is often complicated by convulsions and there is an argument for the prophylactic use of the intravenous phenytoin or phenobarbitone. Inappropriate anti-diuretic hormone release often accompanies intracranial problems and can lead to hyponatraemia which may be prevented by careful restriction of intravenous and oral fluids. Subdural effusions are probably frequent but the majority are small and insignificant. Occasionally, an enlarging head circumference and bulging fontanelle suggest a larger accumulation. This may be visualised by transilluminating the skull, or ultrasound or CT scanning, and confirmed by performing a subdural tap when a fluid containing a high protein content can be aspirated. A rapidly increasing head circumference may also be a consequence of hydrocephalus due to inflammatory obstruction of the CSF pathways. About 10% of all children surviving meningitis have long-term neurological abnormality; convulsions, deafness, spasticity, mental handicap or other learning difficulties.

Recurrent meningitis raises the possibility of a congenital mid-line sinus, or a post-traumatic dural defect providing communication with an air sinus. An immune deficiency should also be considered.

Neonatal meningitis. This affects one in every 4000 babies. It is a very serious illness and is usually due to gram negative bacilli or group B haemolytic streptococci. It has a high mortality and a majority of survivors have some neurological sequelae. Therapy must be directed towards the ventriculitis which is often associated. Systemic treatment must be with drugs like chloramphenicol or cefotaxime which are known to produce good concentrations in ventricular CSF.

Viral meningitis

Viral meningitis is commoner than it is realised. It may be accompanied by a macular rash or preceded by upper respiratory tract or gastrointestinal complaints. The symptoms of viral meningitis are usually less abrupt and milder than with acute purulent meningitis. Cerebrospinal fluid examination and culture is obviously essential to make the distinction. Serial viral titres, nasopharyngeal and rectal swabs may identify the virus.

Tuberculous meningitis

Tuberculous meningitis must be considered in every case of aseptic meningitis or encephalitis. It follows the rupture of a tubercle (Rich focus) into the cerebrospinal fluid and evolves as the resulting inflammatory reaction and arteritis develops. The cerebrospinal fluid examination is not always diagnostic in early cases. A tuberculin skin test is positive in 75% and a chest X-ray shows a suggestive lesion in 80%. Treatment is dealt with in the section dealing with tuberculosis.

Brain abscess

This is a relatively rare condition, there is usually a predisposing cause. Although it is essential to consider lumbar puncture in every child at risk of having intracranial infection, this procedure should be deferred if there are features of raised intra-cranial pressure. A neurosurgical opinion must be sought.

Brain abscess: aetiology, clinical features and treatment

Encephalitis

Encephalitis produces [1] fever, [2] disturbed consciousness, [3] convulsions and [4] focal neurological signs. The majority of cases are viral and there may also be features of meningitis or spinal cord involvement (meningoencephalitis and encephalomyelitis). Viral invasion of nervous tissue may result in immediate inflammation and destruction, mainly of grey matter, or may provoke a delayed immunologically mediated demyelination of white matter.

An encephalitis-like illness without fever or aseptic meningitis raises the possibility of a 'toxic' or metabolic encephalopathy. Lead poisoning and drug ingestion must always be considered.

Herpes simplex encephalitis. This is the most common sporadic severe encephalitis. Only 10 to 15% have associated herpetic gingivostomatitis or skin lesions. Focal seizures and neurological signs are frequent and may suggest a temporal lobe space occupying lesion. The mortality rate is 70% and neurological

Viral meningoencephalitis

Infectious		Post-infectious

Enterovirus
  coxsackie
  poliomyelitis
  echo		

Myxovirus
  mumps
  rabies
		measles 1 : 1000
		rubella 1 : 5000

Herpes virus
  h. simplex
  h. zoster
		varicella 1 : 1000

Arthropod-borne
  yellow fever
  dengue fever		

Other viruses
  lymphocytic choriomeningitis
  psittacosis
		pox virus
		vaccinia 1 in 100,000

sequelae are frequent in the survivors. The cerebrospinal fluid contains a variably elevated white cell count and may be blood stained. Electroencephalography and computerised axial tomography help to distinguish this encephalitis from a cerebral abscess or tumour. The development of potentially successful anti-viral therapy, acyclovir, has emphasised the need for prompt treatment whenever the disease is suspected. Retrospective diagnosis can be made later by showing increasing antibody titres to *H. simplex* in blood and CSF.

Post-infectious encephalitis
The more common varieties have the following frequencies; measles 1 in 1000; varicella 1 in 1000; rubella 1 in 5000, vaccinia 1 in 100 000.

Measles encephalitis. This commences with irritability, drowsiness and multiple seizures two to four days after the appearance of the rash. The EEG shows a severe diffuse abnormality. The course varies from complete recovery in a few days to death in status epilepticus or grossly impaired recovery. There is no specific treatment.

Subacute sclerosing panencephalitis (SSPE). SSPE is a prototype of human slow virus infection which is now recognised as a late complication of measles. The disease may progress over a period of years or death can occur as soon as six weeks after onset. The persistence of virus in the brain may be due to a defective immune response when measles is acquired at an early age. It enters the differential diagnosis of degenerative brain disorders.

Varicella. This causes a relatively benign encephalitis, often an acute self-limiting cerebellar ataxia.

Reye syndrome. This refers to the association of acute encephalopathy with brain swelling and diffuse fatty infiltration of the liver. Viral infections, particularly influenze B and varicella, have been linked to certain epidemics but the aetiology of this condition is largely a mystery. Vomiting or symptoms of an upper respiratory infection often precede the onset of lethargy and seizures and hyperventilation frequently accompany the increasing coma. A CT scan shows cerebral oedema and the CSF cells and protein are normal. Clinical jaundice does not occur but a prolonged prothrombin time and elevated aminotransferases and ammonia in the blood give evidence of liver involvement. Blood and CSF glucose levels are sometimes reduced. The treatment of Reye syndrome is aimed at reducing the raised intracranial pressure by hyperventilation, hypothermia and osmotherapy. Mortality is 40% but the majority of survivors are neurologically intact (see p. 164).

EPILEPSY AND CONVULSIONS

The definition of terms is important when discussing epilepsy and other causes of transient loss of consciousness in children. The diagnosis of epilepsy has major medical and social implications. Unfortunately it is common for the diagnosis to be made in error and for inappropriate drug regimens to be initiated.

Epilepsy implies a primary disorder of the brain producing recurrent electrical disturbances and resulting in epileptic attacks. It can only be diagnosed if there has been more than one epileptic attack. A child who has only had one convulsion cannot be said to have epilepsy because he may never have another. The prevalence of epilepsy amongst schoolchildren is in the order of eight per 1000.

A convulsion is a non-specific term and refers to all major motor attacks both epileptic and non-epileptic. The terms fit and seizure are also used in this context.

The differential diagnosis of convulsions

Non-epileptic convulsion	Epilepsy
1. Febrile	Idiopathic
2. Metabolic: hypoglycaemia hypocalcaemia hypomagnesaemia hypo/hypernatraemia	Secondary: cerebral malformation cerebral tumour cerebral degeneration cerebral damage
	Differential diagnosis: faints or syncopies breath holding benign paroxysmal vertigo
3. toxins, poisons	migraine nightmares
4. inflammatory	nightmares
5. trauma	tics

Clinical types of epilepsy

Major motor or grand-mal epilepsy. Major motor epilepsy is by far the most common type and consists of loss of consciousness, falling, an initial transient stiffness or tonic phase which may be associated with cyanosis, and then generalised rhythmic jerking, the clonic phase. The attack is usually over a few minutes and is followed by a period of post-ictal drowsiness. If the clonic phase

Febrile Convulsion:

4% of children.

rarely < 6/12   (N) 1-2 yrs.

+ve J. Hx.

Unwell, hot.
   ⤷ Seizure (mins)

Pyrexial.

URTI. - often!.

? UTI   } - esp if < 6/12.
? Meningitis }

Benign => <10 Mins - Good Prog.

Recurrences Common -   Tepid Sponging
                          Diazepam Suppositories

Risk > epilepsy :   2%.   of Benign
                     4%.   of atypical / Prolonged
                     6%.   of Pre-existing Neurological
                                            abnormality

Fits in the Newborn Period

* Hypoxia
* . Hypoglycaemia .   , Hyponatraemia .
* . Hypocalcaemia .   Hypernatraemia .
* . Infection .
  Kernicterus
  Haemorrhage (Cerebral) .
  Cerebral defects + Malformation .
  Narcotic withdrawal Syndrome .

Rare Metabolic Syndromes

        Apnoea ___ obstructive .   Migraine
                                                     Syncope
        Aspiration   —   Hysteria
                                                     Tourette
                                                     (epilepsy)

Infancy: Reyes Syndrome .
           Near-Miss SIDS — (gas exchange)
           Drugs : Antihistamines .
           Pertussis —   (± whoop)
           Epilepsy — Infantile Spasms .

Toddlers: Benign Febrile Convulsions .
           Breath holding .
> 5yrs: Epilepsy   (Hysteria / Malingerin

is prolonged beyond 20 minutes the child is said to be in status epilepticus. This is a medical emergency as it may lead to death from asphyxia or exhaustion.

Focal motor epilepsy. Focal motor epilepsy consists of twitching or jerking of one side of the face, one arm or one leg. Consciousness is usually retained or only slightly impaired and the child does not usually fall. Sometimes jerking can be seen to spread across one side of the face or along a limb; this is called a 'Jacksonian march'. A focal motor attack may proceed to a major motor attack with loss of consciousness, falling and generalised convulsions. Focal motor epilepsy often falls into the secondary or symptomatic category.

Psychomotor or temporal lobe epilepsy. This is often difficult to diagnose in children because the child finds it hard to describe the complex sensory phenomena. Any stereotyped episodic behaviour such as lip smacking or well organised motor phenomena associated with momentary loss of awareness may represent temporal lobe epilepsy.

Myoclonic epilepsy. This is characterised by single or repetitive contractions of muscles or groups of muscles. Myoclonic seizures are usually due to underlying brain damage, for example the result of perinatal hypoxia. A variant of this form of epilepsy, akinetic attacks, results in sudden loss of body tone and a fall to the ground. ⌐Drop attacks.

Infantile spasms. Infantile spasms represent a rare form of epilepsy seen only in young children. It usually commences between three and eight months of age. The majority show typical flexion, jack-knife or salaam spasms, which may occur as often as several hundred times a day. The spasm involves sudden flexion of the neck, trunk and limbs and lasts one to three seconds. It may be preceded by a cry. Although treatment may control the spasms, it often does not affect the associated mental deterioration, and many children are left severely handicapped.

Petit-mal attacks. These consist of episodes of impaired consciousness without falling or involuntary movements. The child stops whatever he is doing and looks vacant for 5 to 20 seconds and then continues as if nothing had happened. Characteristically petit-mal attacks can be induced by hyperventilation. They are not seen under the age of two years, have their peak incidence between five and nine years, and seldom persists into adult life. Petit mal epilepsy with diagnostic three cycle per second spike-wave discharges on EEG is a relatively rare condition. Petit mal-like attacks without this specific EEG finding are much more common.

Assessment. All children with suspected epilepsy should be fully assessed. A careful and detailed history from someone who has witnessed the attacks is of the utmost importance. General examination with special emphasis on developmental and neurological aspects is also required. A skull X-ray and fasting blood sugar and calcium estimations are often indicated.

An EEG may help to decide if doubtful attacks are epileptic or not, and may give some help in deciding the kind of epilepsy present. Caution is necessary as a normal EEG is seen in a number of children with attacks highly suggestive of epilepsy, and conversely abnormal discharges may occasionally be seen in EEGs from children who have never had an attack of any kind. A child with infantile spasms usually has a very severe EEG abnormality termed hypsarrhythmia. Some children have photosensitive epilepsy induced for example by a flickering television screen, and this may be confirmed by the EEG. Focal motor and psychomotor attacks are associated with cortical spike foci. There is no single EEG pattern which characterises major motor convulsions and many kinds of EEG abnormality may be seen.

A CT head scan may be required if there are clinical grounds to suspect a structural lesion of the brain or if the EEG shows a persistent slow wave focus.

Management. Children with epilepsy require regular drug therapy in an attempt to prevent further convulsions. Experience has shown that certain categories of epilepsy respond best to particular groups of anticonvulsants.

Drug therapy in epilepsy

Type of epilepsy	Drug of first choice	Other drugs
Grand mal epilepsy	Sodium valproate	Phenytoin Carbamazepine
Focal epilepsy	Carbamazepine	Phenyton
Temporal lobe epilepsy	Carbamazepine	Phenytoin
Petit mal epilepsy	Ethosuximide	Sodium valproate
Myoclonic epilepsy	Clonazepam	Sodium valproate Ketogenic diet
Infantile spasms	ACTH or corticosteroids	Clonazepam
Status epilepticus	Diazepam i.v.	Paraldehyde i.m.

Optimal drug dosage and susceptibility to side-effects vary from individual to individual, and serum anticonvulsant levels are valuable in assessing therapy. The regimen should be kept as simple as possible and it is seldom necessary to use more than two drugs.

A diagnosis of epilepsy raises considerable fears not only in the family but among school teachers and social contacts. Children with epilepsy do not require much limitation of their activities. For obvious reasons they are advised not to cycle in traffic but they may swim provided there is a responsible adult in attendance. Learning difficulties are more common than in other children but the majority of children with epilepsy attend ordinary schools and are average scholars. More than 60% of children diagnosed as having epilepsy seem to 'grow out' of their seizure tendency during childhood and anticonvulsant therapy can be discontinued if they have been free of convulsions for two to three years. A very small minority of children continue to have frequent epileptic attacks despite anticonvulsant therapy. The overall prognosis for childhood epilepsy is good with modern management.

Treatment of status epilepticus. It is unfortunate that many children await arrival at a casualty department before any attempt is made to stop status epilepticus. Every family doctor should be prepared to terminate these attacks as promptly as possible. The child should first be placed in a position which assures

Anticonvulsants: dosage and side-effects

Drug	Side-effects Common	Rare
Phenytoin 4–8 mg/kg/day	Cerebellar ataxia** gum hyperplasia hirsutism, rashes	rickets toxic encephalopathy facial coarsening
Carbamazepine 10–20 mg/kg/day	rash* fatigue* dizzyness*	bone marrow depression hepatic toxicity
Sodium valproate 20–40 mg/kg/day	drowsiness* nausea*	thrombocytopenia (high dosage) hair loss*; hepatic toxicity, pancreatitis
Phenobarbitone 3–6 mg/kg/day	irritability** overactivity**	rickets
Ethosuximide 20–40 mg/kg/day	nausea* rashes	bone marrow depression
Clonazepam 0.05–0.2 mg/kg/day	drowniness** salivation**	

* Transient if drug continued
** May settle with slight dose reduction

patency of the airway. Diazepam given intravenously, 0.2 to 0.3 mg per kg, is the drug of choice as it acts almost immediately. There is a risk of provoking apnoea if it is injected too quickly or if an excessive dose is administered. It is ineffective if given intramuscularly, but diazepam can be given rectally in a dose of 0.5 mg/kg. Paraldehyde given intramuscularly, 0.15 ml per kg, is a satisfactory alternative. A plastic syringe is safe as long as the injection is used promptly. Intramuscular phenobarbitone is too slow acting to be useful.

Febrile convulsions
Febrile convulsions are very common and affect some 4% of all children, most often in the second year of life. They are strongly age-related and hardly ever occur before six months or after six years of age. The usual history is that the child is noticed to be unwell and hot and then has a major seizure lasting a few minutes. There is often a family history of febrile convulsions. On examination the child has a high temperature, and frequently evidence of upper respiratory tract infection. More serious conditions such as meningitis or urinary tract infec-

Febrile convulsions: age incidence and recurrence rate

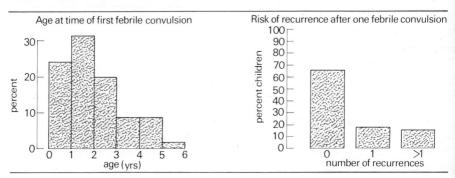

tions must always be excluded. The attacks are considered to be benign if they last less than 10 minutes and there are no persisting neurological signs. The prognosis for benign febrile convulsions is good, although recurrences are common. The risk of recurrence may be minimised by advising the parents to use tepid sponging and antipyretics whenever the child becomes febrile. Diazepam suppositories 0.5 mg/kg given at the time of fever further reduce the risk of recurrence and may be indicated.

Regular prophylaxis with sodium valproate 20–40 mg/kg/day or phenobarbitone 4–5 mg/kg/day reduces the risk of recurrence. The latter can be given as a single dose at night but unfortunately causes significant behavioural problems in some children. Such regular drug prophylaxis is not usually commenced until a child has had more than two febrile convulsions, unless there is preexisting neurological abnormality or the convulsions have been prolonged or atypical in some way. In either of these events there is an increased risk of recurrence of febrile convulsions.

The risk of developing epilepsy after one or more febrile convulsion of any kind is only 2%, but this is increased to 4% if any of the febrile convulsions were prolonged or atypical, and to 6% if there was preexisting neurological abnormality.

Other causes of transient impairment of consciousness

Breath holding attacks. These are common in toddlers and are usually precipitated by 'not getting his own way'. The child cries, holds his breadth and goes blue. The attack usually stops at this point but loss of consciousness sometimes occurs. Drug treatment is not necessary and the attacks cease spontaneously.

Reflex anoxic seizures. These occur in infants who have very sensitive vagal cardiac reflexes. Attacks are usually brought on by pain especially unexpected bangs to the head. This causes reflex cardiac asystole with immediate loss of posture, deathly pallor and floppiness. The heart recommences beating itself and the child then recovers.

Syncope or fainting. This is not uncommon among older children. Careful history reveals likely predisposing factors such as immobility or fear, and rapid recovery without any post-ictal phase.

Benign paroxysmal vertigo. This may present as sudden attacks of falling, swaying or dizziness but consciousness is not lost. Impaired vestibular function is revealed by caloric tests. No treatment is indicated as these attacks are brief and disappear spontaneously.

Migraine, day dreams, night terrors, hysteria and masturbation. These also enter the differential diagnosis.

Tics or habit spasms. These are irregular contractions of muscle groups, for example blinking and jerking or facial grimacing. They can be controlled voluntarily but feelings of tension increase until the movement has to be repeated. They are often a reflection of underlying emotional disturbance and should not be confused with focal epilepsy.

NEUROMUSCULAR DISORDERS

Muscle and lower motor neurone disorders present as floppiness, delayed motor milestones, abnormal gait, clumsiness or progressive muscle weakness.

Muscle disorders

The muscular dystrophies. These are characterised by progressive degeneration of certain groups of skeletal muscles and are frequently hereditary. A number of different forms have been distinguished on clinical and genetic grounds. Muscular dystrophy is the commonest cause of muscle disease in childhood.

Duchenne muscular dystrophy. This is the commonest and most serious type of muscular dystrophy with 30 per 100 000 live born males affected. Inheritance is as a sex-linked recessive but mutations are frequent and said to be responsible for 30% of isolated cases. The female carriers are usually asymptomatic. Symptoms appear in the first five years of life and consist of delayed walking, frequent falls, a lordotic waddling gait and difficulty climbing stairs. Prominence of the calf muscles is an early feature and is called 'pseudo-hypertrophy' because the muscles although enlarged are weak. Due to weakness of the gluteal muscles, boys with this condition climb up their legs when they rise from the lying position, Gower sign. The diagnosis of Duchenne dystrophy is made by finding a serum creatine kinase 30 to 200 times higher than normal, myopathic changes on electromyography and characteristic muscle biopsy features. It is important to consider Duchenne dystrophy in any boy with unexplained generalised developmental delay or delayed walking past 18 months. The serum creatine kinase is always very elevated before muscular weakness becomes clinically evident and is a useful screening test in such cases.

Most of these boys are unable to walk by the age of 8 to 11 years and are confined to a wheelchair. They often develop scoliosis and an equinus deformity of the feet due to muscular weakness and imbalance. The pseudo-hypertrophy

Duchenne muscular dystrophy: early and late clinical features, and the muscle biopsy appearance

Early

Gower sign

Late

generalised wasting

kyphosis
with
thoracic deformity

hip and ankle
contracture

variation in fibre size;
internal nuclei; splitting
and degeneration of fibres

is replaced by muscle wasting. Respiratory infections precipitate death by age 15 to 25. Intellectual development is usually normal but there is a slightly increased frequency of mental handicap.

Genetic counselling is important in Duchenne dystropohy, and female carriers may be detected by finding a moderately raised serum creatine kinase. Where women are carriers, the prospective parents may elect to have all male pregnancies terminated because of the 1 in 2 risk to the fetus. A gene probe is being developed and when available will be invaluable for carrier detection and prenatal diagnosis.

Becker muscular dystrophy. This is milder form of sex-linked recessive muscular dystrophy with a later onset of clinical muscle weakness.

Facioscapulohumeral muscular dystrophy. This has an autosomal dominant pattern of inheritance and presents in late childhood or early adolescence. There may be a marked variation in the severity of the disease within affected families. Shoulder girdle weakness is an early feature followed by facial involvement and inability to close the eyes tightly. Winging of the scapulae is another feature. This condition has a very slow progression and may be compatible with a normal life span.

Limb girdle dystrophy. This also presents in later childhood or early adult life. The pelvic girdle muscles are most affected. It has autosomal recessive inheritance.

Myotonic dystrophy. This was previously considered to be a disease of adult life but it is now realised that onset in childhood is not uncommon. It differs from the other muscular dystrophies, not only in the presence of myotonia, but also because of the widespread involvement of other tissues. Both males and females are affected and the inheritance is of an autosomal dominant. The muscle weakness characteristically involves the facial and neck muscles producing a myopathic facies, ptosis, an open mouth and a sagging jaw. Myotonia is seen as delayed opening of the eyes after closure or difficulty in relaxing the grasp. Distal limb weakness may also be present. Other features include cardiac involvement, cataracts, testicular atrophy and adrenal dysfunction.

In the congenital form infants have feeding and respiratory difficulties. Many die in the newborn period but those who survive show considerable recovery. The majority are, however, educationally subnormal. It is interesting that in every congenital case the mother is the affected parent.

Congenital myopathies. These are a complex group of disorders which can only be characterised after detailed examination of muscle obtained at biopsy, for example central core disease and nemaline myopathy.

Metabolic myopathies. Type II glycogen storage disease, acid maltase deficiency, is an autosomal recessive condition in which muscle weakness is a major feature. In the infantile form (Pompe disease) infants present with cardiac failure, hepatomegaly and gross hypotonia. The majority die before 18 months.

Acquired muscle disease

Dermatomyositis. Dermatomyositis, an inflammatory disorder of muscle, is rare in childhood. It is characterised by generalised proximal, asymmetrical muscle weakness and a violaceous discolouration of the skin, especially over the butterfly area of the face, eyelids, elbows, knees and knuckles. The child is usually miserable and may be febrile. Blood creatine kinase is elevated and the ESR is sometimes raised. EMG show myopathic changes and an inflammatory cell infiltrate is seen in muscle obtained at biopsy. Treatment with corticosteroids often produces a permanent remission.

Neuromuscular junction disorders

Myasthenia gravis. This is now recognised as being an autoimmune disorder and is associated with circulating antibodies to acetylcholine receptors. It is more common in girls. The onset is usually gradual with ptosis, strabismus, difficulty in chewing, loss of facial expression and arm weakness being common manifestations. The weakness may be very variable and is characteristically induced by fatigue. The diagnosis is confirmed by showing prompt improvement after an intravenous injection of edrophonium. The treatment of myasthenia involves the use of long-acting anticholinesterase drugs such as neostigmine or pyridostigmine. Thymectomy may have a place. Infants born to mothers with myasthenia gravis are susceptible to a transient form of the illness due to transplacental antibody transfer.

Neuromuscular disorders

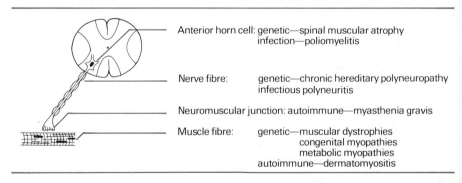

Anterior horn cell: genetic—spinal muscular atrophy
infection—poliomyelitis

Nerve fibre: genetic—chronic hereditary polyneuropathy
infectious polyneuritis

Neuromuscular junction: autoimmune—myasthenia gravis

Muscle fibre: genetic—muscular dystrophies
congenital myopathies
metabolic myopathies
autoimmune—dermatomyositis

Nerve fibre disorders (neuropathies)

Infectious polyneuritis (Gullain-Barré syndrome). This presents as a rapidly evolving symmetrical flaccid paralysis of the legs but trunk and arms are usually also involved. Respiratory and facial muscles may be affected. The weakness is commonly preceded by symptoms suggestive of viral infection. The cerebrospinal fluid often shows a considerable elevation of protein but no cellular response. The weakness progresses over a matter of days and then remains stationary for some weeks before entering a slow recovery phase. There is no specific treatment but a period of ventilation is required for respiratory paralysis in 10% of cases. Most children make a full recovery but this can take up to a year. It is essential to

Acute Werdnig Hoffman disease: clinical features and muscle biopsy appearance

group atrophy of fibres

alert facial expression
  fasciculation of tongue

deformed chest
  see-saw respiration

frog position
  absent reflexes

distinguish spinal cord problems which may need surgical evaluation from acute infectious polyneuritis.

Anterior horn cell disorders

Acute Werdnig-Hoffman disease (spinal muscular atrophy Type I). This is the early infantile form, has an autosomal recessive recessive inheritance, and an incidence of 1 in 20 000 births. Mothers may notice a lack of fetal movements and the infants can be floppy and weak at birth. Symptoms are always present within the first few months of life. In spite of the extreme muscle weakness, the infants are alert and watchful. Muscle fasciculation, especially in the tongue, is a feature. The diagnosis is made by electromyography and muscle biopsy. The condition is progressive and usually leads to death from respiratory failure before 18 months of age.

There are milder forms of spinal muscular atrophy with later onset, for example the Kugelberg-Welander form.

Floppy infant syndrome

The term floppy infant is reserved for babies who have marked hypotonia. A

Paralytic and non-paralytic causes of floppiness in infants

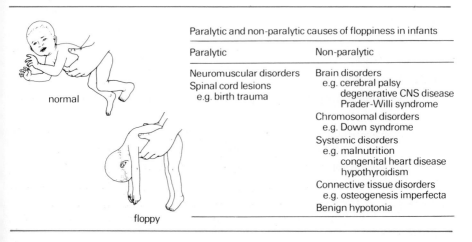

normal

floppy

Paralytic and non-paralytic causes of floppiness in infants

Paralytic	Non-paralytic
Neuromuscular disorders	Brain disorders
Spinal cord lesions	e.g. cerebral palsy
e.g. birth trauma	degenerative CNS disease
	Prader-Willi syndrome
	Chromosomal disorders
	e.g. Down syndrome
	Systemic disorders
	e.g. malnutrition
	congenital heart disease
	hypothyroidism
	Connective tissue disorders
	e.g. osteogenesis imperfecta
	Benign hypotonia

useful test is to hold the baby in ventral suspension. A baby with a paralytic cause of floppiness shows much less movement than one with a non-paralytic cause.

Benign hypotonia. This is a term applied to initially floppy but otherwise healthy infants who eventually regain normal tone and motor development. The recognition of subtle histological variants in muscle cell structure is gradually replacing this nonspecific category.

TUMOURS OF THE NERVOUS SYSTEM

Intra-cranial tumours are second only to leukaemia in the list of childhood neoplasia (three to five per 100 000 per year below 15 years of age). Infratentorial neoplasms predominate in this age group.

Computerised axial tomography has revolutionised the investigation of suspected brain tumours. Ideally, neurosurgical management is aimed at total resection of the tumour although this is not always possible because of infiltration or critical location. Radiotherapy has a valuable role and chemotherapy is now being introduced. Other aspects of management include ventriculo-atrial shunt insertion to control obstructive hydrocephalus, anticonvulsant therapy and dexamethasone for short-term control of related cerebral oedema. In general terms the older the child and the less malignant the tumour the better the prognosis.

Intra-cranial tumours: clinical features

Focal neurological signs	Raised intra-cranial pressure	Endocrine effects
Cerebellar	headache	short stature
ataxia	vomiting	hypogonadism
nystagmus	mood change	precocious puberty
diplopia	papilloedema	diabetes insipidus
Brainstem	VI nerve palsy	
facial weakness	head tilt	
swallowing problems		
ocular palsies		
spasticity		
Cerebral		
seizures		
spasticity		

Infratentorial tumours

Cerebellar astrocytoma. This is slow growing cystic tumour of the cerebellum. It presents with slowly increasing intra-cranial pressure and ataxia. Operative resection is very successful.

Medulloblastoma. This is a rapidly growing and highly malignant tumour with a more acute presentation. Complete resection is rarely possible but radiotherapy and chemotherapy are having some impact on the dismal prognosis.

Brain stem gliomata. These occupy a critical position in the brain stem and produce signs and symptoms of cranial nerve and long tract involvement. They are not amenable to surgery but may show long-term remission after radiotherapy.

Location of brain tumours

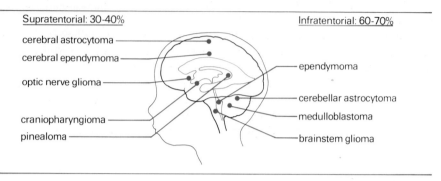

Supratentorial: 30-40%

cerebral astrocytoma

cerebral ependymoma

optic nerve glioma

craniopharyngioma

pinealoma

Infratentorial: 60-70%

ependymoma

cerebellar astrocytoma

medulloblastoma

brainstem glioma

Supratentorial tumours

Gliomata of the cerebral hemispheres. These show a spectrum of malignancy from the more benign slow growing astrocytoma to the rapidly growing glioblastoma. They may present with focal convulsions refractory to therapy, hemiparesis and mental disturbances.

Optic nerve gliomas. These produce optic atrophy with slowly progressive visual loss in one or both eyes. They are more common in children with neurofibromatosis.

Craniopharyngioma. These present as expanding suprasellar lesions with delayed growth from hypopituitarism, visual failure and headache.

Pinealomas. These produce early paralysis of upward gaze and hydrocephalus.

Tumours of the spinal cord. These are rare but important to recognise as the majority are benign and prompt recognition may avoid irreversible cord damage. Cord compression should be suspected in any child with gait disturbance, impaired sphincter function or back pain.

Leukaemic infiltration must also be considered in the differential diagnosis of suspected intracranial or spinal tumours.

HEADACHE

Headache is a relatively common complaint among older children. Mild, self-limiting headaches are frequent in febrile illness but a severe headache of acute onset raises the possibility of intra-cranial inflammation, subarachnoid haemorrhage, leukaemic infiltration or an intra-cranial tumour.

Intermittent headaches may originate from a variety of problems; sinusitis, dental caries, intra-cranial tumours and hypertension. The majority have no obvious organic explanation and may fall into the category of periodic syndrome or tension headaches.

Migraine

Migraine affects about 5% of all children at some time. A family history and the characteristic symptoms of throbbing headache, visual disturbance, photophobia and nausea make the diagnosis relatively straightforward in the older child. There may be problems in the recognition of migraine in the preschool child and it may be manifest by acute periods of distress, pallor and nausea. Attacks resulting in ophthalmoplegia or hemiparesis may occur. An underlying vascular malformation is rare association. Treatment is initially with simple analgesics such as paracetamol. More severe cases may benefit from non-ergotamine anti-migraine preparations. Recently there has been renewed interest in the relationship between food allergy and migraine. Some children benefit from the exclusion of cheese, chocolate or citrus fruits from their diets. More severe exclusion diets (oligo-allergenic diets) have been tried with success in some children with difficult migraine.

Ocular headaches
Ocular headaches result from constant muscular activity attempting to correct a latent squint or refractive error, usually long sightedness or astigmatism.

Benign intra-cranial hypertension
This term is used for an illness with raised intra-cranial pressure of unknown cause. It usually presents with vomiting, headache and papilloedema. CT scan shows small or normal sized ventricles and no space occupying lesion. It may be a complication of otitis media or occur after a non-specific viral illness; rarely it develops from too rapid reduction in corticosteroid therapy. Treatment is directed towards reducing the intra-cranial pressure in order to avoid secondary optic atrophy. A course of corticosteroids is usually successful but rarely may have to be complemented by repeated lumbar punctures.

ATAXIA

Ataxia refers to a disorder of movement manifest by incoordination, clumsiness and poor balance. In the young child, hypotonia and delayed motor development may be the only obvious signs.

Ataxic cerebral palsy
This is caused by malformation or damage of the cerebellum or its connections. The commonest cause is cerebellar hypoplasia which may be inherited as an autosomal recessive. Dandy-Walker syndrome refers to congenital absence of the foramina of Majendie and Luschka with resulting cystic dilation of the IV ventricle. Affected children have a characteristic prominence of the occipital region and are often ataxic.

Acute ataxia
In older children this may be due to intoxication with drugs, for example solvent abuse, phenytoin or alcohol. If the history does not reveal a cause, the rapid recovery certainly suggests it. Cerebellar ataxia may also be a manifestation of viral encephalitis, especially that caused by varicella. The differential diagnosis includes an acute presentation of a cerebellar tumour such as medulloblastoma, but the subsequent progression determines the need for neurosurgical investigation.

Friedreich ataxia

This is the most common of the hereditary ataxias, and is an autosomal recessive condition initially characterised by pes cavus and a relatively clumsy gait. Examination reveals ataxia, loss of postural and vibratory sensation, and impaired leg tendon reflexes. There may, in addition, be optic atrophy and cardiomyopathy. The patients become increasingly handicapped and may be wheelchair-bound by early adult life.

Ataxia telangiectasia

Ataxia telangiectasia is inherited as an autosomal recessive. In addition to slowly increasing cerebellar ataxia, there are characteristic telangiectasia obvious over the bulbar conjunctiva and face. There is an associated impairment of cellular *IgA* immunity which increases susceptibility to infection and may also be related to the predisposition to neoplasia.   *Die in 2nd decade – due to infec.*

There are rare metabolic disorders which result in ataxia; Hartnup disease in which there is a derangement of tryptophan metabolism, and Refsum disease in which phytanic acid accumulates.

CEREBRAL PALSY

Cerebral palsy is the leading cause of crippling handicap in children (2 per 1000). In using the label cerebral palsy, it is necessary to appreciate that the underlying lesion is permanent and non-progressive. In a developing child, however, the resulting clinical picture will not be static. The lesion is localised in the brain and, as it arises in early life, it interferes with normal development. The main handicap is one of disordered movement and posture, but it is often complicated by other neurological and mental problems.

Aetiology

Cerebral palsy is due to brain damage or malformation affecting those areas involved in motor functions. The brain is usually damaged in fetal life or in the early postnatal period. In some cases the cause be multiple, for example birth trauma and hypoxia complicated by hypoglycaemia. Congenital malformations of the brain include congenital cysts, fusion defects, failure of normal migration of grey matter, and aplasias.   *– See last pg – 275 :*

Causes of cerebral palsy

Cerebral malformation		Hypoglycaemia
Trauma:	NON-PROGRESSIVE LESION	Infection
birth		
postnatal		Cerebrovascular accident
Hypoxia		Poisoning
Kernicterus		Toxins

Spastic cerebral palsy

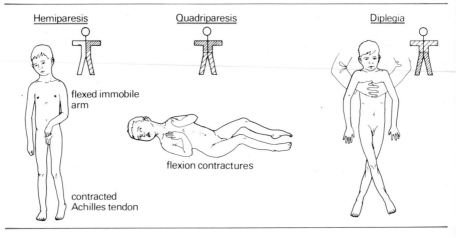

Classification

Spastic cerebral palsy. Spastic cerebral palsy which accounts for 70% of cerebral palsy cases, involves damage to the cerebral motor cortex or its connections, producing clasp-knife hypertonia, abnormally brisk tendon jerks, ankle clonus and extensor plantar responses. Hemiparesis affects just one side of the body and the arm is involved more than the leg. Quadriparesis affects both sides of the body, the arms being affected as much or more than the legs. In spastic diplegia both legs are spastic and the arms are less affected or not affected at all.

Dyskinetic cerebral palsy or choreoathetosis. Ten per cent of cases are characterised by irregular and involuntary movements of some or all muscle groups. These may be continuous or occur only on voluntary active movement. Athetosis is the commonest form with slow purposeless distal muscle movement. Choreic movements are quick, jerky and more proximal. _Hypotonia → ↓ f_

Ataxic cerebral palsy. This is associated with hypotonia, weakness, uncoordinated movements and tremor and accounts for 10% of cerebral palsy. _intention tremor._

Mixed cerebral palsy. These form the remaining 10% of cases.

Clinical features

Infants who show poor sucking ability, increased or decreased muscle tone, abnormal reflexes, irritability, convulsions or drowsiness in the newborn period are at risk of developing cerebral palsy. However, many such infants do develop normally and great care must be exercised in anticipating future development. Usually cerebral palsy is not diagnosed until several months have passed, and when it becomes obvious that motor development is abnormal or delayed. For example, the infant may be brought to the doctor because at three months of age he is not showing real head control or at 10 months of age he is not yet sitting alone. His mother may say that he seems stiff on handling. An infant with spastic hemiplegia is sometimes noted to have developed arm and hand preference before one year. The persistence of primitive reflexes, such as the asymmetric tonic neck reflex, beyond the time they usually disappear is suspicious. The characteristic involuntary movements of choreoathetosis are not usually obvious until near the end of the first year of life or even later. Affected children are usually very floppy and show delayed motor development in infancy. Children with ataxic cerebral palsy are also hypotonic and delayed in motor development but subsequently show an intention tremor.

Management

The child with cerebral palsy requires a multi-disciplinary assessment initially to define the problem, and then to develop a structured treatment programme. Physiotherapy aims to encourage normal motor development, to inhibit abnormal motor development and to prevent contractures. The parents are taught to perform the exercises at home.

Some degree of mental handicap is seen in about 60% of children with cerebral palsy. However, it should not be forgotten that children with severe cerebral palsy may have normal intelligence; this applies particularly to the dyskinetic group. Epilepsy occurs in approximately 30% and is symptomatic rather than idiopathic. Visual impairment due to errors of refraction, diffuse ambliopia or optic atrophy occurs in 20%. Squint due to external ocular muscle imbalance or paralysis is present in 30%. Twenty per cent have a degree of hearing loss which is often of the sensorineural type. Children with choreoathetosis are particularly liable to have associated deafness. Speech disorders are common and are due to a variety of causes including hearing loss, perceptual defects, mental handicap and incoordination of tongue, palate, and lip muscles.

Children with cerebral palsy often do less well in school than would be expected by their estimated abilities. One reason for this is the high frequency of perceptual defects. Behaviour disorders may be due to the frustrations of being handicapped, to strained family life brought about by the presence of a handicapped child, and to the hyperactivity which may be associated with brain damage.

Even with adequate physiotherapy, long-standing muscle weakness or spasticity is likely to produce orthopaedic deformities. These are more common in spastic cerebral palsy where the involved muscles develop fibrotic contractures. Spasticity in the adductors of the thigh may lead to dislocation of the hips and operation may be necessary to correct this. Spasticity and contracture in the calf muscle produce a fixed equinus deformity of the ankle which requires a tendo-achilles lengthening operation to allow the heel to be used for walking and weight bearing. Neglect of these deformities may lead to painful osteoarthritis.

Drugs have a limited role in the management of cerebral palsy, apart from the treatment of epilepsy. Schools for the physically handicapped provide physiotherapy and speech therapy, and they have specially trained staff and equipment. There is, however, a deficiency of opportunity for the handicapped school leaver. The overlap between the pathology of cerebral palsy and mental handicap is such that many children in schools for the severely educational subnormal also have cerebral palsy.

BIBLIOGRAPHY

General
Brett E 1983 Paediatric Neurology. Churchill Livingstone, Edinburgh

Intracranial infection
Davies P A 1977 Neonatal bacterial meningitis. British Journal of Hospital Medicine 18: 425–434
Goldacre M J 1976 Acute bacterial meningitis in childhood. Lancet i: 28–31
Hambleton G, Davies P A 1975 Bacterial meningitis: some aspects of diagnosis and treatment.
    Archives of Diseases Childhood 50: 674–684
Illis L S 1977 Encephalitis. British Journal of Hospital Medicine 18: 412–422

Epilepsy
Bower B 1978 The treatment of epilepsy in children. British Journal of Hospital Medicine
    19: 8–19
Nelson K B, Ellenberg J H 1978 Prognosis in children with febrile seizures. Pediatrics
    61: 720–727
O'Donohoe N V 1979 Epilepsies of childhood. Butterworths, London

Neuromuscular disorders
Dubowitz V 1978 Muscle disorders in childhood. Saunders, Philadelphia
Gardner-Medwin D 1977 Children with genetic muscular disorders. British Journal of Hospital
    Medicine 17: 314–340

Neural tube anomalies
Lorber J 1975 Ethical problems in the management of myelomeningocele and hydrocephalus.
    Journal of the Royal College of Physicians 10: 47–60
Stark G D 1977 Spina bifida. Problems and management. Blackwell, Oxford

Tumours of the nervous system
Till K 1975 Paediatric neurosurgery. Blackwell, Oxford

Cerebral palsy
Blencowe S M 1969 Cerebral palsy and the young child. Livingstone, Edinburgh
Christensen E, Melchior J C 1967 Cerebral palsy. A clinical and neuropathological study. Clinics
    in developmental medicine No. 25. Spastics Society, London
Scrutton D (ed) 1984 Management of motor disorders of children with cerebral palsy. Spastics
    International Medical Publications, London

Prenatal Factors:
1. Sm for dates
2. Consanguinity
3 Obv. Congen defects.

Emboli · micro.
→ filtered ... → brain

Trauma to Mother
↓ BP → Hypoxia
periventricular Haem.
        outreg.

Infections - TORCH
Malformations - Cysts.

Perinatal (labour - 7 Days)
premature birth.
Difficult labour.
Mechanical injury during
        birth
LBW babies.

Postnatal Factors:
Hypoglycaemia
Kernicterus.
Genetic - Synd.
Obv. Brain damaging event
    between 7/7 - 2/yrs.

19
Vision, Hearing, Speech

VISION

Vision is the most highly evolved of man's special senses. Binocular stereoscopic perception and interpretation requires not only an exact optic mechanism but also complex neural interconnections. The retina and eye are relatively mature at birth, and 75% of postnatal ocular growth occurs in the first three years of life. Myelination of the optic pathways is, however, still incomplete at term, and experimental work has recently confirmed the clinical impression that normal development of the optic radiation and visual cortex is dependent on undistorted light reception. It is therefore essential to act promptly when, for example, a severe ptosis or a cataract threatens the visual development of a newborn infant.

Assessment of vision

Before the age of six months, vision may be assessed by the response to a moving face, a slowly moving ball and by attention to hand-eye skills. Vision must always be considered in the context of general development. Quantification of visual acuity is possible in infancy using a preferential looking test in which the baby is presented a striped and a uniformly grey target simultaneously. Targets with

The development of vision

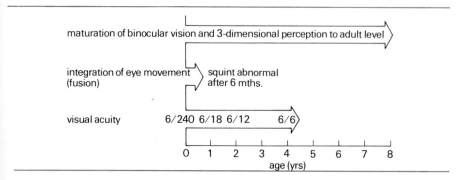

narrower stripes are presented until the baby no longer gives them preferential attention compared with the uniformly grey target. After three years single letter Stycar letter matching cards and after five years Stycar letter charts can be used. The Stycar letters have been specially selected as those which cause young children least confusion. Adult type Snellen charts can be used after seven years.

The assessment of vision

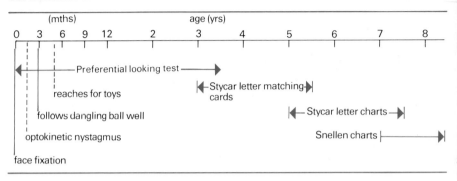

Squints

Squints are common in early childhood. All fixed squints and any squint which persists to age five or six months requires careful evaluation. Having detected a squint, expert assessment involves full examination of the eyes to exclude, for example corneal opacities, cataracts, and refractive errors. The usual cause of infantile strabismus is an ill-understood failure to develop binocular fusion at the normal time. Other important causes include refractive errors, particularly hypermetropia and astigmatism, neurological disorders which interfere with the normal function of the extraocular muscles, and eye diseases such as cataracts or retinoblastoma. Whatever the cause, the image of the squinting eye is suppressed, thereby avoiding diplopia and, if neglected, this may lead to an irreversible failure of development of the visual pathways from the squinting eye (amblyopia).

Testing for a squint

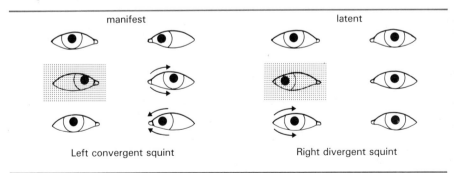

The blind child

For educational purposes a child is defined as blind if he requires education by methods which do not involve sight, for example Braille, and as partially sighted if he requires special educational consideration but can use methods which depend on sight. In practice, most blind children have some vision even if it is only recognition of light and dark, or perception of shapes.

In the U.K. about 500 children each year are newly registered blind or partially sighted, an incidence of approximately 1 in 2500 children. As many as 50% of blind children have additional handicap; physical disability, low intelligence, hearing and language difficulties. In their survey of visual handicap, Schappert-Kimmijser et al. (1975) reported that the main causes of visual handicap in childhood were optic atrophy (18%), congenital cataracts (16%), and choroidoretinal degenerations (15%). Overall the conditions causing blindness were genetically determined in 45% of children and due to some perinatal disturbance in 33%. The incidence of retrolental fibroplasia dramatically decreased in the early 1960s, possibly due to greater care when giving oxygen therapy in the newborn period.

Causes of childhood blindness (after Schappert-Kimmijser et al 1975)

Blindness must be suspected where there is a pendular nystagmus or roving, purposeless eye movements. Normal children cease to show random, uncoordinated eye movements after six weeks of age. Blind infants also tend to poke their eyes in a characteristic fashion, probably to produce pleasurable visual hallucinations of retinal origin.

With the exception of cataracts, most causes of blindness in children are not amenable to medical treatment. Recent advances in cataract surgery allow their early removal in congenitally acquired cases and the infant is immediately provided with constant-wear, thin, soft contact lenses to reconstitute the optic mechanism and thereby avoid stimulus deprivation amblyopia. The results are still frequently unsatisfactory.

Parents of a blind child need expert, sympathetic advice from a very early stage. Peripatetic preschool teachers from the Royal National Institute for the Blind often fulfil this role in the U.K. The parents must be taught to stimulate their infant using non-visual means, touch and speech. The home should be adapted so that the child can explore his environment safely. Residential school is often necessary for the blind child who needs to learn Braille. The child with partial sight may cope in an ordinary school with the help of special equipment.

HEARING

Hearing refers to the reception of noise, its transduction to nerve impulses and their transmission to the relevant areas of the cerebral cortex. A higher appreciation of sounds and their interpretation, listening, is integral to language development. The fetus is sensitive to noise and from the moment of birth there is an important sound interplay between mother and infant. Hearing provides for emotional contact, language development, identity with the environment and assists in the awareness of posture and body orientation. All children should be screened for deafness by tests which are appropriate to their stage of development and it is usual for these tests to be performed at six to nine months of age, and again at the preschool examination.

The assessment of hearing

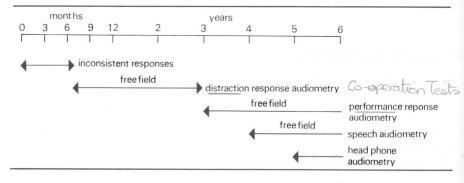

Co-operation Tests

Assessment of hearing

Babies up to about seven months show inconsistent responses to noises and reliable testing can only be done with sophisticated apparatus such as the Bennett cradle or brainstem evoked response audiometry. From seven months infants will turn their head and eyes towards the source of a quiet sound (distraction responses). It is essential to have a contented child in a quiet room. The examiner stands one to three feet to the side of the child and just outside his range of vision. The sound stimulus should be given at ear level. Sound makers employed are a high pitched rattle, spoon in cup, tissue paper, hand bell and selected speech sounds, for example 'oo' and 'ss'. A free field pure tone audiometer may be used to generate the sound stimuli. From three years, a child will play a game of putting a toy in a box whenever he hears the sound (performance responses). From four years, picture cards or toys can be used. The child is asked in a quiet voice to show the examiner a certain picture or toy from an array in front of him (speech audiometry). Most children of five years and over will tolerate wearing headphones and give reliable pure tone audiograms showing both air and bone conduction thresholds. The final proof of adequate hearing is the comprehension and imitation of normal speech. Although pure tone audiometry has a place in defining the hearing of children, it cannot replace clinical speech tests.

Causes of childhood deafness

Conductive deafness (4% of all children)	Sensorineural deafness (0.3% of all children)

Glue ear, following otitis media (almost all cases)	• Genetic — various types 50%
	• Intrauterine (8%)
	    congenital infection, e.g. rubella
	    maternal drugs, e.g. streptomycin
	• Perinatal (12%)
	    birth asphyxia
	    severe hyperbilirubinaemia
	• Postnatal (30%):
	    meningitis
	    encephalitis
	    head injury

Types of deafness

Whereas hearing loss of less than 20 dB normally has no effect on the child's development, a loss of over 40 dB creates problems in the development of ordinary speech. Testing over a range of frequencies may show a widespread loss or a loss purely in the high frequency zone. Deafness is classified into two categories, sensorineural and conductive. In sensorineural deafness there is damage to the cochlea or auditory nerve whereas in the conductive type there is middle ear dysfunction. Most severe deafness in children is sensorineural in type and is present from birth. The two types of deafness can be distinguished in older children by pure tone headphone audiometry. In the sensorineural type, there is equal impairment of bone and air conduction of sound; in the conductive type, there is an air bone gap with bone conduction hearing better than air conduction.

Audiograms: three patterns of hearing loss

air conduction ×   bone conduction ⌐

Forty per 1000 schoolchildren have mild deafness, usually a conductive middle ear deafness due to glue ear. Two per 1000 children have moderate deafness sufficient to require them to use a hearing aid, and one per 1000 children is severely deaf and requires special education.

Treatment of deafness

More careful management and follow-up of children susceptible to otitis media may reduce the incidence of glue ear. In established cases of glue ear the deafness is usually reversed by aeration of the middle-ear by means of a grommet inserted in the tympanic membrane, or by removal of the hypertrophied adenoids which often block the Eustachian tubes.

There is no specific therapy for sensorineural deafness but if there is some residual hearing, a hearing aid is useful. This is simply a device for amplifying sounds within the frequency range of the spoken voice. There are problems in that the receiver is not selective and is liable to cause distressing exaggeration of environmental and background noises, for example rustling clothes. Careful instruction in its use is required as well as attention to such items as the ear piece. It must be emphasised that the provision of an aid is only part of a more general process of rehabilitation and education. Parents of the young deaf child need expert guidance on how to encourage him to talk and develop language. Such help is given by the peripatetic teacher of the deaf. Many moderately deaf children can attend a normal school, but the more severely affected require specialist education, either at a school for the deaf or in a partially hearing unit attached to a normal school. As genetic causes are present in 50% of children with sensorineural deafness, genetic counselling if often indicated to try to prevent further cases occurring in the family.

SPEECH AND LANGUAGE

Language is essential to our culture as it provides the symbolic code for communication and for our thought process. The early development of vocalisation (exploratory sounds) and verbalisation (meaningful sounds) is closely linked to the mechanisms of hearing and listening.

There is a wide age range among normal children for the development of vocabulary. Some may be excellent at non-verbal communication and clearly have a well developed inner language. In others, the physiological basis of speech development is intact but is hindered by detrimental family relationships, social factors or psychiatric disturbances. It is also recognised that children in institutional care have delayed speech development and this is probably due to a less intense interpersonal relationship.

Assessment of speech

Speech development must be considered in the context of the wide range of normal development. The parents of the two-year-old boy with obviously normal development but a vocabulary of only 10 to 20 words may be comparing him with the little girl of similar age down the road with a vocabulary of 200 words. Both are within the normal range. Assessment must consider general development as well as environmental factors. Comprehension and free conversation during play are useful guides before embarking on more specific diagnostic exercises. An experienced speech therapist plays a valuable role in assessing and treating these children, and will be able to make a distinction between comprehension and expressive language delay. It is essential to make sure hearing is normal in any child who is showing delayed speech development.

Causes of speech delay

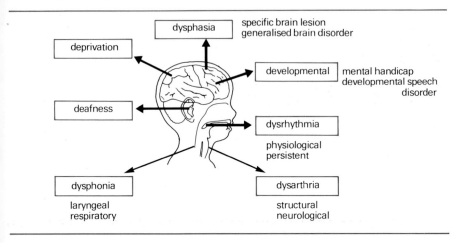

The developmental speech disorder syndrome

About 6% of three to four-year-old children show significant delay in speech development. In half of these children the cause is mental handicap, cerebral palsy or deafness. The remainder have a developmental speech disorder syndrome. It is more common in boys and there is often a family history. With speech therapy help the majority eventually catch up with speech and language development but some of these show later difficulties with reading and spelling (dyslexia). Only a minority, perhaps 1 in 1000 of all children continue, to have major problems with speech and language in later childhood, and the term developmental dysphasia is sometimes used for them. Such children require specialised teaching and may benefit from learning a non-verbal form of communication such as the Bliss or Paget-Gorman systems.

Dysrhythmia

It is common for children between three and four years of age to have a so-called physiological stammer. This corrects itself spontaneously and must not be made a focus of attention. A more persistent stammering or stuttering has a familial predisposition. In younger children, therapy is largely directed towards diverting attention away from the speech difficulty with the expectation of spontaneous improvement. In older children, more formal exercises such as syllable timed speech may be necessary for the most disruptive cases.

BIBLIOGRAPHY

Drillien C M, Drummond M B 1977 Neurodevelopmental problems in early childhood. Blackwell, Oxford
Fraser G R 1976 The causes of profound deafness in childhood. John Hopkins University Press, Baltimore
Holt K S, Reynell J K 1967 Assessment of cerebral palsy ii. Vision, hearing, speech, language, communication, and pyschological function. Lloyd-Luke, London
Moreley M E 1972 The development and disorders of speech in childhood. 3rd edn. Churchill Livingstone, Edinburgh
Schappert-Kimmijser J, Hansen E, Haustrate-Gosser M M, Lindstedt E, Skydsgaard H, Warburg M 1975 Documenta Ophthalmologica 39:213

20
Mental Handicap

The level of medical care provided within a community may be assessed by the prevalence, identification and care of those who are severely mentally handicapped. Better services result in fewer people being affected, and the early recognition of those that are in the lower range due to the effects of deleterious genetic, environmental and social factors. The care offered must also be as supportive and humane as the community can afford.

The words used to describe the mentally handicapped have changed with the years for they quickly become terms of derision (e.g. moron, idiot, cretin, mongol); and currently 'mentally retarded' is being abandoned. As a group, however, these children may be defined as having a low mental ability and learning problems. The severely handicapped have difficulty in learning to walk, dress and communicate. The more mildly affected have difficulty acquiring skills to look after themselves, and earn a living.

Aspects of mental ability or intelligence can be measured by a variety of tests.

The population distribution of intelligence and current classifications of mental handicap

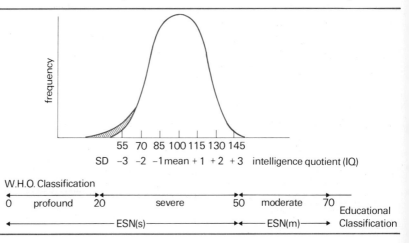

The prevalence and social class distribution for mental handicap (after studies of Rutter et al 1970 and Birch et al 1970)

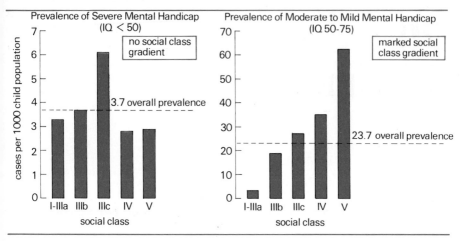

They measure what an individual has achieved at the time of the assessment and, although they may be a guide to what he might achieve, they do not necessarily measure his potential. The results of the tests are expressed as a quotient, the child's 'mental' age over chronological age. The distribution of intelligence follows a Gaussian or normal distribution with a distortion in the lower range due to the effects of deleterious environmental and social factors. Fetal and early infant death counteracts some of this excess.

It is helpful to divide those with low intelligence and who require special education into two groups, mild and severe. The mildly handicapped are composed largely of those in the lower range of the normal distribution, with IQs in the 50 to 70 range. They often come from families of low intelligence and poor social background. The severely handicapped with IQs below 50 usually have some organic disorder; a recognised inherited disorder, a brain deformity or have suffered a severe injury which has permanently damaged the brain. Obviously

Causes of mental handicap (after studies of Rutter et al, 1970 and Birch et al, 1970)

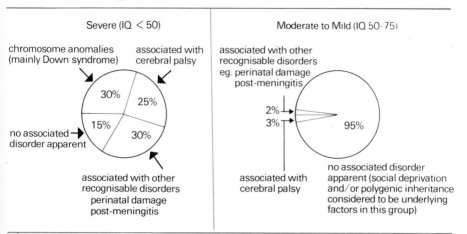

there is some overlap between the two groups.

The classification in the table below emphasises the extensive list of disorders which may contribute to mental handicap; each chapter in this book contains problems which may produce this end result. The diseases discussed in the second half of this chapter warrant a separate section, not because of their frequency, but because they do not fit conveniently into other categories.

A classification of the recognised causes of mental handicap

Causes of mental handicap	Examples
A Genetic	
• Chromosomal disorder	Trisomy e.g. Down syndrome
	Deletion e.g. cri du chat syndrome
	Sex chromosome anomaly
	e.g. Fragile X syndrome
• Metabolic disorder	Aminoacid e.g. phenylketonuria
	Carbohydrate e.g. galactosaemia
	Organic acid e.g. isovaleric acidaemia
• Cerebral degenerative disorder	Gangliosidoses
	Lipidoses
	Complex carbohydrates
	Mucopolysaccharidoses
	Leucodystrophies
• Structural disorders	Tuberose sclerosis
	Familial hydrocephalus
B Intrauterine	
• Congenital infection	Cytomegalovirus
	Rubella
	Toxoplasmosis
• Drugs	Phenytoin, alcohol
• Cerebral malformations	Hydranencephaly, porencephaly
C Perinatal	
• Problems during pregnancy	Pre-eclamptic toxaemia
	Antepartum haemorrhage
	Premature onset of labour
• Problems during labour and delivery	Prolonged labour
	Fetal distress
	Trauma
	Asphyxia
• Neonatal problems	Intraventricular haemorrhage
	Hypoglycaemia
	Infection e.g. meningitis
	Jaundice
D Postnatal	
• Trauma	Accidental or non-accidental injury
• Infection	Encephalitis, meningitis
• Anoxia	Asphyxia, status epilepticus
• Metabolic and endocrine	Hypoglycaemia, hypernatraemia,
	Hypothyroidism
• Poisoning	Lead
• Psychological	Infantile psychosis/autism

The identification and treatment of mentally handicapped children

Developmental assessment should be available for all infants, and for those where suspicion arises there must be ready access to the skills of a multi-disciplinary assessment team. It is important that prompt, confident reassurance is given to the parents of children who demonstrate innocent variation of development, and that sensitive explanation is provided where abnormality is likely. Many local authorities keep 'at-risk' registers of children with complicated birth histories, but at least 30 to 40 per cent of eventually handicapped children are not included.

Following careful assessment, the cause of severe mental handicap will be found in 85% of cases. The history, examination and investigations may all contribute to the diagnosis (see table). Cerebral palsy although strictly not a cause of mental handicap is an associated finding in 25% of severely mentally handicapped children. A number of conspicuous malformation syndromes are associated with handicap. It is also important to document minor anomalies for these may also provide clues to underlying major disorders. A single minor anomaly is relatively common, 14% of newborn infants, but the presence of three or four anomalies carries a 90% risk of an associated major defect. Particular attention should be paid to eyes, ears, palate, hair pattern, hands and feet. There are invaluable reference atlases which link malformations with defined syndromes. Lead intoxication is rarely a primary cause but many mentally handicapped children show pica and are at risk of ingesting paint flakes or contaminated soil. Hypothyroidism and aminoacid disorders, particularly phenylketonuria, are readily excluded by appropriate biochemical tests. Progressive deterioration in performance emphasises the need to look for metabolic, storage or neurodegenerative disorders. Modern techniques and the identification of specific enzyme deficiencies have improved the yield of such investigations. There is almost no place for brain biopsy.

Features on history, examination and investigations which may identify the cause of mental handicap

Historical items

• Family history of affected males	Fragile X syndrome
• Maternal alcoholism	Fetal alcohol syndrome
• Light-for-dates	Placental dysfunction, congenital infections, fetal alcohol syndrome
• Pica	Lead poisoning
• Deterioration	Cerebral degenerative disorder

Clinical findings

• Floppy infant	Prader-Willi syndrome, congenital myotonic dystrophy, Down syndrome
• Obesity	Pseudohypoparathyroidism, Prader-Willi syndrome
• Funny smell	Organic acidurias, maple syrup urine disease
• Cerebral palsy	Perinatal asphyxia
• Hepatosplenomegaly	Niemann-Pick disease, Gaucher disease, Hurler syndrome
• Cardiac abnormalities	Down syndrome, congenital rubella, infantile hypercalcaemia
• Coarse facies	Hypothyroidism, mucopolysaccharidoses

• Deafness	Congenital rubella, mucopolysaccharidoses
• Large head	Soto syndrome, hydrocephalus, neurofibromatosis, mucopolysaccharidoses
• Microcephaly	Congenital infections, maternal phenylketonuria, fetal alcohol syndrome, Smith-Lemli-Opitz syndrome, perinatal asphyxia, genetic microcephaly
• Large fontanelles	Pseudohypoparathyroidism
• Hypertelorism	Agenesis of the corpus collosum, cri du chat syndrome
• Hypotelorism	Holoprosencephaly
• Slanted palpebral fissures	Down syndrome
• Synophrys (eyebrows meeting in midline)	DeLange syndrome
• Congenital ptosis	Smith-Lemli-Optiz syndrome
• Cataracts	Congenital rubella, galactosaemia
• Corneal opacity	Mucopolysaccharide disorder
• Lens dislocation	Homocystinuria
• Retinal pigmentation	Laurence-Moon-Biedl syndrome, congenital rubella, Leber's amaurosis
• Hypopigmented macules	Tuberous sclerosis
• Café au lait patches	Neurofibromatosis
• Port wine naevus on face	Sturge-Weber syndrome
• Pigment whorls	Incontinentia pigmenti
• Hirsutism	DeLange syndrome, mucopolysaccharidoses
• Polydactyly	Laurence-Moon-Biedl syndrome
• Small hands and feet	Prader-Willi syndrome
• Large hands and feet	Soto syndrome
• Broad thumbs	Rubenstein-Taybi syndrome
• Simian creases	Down syndrome, DeLange syndrome, Smith-Lemli-Opitz syndrome
• Joint contractures	Mucopolysaccharidoses, sex chromosome disorder
• Cryptorchidism	Smith-Lemli-Opitz syndrome, Prader-Willi syndrome
• Hypospadias	Smith-Lemli-Opitz syndrome

Investigations

Thyroid function tests	Hypothyroidism
Serum and urine amino acids	Aminoacidurias
Blood lead level	Lead poisoning
Blood calcium	Pseudohypoparathyroidism
Blood acid-base balance	Organic acidurias
Urine mucopolysaccharide screen	Mucopolysaccharidoses
Urine organic acids	Organic acidurias
Chromosome studies	Chromosomal abnormalities
Skull x-ray	Intracranial calcification
CT scan	Cerebral malformation, hydrocephalus, leucodystrophy
White blood cell enzymes	Cerebral degenerative disorders

METABOLIC AND OTHER CEREBRAL DEGENERATIVE DISORDERS

Phenylketonuria (autosomal recessive)

Phenylketonuria causes severe mental deficiency, microcephaly and seizures. It results from a block in the hepatic conversion of phenylalanine to tyrosine. Infants with classical PKU have less than 1% of normal phenylalanine hydroxylase activity. Less severe variants have milder deficiency, 1 to 5 per cent. A rare subgroup lack an essential cofactor, tetrahydrobiopterin (BH_4), and have a severe progressive disease refractory to the usual dietary measures but possibly amenable to neurotransmitter replacement.

PKU is a relatively rare disorder, 10 cases per 100 000 births, but the effectiveness of prompt therapy justifies routine neonatal screening of blood phenylalanine levels. This is conveniently performed on capillary blood using the Guthrie bacterial inhibition technique in which a specific strain of *B. subtilis* can multiply only in the presence of phenylalanine. To be valid the infant has to be established on milk, and the test is conventionally performed on samples collected at the end of the first week of life. 3 Days !

Dietary phenylalanine restriction must be established promptly and has to be carefully monitored to meet the twin aims of brain protection while allowing sufficient quantities of this essential aminoacid for growth. The overall results of careful treatment are good with 75% of the U.K. 1974–78 cohort attending normal schools albeit with a higher incidence of behavioural and psychometric problems. Debate surrounds the issue of when and how to withdraw dietary restriction. Beyond the age of 6 to 8 years the nervous system is less vulnerable to elevated phenylalanine levels, and compliance certainly falls.

Maternal phenylketonuria is now increasing as a problem, and has devastating effects on the fetus, causing microcephaly, severe handicap and other structural anomalies. This emphasises the long-term responsibilities of the health-care team who must maintain patient contact, attempt guidance for planned conception and reintroduce dietary restriction.

Gangliosidoses

Tay-Sach disease. Tay-Sach disease is the most frequent of these rare disorders. It is due to the abnormal accumulation of ganglioside GM_2 in the grey matter. The developmental regression is usually obvious by six to nine months of age with increasing motor weakness. An exaggerated startle response to sound, hyperacusis, is an early sign. Visual inattention and social unresponsiveness are part of the deteriorating course which includes convulsions and difficulties in swallowing, and ends in death by three to five years. A cherry red spot at the macula is characteristic of this degenerative disorder. The diagnosis may be confirmed by measuring serum hexosaminidase activity. Prenatal detection is possible, but as 80% of cases mark the first appearance of the condition in families, it is far more valuable to identify at-risk couples before they reproduce. The high frequency of the heterozygote in Ashkenazi Jewish populations has been a stimulus to successful voluntary detection programmes.

Other gangliosidoses include a generalised form with hepatosplenomegaly and

The biochemical basis of Tay-Sach, Gaucher and Niemann-Pick disease

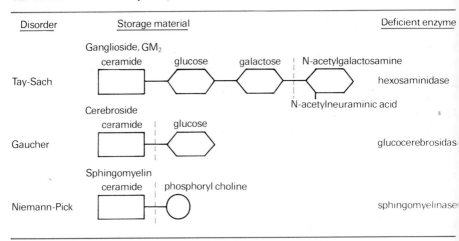

skeletal deformities, generalised gangliosidosis, and a variety with later onset neural presentation, juvenile Tay-Sach disease. The measurement of specific enzyme activity enables precise identification.

Neural lipidoses

Gaucher disease. Gaucher disease may be classified into neuronopathic and non-neuronopathic or visceral varieties. The former presents in infancy with feeding problems, stridor, and spasticity. There is prominent hepatosplenomegaly and Gaucher cells can be identified in marrow or liver biopsy. Death occurs within months. The non-neuronopathic form presents later in childhood or early adult life with hepatosplenomegaly, pancytopenia and bone involvement. It is compatible with a reasonable life span.

Niemann-Pick disease. Niemann-Pick disease also causes abnormal storage in the reticuloendothelial system and two of the four recognised varieties are neuronopathic. It may resemble Tay-Sach disease and have a cherry red macular spot. It can also present in the differential diagnosis of neonatal hepatitis. Typical foam cells can be found in marrow and liver biopsy.

Mucopolysaccharidoses

These complex carbohydrate storage disorders typically cause abnormal accumulation in fibroblasts and chondrocytes resulting in coarsened skin, corneal clouding, skeletal dysplasia and hepatosplenomegaly. The manifestations vary and not all have neural involvement. There are currently seven or eight varieties which can be distinguished by the enzyme defect and the major storage substance, dermatan, heparin or keratan sulphate and its excretion in the urine.

Hurler syndrome. This is the best recognised form and results from the deficiency of α-L-iduronidase.

The mucolipidoses. The mucolipidoses resemble the mucopolysaccharidoses but lack the urine products. Sophisticated biochemical studies are required for

Hurler syndrome

---

grossly retarded development

coarse facies
hazy corneas
enlarged tongue

cardiac abnormalities

hepatosplenomegaly
umbilical hernia
claw hand
joint deformities

urine:
    dermatan sulphate
    heparan sulphate

---

their precise identification.

White matter degenerative disorders

These present with progressive motor deterioration and spasticity. There is associated intellectual loss, progressive blindness due to optic atrophy, and convulsions.

Metachromatic leucodystrophy. This is the most commonly recognised variety and usually becomes obvious in the second year. Sulphatides accumulate in nervous and other tissues due to deficiency of the enzyme, aryl sulphatase. The diagnosis is made by demonstrating metachromatic material in urinary sediment or tissue biopsy, and establishing deficient aryl sulphatase activity in white cells or cultured fibroblasts.

Specific treatment

Dietary manipulation assists a small but important group of children with inherited disorders of carbohydrate, aminoacid or organic acid metabolism. We have not yet devised a satisfactory means of replacing deficient enzymes within the tissues, and

Inborn errors of metabolism: possible therapy

the blood-brain barrier may prove to be an impenetrable obstacle. Prevention through accurate diagnosis of index cases and genetic counselling provides the only successful method of control in the majority of these disorders.

General management

Handicapped children and their families require the resources of a multi-disciplinary approach. In addition to general assessment, the child's social, motor, language, hearing and visual abilities must all be considered. A therapeutic programme must begin as early as possible with parents playing an active role together with physiotherapists, speech therapists, and play counsellors. Health visitors and social workers assist the parents in coming to terms with their problems and advise on financial and equipment help. Seizure disorders and behavioural problems may require specific drug therapy.

The Education Act of 1970 legislated for special schools to be available for all handicapped children. More recently the 1981 Education Act established the basis for a more enlightened framework, evolving away from traditional categories of handicap and promoting integration with normal schoolchildren. Although schools are classified as dealing with the E.S.N. (M) or E.S.N. (S) categories the system has to be flexible to accomodate co-existing physical problems. Children in the IQ range 50 to 70 often achieve some independence and benefit from the high staff: pupil ratio available in E.S.N. (M) schools. Eighty per cent are capable of an open occupation and the remainder are provided with employment in sheltered workshops, adult occupation centres. Children with IQ below 50 are rarely independent and often need to be dressed and fed. They may not be able to speak and require constant attention. Education at E.S.N. (S) schools is essentially aimed at training the children to do simple social tasks. As these children become older the parents find it increasingly difficult to look after them. Up to the age of 14, only a minority are in residential care but after this age the proportion increases rapidly. Residential facilities vary considerably but there is a tendency towards smaller units which attempt to retain the family structure and links with the surrounding community. Those remaining at home when they leave school usually attend an occupational centre run by the local social work department.

BIBLIOGRAPHY

Birch H G, Richardson S A, Baird D, Horobin G, Illsley R 1970 Mental subnormality in the community. A clinical and epidemiological study. Williams & Wilkins, Baltimore
Griffiths M 1973 The young retarded child. Churchill Livingstone, Edinburgh
Hewett S 1970 The family and the handicapped child. Allen & Unwin, London
Kershaw J D 1973 Handicapped children. Heinemann, London
Kirman B H 1972 The mentally handicapped child. Nelson, London
Mackay R I 1976 Mental handicap in child health practice. Butterworths, London
Rutter M, Graham P, Yule W 1970 A neuropsychiatric study in childhood. Spastics International Medical Publications. Heinemann, London

21
Behaviour

Until recent years, doctors treating children tended to ignore unusual or deviant behaviour, believing its correction to be the responsibility of the parents or, if the problem was particularly troublesome, the psychiatrist, social worker, teacher, or the welfare services. However, it is a mistake for a family or hospital doctor caring for children not to have studied the behavioural disturbances, for on the one hand many childhood illness are associated with some disturbance in behaviour, indeed some organic disease may present with a behaviour problem, and on the other hand children at conflict with themselves or their family or their surroundings may present with symptoms which mimic organic diseases.

In the first part of this chapter, behavioural problems which are thought to be due to brain damage, brain dysfunction or a delay in brain maturation are discussed. In the second part the interactions between the child, his family and his surroundings which might produce conflicts are outlined and illustrated. In the third part some of the effects on the child of deviant behaviour by the parent are considered. Overlap between the sections is inevitable.

PHYSICAL ILLNESS

Diseases affecting the brain

General. It is obvious that any illness which affects the brain might alter a child's personality and affect his behaviour. One parent, a bird-watching enthusiast, recognised unusual behaviour in his own youngster some weeks before his child was admitted semiconscious with diabetes. The list of diseases, metabolic, traumatic, infective, neoplastic which may affect the brain and its function is endless, all may have associated behaviour problems, some of which are easily recognised and understood, but others, for example the odd behaviour of a child with a cerebral tumour, may be overlooked for some time. Their precise relationship to the physical illness is not always clear. There are, for example, many reasons why a child after severe head injury might be unfriendly and withdrawn. Children with perceptive problems, deafness and blindness, may develop their

A classification of the recognised causes of mental handicap

| • Diseases which interfere with vital supplies to the brain:
 • Perceptive disorders
 • Brain pathologies:
    epilepsy
    mental retardation | • Developmental delays:

 in motor control <br> in speech <br> in reading <br> in bladder control | • Psychiatric syndromes:

 tics <br> hyperkinetic syndrome
 'minimal brain damage'
 autism |

own patterns of behaviour which to others appear odd and sometimes unacceptable. However the main subjects of this section are not the variations in behaviour which occur in children with organic disease or of children with perceptive problems, important though these are, but brain conditions which present and are recognised by the peculiar behaviour patterns they produce.

Epilepsy is due to an involuntary, uncontrollable activity from the brain which produces a seizure. The usual forms of seizures include grand mal, focal epilepsy, and petit mal seizures and have been discussed elsewhere. Temporal lobe seizures may occur with clouding of awareness, confusional states, automatic motor behaviour patterns and angry or terrified outbursts. Epilepsy of whatever form is associated with an increased incidence of behaviour disturbance. This might be related to the brain dysfunction or to the drugs used to control the fits or to the handicap epilepsy brings to the child in his relationships.

Mental handicap. Mental handicap whether due to obvious brain injury or to an uncertain mix of genetic and early environmental factors may present primarily with behaviour difficulties. These disturbances may be more of a burden to the child, his parents and his teachers, than his basic learning problem. Whether, for example, aggressiveness, negativism, self-destruction or repetitive behaviour in retarded children is due to their abnormal brain function or a consequence of how they are handled in early life is an important question to be considered if appropriate management programmes are to be devised.

Maturational delay

Children with mental handicap have a generalised delay in development and usually end up with reduced abilities in all areas, so-called global retardation. However the delay may be in one area only and with time, the child may learn to overcome the difficulty or to bypass it. Thus the child may have a functional delay in motor control, hearing, speech, bladder control etc. As we all develop in different ways and at different rates, and end up with different levels of ability, each identified group contains children in the extremes of the normal range, children held back for a variety of reasons, as well as specific functional disorders.

Clumsiness or motor dyspraxia. Clumsiness in its severe form may result in a child being so uncoordinated that he has problems at home, at school and at play. His school work is untidy as a result of poor eye-hand coordination, and he performs badly at sports, particularly ball games. Such children are delayed in learning to dress themselves and have difficulty in keeping themselves tidy. They continually knock things over and frequently fall over themselves. The academic and social difficulties which follow can cause the child considerable unhappiness and lead to behavioural problems if they are not recognised and dealt with sympathetically. Specific physiotherapy programmes may help.

Specific reading retardation. Reading is a complex activity which requires a great number of skills, and therefore reading difficulties might be due to a variety of factors. For example children with a general learning problem are slow to read, children who are understimulated or badly taught are slow to read, and children who have a perceptive problem are slow to read. But apart from those in which a reading delay might be anticipated, there are many otherwise normal children, who have specific reading retardation. Some experts consider that 4 to 8% of schoolchildren have such a problem. Boys are more often affected than girls and there is often a family history. Usually the children are a little slow to develop speech and characteristically they have even more difficulty with spelling than with reading so that, for them, dictation is a nightmare. They may also have difficulty with handedness. There is an argument for screening all children for specific reading retardation not only so that their reading exercises can be approached with insight and sympathy but also to ensure that their general education is not hampered by their limited reading ability. Dyslexia and 'word blindness' have been names given to the most overt form of this problem.

Specific speech and language delay. Hearing, intellectual, or psychosocial impairment are more common factors leading to speech delay than a specific developmental disorder. Nevertheless there are a small group of children, around 2%, of those with speech delay, who have normal intelligence and hearing and come from a happy, stimulating environment but who are unable to speak clearly. They require a personal educational programme.

Nocturnal enuresis. Involuntary emptying of the bladder during sleep is a common and troublesome problem. In round terms the majority of children are dry at night by 3 years of age, some 10% plus regularly wet the bed at 5 years of age, and somewhat less than 5% still do so at 10 years of age. One or two in every hundred will have an organic problem, either a congenital abnormality of the urinary tract, a urinary infection, polyuria or neurogenic bladder. A careful history, thorough examination and urine examination for glucose, infection and specific gravity should exclude these possibilities. Only rarely on the history of nocturnal enuresis alone is radiological investigation of the renal system justified. In another small percentage nocturnal enuresis will be the presenting symptom of a child emotionally upset. Gentle probing enquiry should bring this to light and point the interview into the appropriate direction.

In the majority, clinical enquiry gives no indication of the aetiology. Often there is a family history and there will be relatively more children from poor and unhappy homes than might be expected. It might be hard to refute the parents' suggestion that their child's bladder capacity is too small or that they pass excess amounts of urine during the night. Some physicians recommended exercises to enlarge the bladder capacity. Physiologists have postulated immature circadian rhythms, psychiatrists on the other hand have suggested that when children, in the mystery of sleep, wet themselves and their bed, they are saying that they want to be comforted like a baby, they are frightened or that they are making a hostile gesture in the security of their bed about something that has happened to them during the day.

Many children improve, some surprisingly quickly with whatever method of management is used, whether it be habit training with star charts, lifting at night, drugs or a pad and bell. Suggestion and encouragement are perhaps the most helpful. Tricyclic drugs, for example, imipramine 25 mg for the child under 30 kg body weight and 50 mg for those over, work at least temporarily in about a third. The greatest claim has been made for the bell alarm which is placed in the child's bed so that the alarm rings when the child wets. It is said to help over two-thirds of those who can be brought to use them.

Faecal soiling. Although it may seem appropriate to discuss faecal soiling after noctural enuresis, as a problem it has more in common with those disorders precipitated by conflict. There is far less reason to believe that, in the majority, it is due to a delay or abnormality in the development of brain function. Faecal soiling usually occurs during the day. Most children are clean by 2½ years of age and soiling may be viewed as abnormal after 4 years of age and certainly by the time the child goes to school.

It may take three fairly distinct forms. In one, sometimes called encopresis, the child has bowel control but passes the formed stool in unacceptable places, for example behind the curtains in the lounge, on the wallflowers in the garden, indeed everywhere except in the toilet. Sometimes the act is performed in a secretive manner and sometimes it is meant to be provocative. Usually the child has problems which cannot be resolved easily and expert advice is required. Children inappropriately or inadequately trained, or who are mentally or socially slow form a second group. In these children a formed stool is passed, sometimes in the toilet but usually in the pants. A firm, consistent training programme should help these patients. Set-backs during bowel upsets whether from inappropriate food or infections are to be expected. Children who are chronically constipated often present with soiling. The insensitive distended rectum cannot stop soft faeces passing round the hard impacted masses and oozing out. These children

Susan

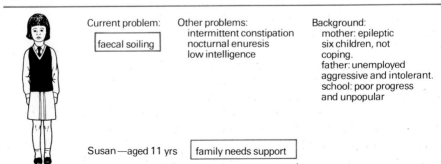

Current problem:

faecal soiling

Other problems:
intermittent constipation
nocturnal enuresis
low intelligence

Background:
mother: epileptic
six children, not
coping.
father: unemployed
aggressive and intolerant.
school: poor progress
and unpopular

Susan—aged 11 yrs   family needs support

continuously soil themselves and always smell. The soiling disappears after the constipation has been corrected.

Tics

Tics are sudden repetitive coordinated movements of no apparent purpose. They can effect any muscle groups but commonly take the form of blinking, facial grimacing, twisting the head, or shrugging the shoulders. The average age of onset is two years and it has been reported that as many as 4% of children develop them at some time. Tourette described a bizarre syndrome where vocal tics, often rude words, accompany gestures which might be equally embarrassing. In 25% of children with tics there is a family history. In some there is evidence of brain damage or other features of delayed maturation. The majority are precipitated by stress. Usually the tics disappear, sometimes in weeks or months, often in late adolescence, and rarely do they persist into adult life.

Hyperkinetic syndrome

In children with the hyperkinetic syndrome there may be a family history, evidence of a developmental delay or a history which suggests that the child might have had 'minimal brain dysfunction' or 'minimal brain damage'. In some there is little evidence to suggest any of these alternatives.

The children are not so much clumsy as apparently overactive. They never sit still, they are distractable, they never settle down, they are destructive, impulsive and excitable. It is when they first go to school that they appear to be at their most difficult and it may be then that their problem first comes to light.

In adolescence, though the hyperactivity is less, their learning difficulties with socially disruptive behaviour may lead to further problems. As adults they are more likely to have trouble with the law, or need psychiatric help.

Management starts with a careful evaluation of the child's problems and continues by full discussions with parents, teachers and anyone else concerned. Each programme is individual. Once the child is under regular sympathetic observation the effects of drugs can be assessed. Brain stimulants, methylphenidate and dextroamphetamine, benefit over half the affected children; the tricyclic antidepressants may also help.

Autism and childhood psychosis

Schizophrenia can begin in late childhood, the symptoms are similar to those found in adults. Adults who develop schizophrenia have often shown unusual behaviour when they were youngsters, but the pattern is not characterisctic and so prediction and maybe prevention is not yet possible. Bizzare or psychotic behaviour is also seen in encephalopathies and in the severely retarded. About half the children with psychosis have a cluster of clinical features which suggest a specific disorder, infantile autism.

Characteristically, autistic children fail to develop social relationships, they are slow to speak and have little non-verbal communication. They also follow ritualistic behaviour patterns and endlessly perform repetitive movements. Parents seek advice because they wonder if the child is deaf and again later because of delay or absence of speech development. Often the infant's behaviour has been unusual from birth and only occasionally is the child's development for the first year or so apparently normal. Over half the children are mentally retarded as well and these have the worst prognosis. Even those with average intelligence have great difficulty coping when they grow up. Only a few manage to be gainfully employed and they rarely marry.

Autism is rare: in a population of one million some 20 to 40 children might be identified. They need to be under the care of experts in special schools but because of its rarity it is difficult to provide this for all children whilst maintaining strong home links. Drugs currently play only a small part in management, they may help if there is an associated sleep problem.

THE INTERACTION BETWEEN THE CHILD AND HIS WORLD

A child may develop symptoms of physical disorder or behaviour problems or educational difficulties due to conflicts and confusion within himself, or with his family, with his peers, with school or with society at large. If a schoolgirl gets stomach-ache because she hates her ballet lessons or dislikes her new step-father, then eliciting that information may be just as important for that child as testing the urine in another suspected of having urinary infection. This section merely points to some of the more obvious factors which might lead to problems.

The child

Acute organic disease. Acute organic disease frightens children possibly more than adults, and they show it in different ways according to their maturity. It can be difficult to distinguish the symptoms and signs due to this reaction from those due to the underlying pathology. A terrified two-year-old with croup may improve dramatically in the arms of a friendly, confident, capable nurse or become even worse if placed on a strange bed surrounded by flashing lights and stainless steel.

Chronic organic disease. Chronic organic disease makes extra demands on the child. Some children cope marvellously well but in others the continuing difficulties are just too much and secondary symptoms or behaviour problems add to their difficulties. The burden of the disease for some children can be very heavy; what, for example, can be said to an adolescent with muscular dystrophy or cystic fibrosis when he learns by one means or another of the prognosis of his condition? Sometimes it is the parents who cannot accept or have difficulty managing the child's condition. It is always sad when a child with asthma exaggerates his bronchospasm, or a child with diabetes deliberately breaks diet to precipitate hyperglycaemia, in order to gain admission to hospital where they feel more secure, and where the pressures of coping either with the family or the outside world are avoided.

Deformity and disability. Deformity and disability present at birth may lead to problems if one or both parents have difficulty accepting their own abnormal child; they feel ashamed about him when they should be showing him off. Later as the child grows up he may have trouble at school, for children go through a period of wanting to be the same and of mocking those who are different. Just being different can lead to problems.

Claire

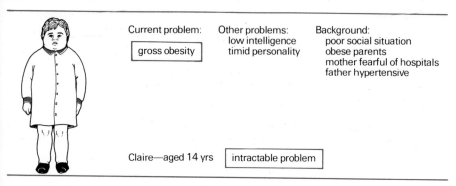

Current problem:

gross obesity

Other problems:
low intelligence
timid personality

Background:
poor social situation
obese parents
mother fearful of hospitals
father hypertensive

Claire—aged 14 yrs   intractable problem

Intelligence. Intelligence is determined by a mixture of genetic and environmental factors. Happily, in the main, parents get children of similar abilities but misfits occasionally occur, a slow child in an academic family, an awkward child in an athletic family, a gifted child in an average family, a swan amongst ducks. All may lead to conflict and result in bodily symptoms, behaviour disturbances and underachieving.

Temperament. Temperament likewise appears to be genetically and environmentally determined. A child's temperament is not only a factor in the risk of disorders developing but may also determine the mode of expression. An outgoing, extrovert child is more likely to develop behaviour problems, while a sensitive, timid child is more likely to internalise conflicts and have disorders of bodily function. The success of any management programme depends on those concerned knowing the child for whom they are making plans.

The family

A great deal has been written recently about the qualities required of parents. A child needs not only food, warmth and physical protection but also to be loved, to feel important, to be stimulated and encouraged to make the most of his abilities, and to be controlled and guided in the ways of his society. It is the privilege and responsibility of parents to meet these needs and most parents delight in the task. Many factors, some beyond anyone's control, can interfere with the relationship between parents and child.

Maternal deprivation. The bond between mother and child is fashioned at birth and secured over the first week of life. If others care for her sick child the mother may not develop that blind love and devotion which is so essential for his early well being. Separation from parents, particularly the young child from his mother, even for brief periods may not only have immediate effects on the infant, for example uncontrollable screaming or quiet withdrawal, but have more lasting effects as well. For most families brief periods of separation are not as harmful in the long term as was originally thought but in the context of certain family relationships they can be. Most children tolerate such events without lasting effect, but clearly they should be avoided if possible, particularly in the early years. If either the mother or her dependent infant needs hospital care, they should be admitted together if it is at all possible. One is often important in the other's recovery.

Family breakdown. Unhappily for children in western societies divorce rates are increasing, couples seeking divorce are tending to be younger and the duration of their marriages is shorter. Illegitimacy rates are also increasing, so are the numbers of mothers with young children who go out to work. Such situations add to the child's problems and may limit the care he receives.

Parental abilities and attitudes. If a parent is sick, what of the child? If a child has stomach ache it is well to ask about the family symptoms. Children are quick to note how adults gain sympathy and avoid the unpleasant, and they assume that there is no reason why they should not use the same tactics. A parent with a chronic illness may add to the child's anxieties and responsibilities and push the child beyond his limit. A parent with a psychiatric disorder, for example, depression, may have a devastating effect on the child. Sometimes it is the child's illness which draws attention to the mother's need. The effect that the death of a parent has on a child varies with his maturity. A disturbed child may be considerably helped by having the opportunity to talk frankly about it with a sympathetic but uninvolved adult.

Even when both parents are well and able to provide a comfortable home, their attitudes and expectations of their children can still lead to difficulties. In the extremes they may over-protect them or over-discipline them or ignore and reject them or they may wish to dominate them, even when they are capable of being independent. On the other hand, they may have unrealistic expectations of their abilities; for example, a mother who expected a six-month-old infant to use a pot, a father who expected his children to move at the blow of a whistle, a professional woman who thought her seven-year-old should realise when she wished to be left alone.

Adoption. The situation of a couple longing for children that they cannot have and adopting into their family an unwanted child has its own peculiar problems. Inevitably the child has those characteristics, appearance, abilities and personality determined by his genetic make-up from his parents but also he is influenced by the environment provided by his new home. As neither parents nor child are perfect, it is not surprising to find that the adopted child is more likely to develop

John

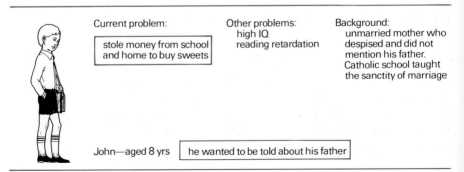

| | Current problem: | Other problems:
high IQ
reading retardation | Background:
unmarried mother who
despised and did not
mention his father.
Catholic school taught
the sanctity of marriage |
| | stole money from school
and home to buy sweets | | |

John—aged 8 yrs | he wanted to be told about his father |

behaviour problems (which may be due in part to inherited characteristics) and the parents must be aware of this. Nevertheless the future of the adopted child is undoubtedly better than if he had not been adopted at all.

Children in care. It has been said that bad parents are better than no parents. This is not true. However, in the absence of a larger family to embrace a child who loses both parents, the best efforts of the social services often fall well short of the child's needs. It is easy to be pessimistic about the long-term prognosis of such children. Professor Michael Rutter, at the conclusion of his book on maternal deprivation, points out that many children build happy and successful lives out of appalling childhoods and recommends that we seek the secrets of their success so that we might more effectively help others to avoid an unhappy outcome.

Environment

Deprivation. Ineffectual parents tend to be poor and to live in bad housing in deprived sections of the towns or country. It is difficult to be sure of the extent that a child's problems are due to his make-up, the care and attitudes of his parents or to his physical surroundings. But there is no doubt that poverty, overcrowding and poor housing, are associated not only with increased rates of illness and death in infancy and childhood but also behaviour problems and school failure. It is so difficult for children from such backgrounds to become good parents themselves. The poor are at a threefold disadvantage; they are more likely to fall ill, they have less family reserves to meet new problems and they are less able to make use of the support the state provides. Even in the U.K. with a National Health Service, the deprived are still at a disadvantage in comparison with the middle classes.

Neighbourhood. Wealth is relative, and poverty as defined in western societies need not bring misery. It has been shown that the prevalence of health and social problems varies considerably from one community to another with apparently similar levels of wealth, housing, and services. In some communities there is stability and mutual responsibility, in others there is aggression, cruelty and conflict. Race, culture, religion, industrial troubles can all lead to a family being rejected by the neighbourhood. Families continually on the move may create

Peter

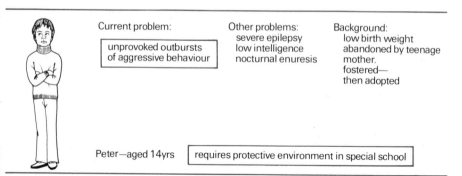

	Current problem:	Other problems:	Background:
		severe epilepsy	low birth weight
	unprovoked outbursts of aggressive behaviour	low intelligence	abandoned by teenage
		nocturnal enuresis	mother.
			fostered—
			then adopted

Peter—aged 14yrs   requires protective environment in special school problems of identity for their children.

School. School is where children go to work, where they make friends and enemies, where they test out their temperament against others, where they find out how other families think and behave. So problems at school may be far more than difficulties with learning. A child who has difficulty with his school such that special education is considered necessary, should have a thorough and expert medical assessment so that the restraint due to a medical condition is reduced to a minimum.

BEHAVIOURAL PROBLEMS

From what has been said so far it can be appreciated that many factors may contribute to the genesis of any particular problem which brings a child to the doctor's attention. The physician is particularly concerned with symptoms which suggest physical disease but have their origins in a psychological disturbance, and with behavioural problems which are a consequence of a physical disorder, either as a direct effect of brain disturbance or indirectly due to the difficulty the child has coping with his illness or handicap.

The preschool child

Feeding problems. Interaction between an uncertain or insecure mother with a healthy baby, or a happy mother with a determined or difficult baby may lead to the baby vomiting, refusing food or failing to gain weight satisfactorily. Sometimes the problem is resolved by patience and counselling either from the health visitor, relative or friendly neighbour but it is not uncommon for a child to have to be admitted to hospital to exclude an organic cause and to reassure both mother and her baby.

Sleep problems. Adults used to a regular biological rhythm differ in their tolerance of the baby's desire for a feed in the middle of the night. Occasionally infants appear to scream and cry through most of the night and this may be tolerated when the baby is young and weak but a playful demanding toddler in the middle of the night can stretch the patience of most parents. The temptation for the parents is to take the child in their bed or for one or other parent to sleep

Jason

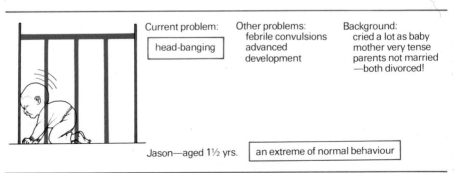

Current problem:
head-banging

Other problems:
febrile convulsions
advanced
development

Background:
cried a lot as baby
mother very tense
parents not married
—both divorced!

Jason—aged 1½ yrs. | an extreme of normal behaviour

with the child to comfort him but this is really no solution and can lead to further problems. Adults without sleep perform poorly in their work and this adds to the strain. In this situation there is an argument for giving the infant a sedative in a doses which ensures that he sleeps well for at least six hours each night. This helps him to establish a normal sleep habit and gives his parents a chance to regain their equilibrium. The sedative should be given in increasing dosage until it is effective and then maintained for some weeks. It is essential to explain to the parents the purpose of the exercise.

Breath-holding attacks. Infants and toddlers quickly find that they can control their parents by refusing to do what they are asked. For example, they may refuse to eat or to go the toilet, but perhaps their most dramatic card is to refuse to breathe. Breath holding attacks to the point of going unconscious, when they may or may not provoke a fit, are not uncommon. They certainly terrify the parents and may reduce them to quivering slaves. From the medical point of view it is important to distinguish the episodes from convulsions due to other causes and to reassure parents about the nature of the attacks. In the vast majority of cases the children come to no harm. These determined, often stubborn youngsters need to be handled firmly and consistently.

Rhythmic behaviour. Head rocking, head banging, thumb sucking, self-stimulation, baby behaviour, and many other variants may all occur during normal development. They are more likely to appear when the child is uncertain, anxious or tired. In the very disturbed, autistic or retarded child they can become bad habits and strategies need to be devised to avoid or suppress them.

Delayed development and regression. Understimulation with or without undernutrition may limit a child's development and growth. It is not surprising perhaps that a child left alone for hours with no toys in a high rise flat is quite withdrawn, apathetic, and has little muscle tone or strength, and delayed motor, social and mental development.

Bowel and bladder control. Again inappropriate training or anxiety and conflict will interfere with the development of bodily control and appropriate social habits. Noctural enuresis which in the main is probably due to a disorder in maturation and encopresis has been discussed in the first part of this chapter.

Schoolchildren

Recurrent abdominal pain. One of the common symptoms which bring children to clinic is recurrent pains usually in the abdomen or head, occasionally in the limbs. A few will have organic disease and so all require a careful clinical evaluation. In others it may be a cry for help, the child having a psychiatric disorder or a terrible domestic situation. But for the majority, the clinical investigations will be negative and there will be no major psychosocial problems. There may have been mild or moderate disturbances in the child's life, or they may not be being as successful as they would like, or fear they cannot maintain the standards expected of them. Often they are children of good ability with greater self-control and sense of responsibility than the average.

A thorough examination and reassurance with explanations will help many.

Jane

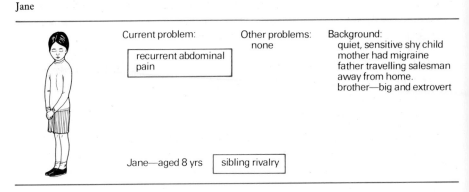

Current problem:

recurrent abdominal pain

Other problems:
none

Background:
quiet, sensitive shy child
mother had migraine
father travelling salesman
away from home.
brother—big and extrovert

Jane—aged 8 yrs   sibling rivalry

However in those referred to hospital, a good percentage continue to have recurrent pains into adolescence and adult life. Headaches rather than abdominal pains tend to persist.

Periodic syndrome. This describes a condition when attacks of abdominal pain are associated with severe vomiting. The vomiting can sometimes result in dehydration to a degree that requires correction by intravenous therapy. In this situation it is difficult to believe that the child has not got an organic disease but so far no pathology has been identified. However in its milder form it merges with the clinical entity of 'recurrent abdominal pain'.

School refusal and truancy. Illness is the commonest reason for school absence. Sometimes children are kept away from school to help in the home. It is important to distinguish these two categories from those children who refuse to go to school because they are anxious, frightened or depressed, or those children who play truant from school because they dislike the atmosphere in which they appear to fail and are subject to ridicule and as they see it, to unfair discipline.

Conduct disorders. Often parents are concerned because their young children are unacceptably aggressive, destructive, cruel or antisocial. Again individual tolerance will depend on the family and the community. In some lively teenagers, outbursts of aggressive, destructive, foolish or antisocial behaviour may be dismissed as high spirits but in others living in inner city areas with mixed cultures and limited outlets it results in delinquency.

Emotional disorders. Children, like adults can get unduly anxious; they may suffer from unreasonable fears and they can have outbursts of hysterical behaviour. By nature, children are optimistic and confident about the future, but occasionally even without obvious cause they can become severely depressed and seriously attempt suicide. These children should have the counsel of a child psychiatrist.

Anorexia nervosa. In this odd condition, young people either just before or during puberty, deliberately avoid food so that they lose weight, and they often go on losing weight till they become tragically thin. It is thought that they have an irrational fear of growing up, of becoming sexually and physically mature.

Alison

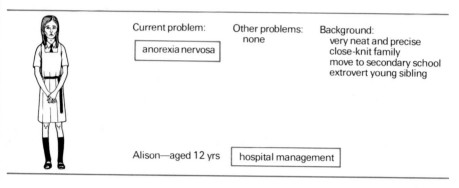

Current problem:

anorexia nervosa

Other problems:
none

Background:
very neat and precise
close-knit family
move to secondary school
extrovert young sibling

Alison—aged 12 yrs   hospital management

Usually they are able youngsters if somewhat obsessional and precise. Rarely are there major psychological problems which need attention.

As they can starve themselves to death, some management must be attempted but as no pathology or avoidable environmental factors are usually identified, it has to be symptomatic. It sounds somewhat crude, but the most effective approach appears to be to remove all the child's privileges and return them one by one as she begins to eat more and more. Antidepressive drugs may help.

Management

The above paragraphs merely list some of the symptoms and problems which children under medical care may have. Management includes recognising them for what they are, identifying the contributing factors and conferring with the other people concerned. The latter may include the family doctor and other members of the primary care team, the health visitor, the school teacher, school health services and school welfare officers, the educational psychologist and social service workers. When, after review, a programme of care has been agreed, it is essential that a person is identified to be responsible for counselling the child and parents, and ensuring that all concerned are properly informed. Being thorough at the outset can avoid many problems later. With the more intractable emotional and conduct disorders a child psychiatrist will be the key person, but the majority will fall within the responsibility of the health visitor or the family doctor or the paediatrician.

THE MALTREATMENT OF CHILDREN

Deviant behaviour by adults may take the form of injuring their children. Child murder, child cruelty, child neglect, child abuse, child molesting and the use of children for pornography all fall into this category. The obvious examples are easily recognised, but defining the limits of child abuse or child neglect is difficult. It might be considered that it is the right of every child to be allowed to develop to his full potential. Child abuse could then be defined as any action or omission by an adult responsible for that child which either temporarily or permanently interferes with that development. In a real world we must settle for something less. What we are able to achieve is a good measure of our success as a society. In this section we will not be concerned with mental or social abuse or educational ineptitude, not because these are unimportant, but because they are not primarily medical problems. Similarly child cruelty and murder will not be considered further.

Child abuse

Clinical features. Non-accidental injuries and other forms of child abuse occur when parents, at their wits end, strike out at their helpless but demanding infant. It also happens when ignorant, inept, cruel, selfish, irresponsible or mentally sick parents do not exert reasonable self-control. Gripping and shaking the baby may produce finger tip bruising on his chest and arms. Forcing his mouth open to

Gripping injuries

finger tip bruises

give food may cause similar bruises on the cheeks. The frenulum may be torn or the palate scratched by objects pushed in the mouth. Slapping and hitting the infant may also cause black eyes or characteristic strap marks. The skin of the attacked infant may also show scratches, bite marks, cigarette burns of scalds. Rough handling may fracture long bones, ribs or skull. Swinging the baby by the legs or arms can cause epiphyseal separation at the end of the long bones. Squeezing the limbs with rotation can separate the periosteum and cause periosteal haematomas. Repeated injuries of the same bone leads to large callus formation. Banging the head not only produces fractures of the skull but haemorrhages in the eyes and occasionally blindness.

Some non-accidental injuries

cigarette burns

scalding

bite marks

Bony injuries

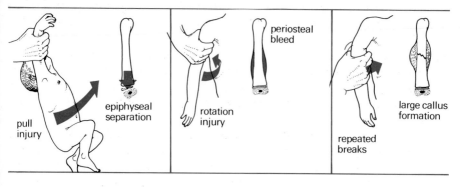

Shaking the head can tear superficial veins over the brain and cause subdural haematomas. The child may weather the initial injury, but the blood clot may then draw in fluid; the infant then develops the clinical features of a space-occupying lesion of slow onset. He may present with vomiting or fits or changes in the level of responsiveness and activity. The fontanelle is full and there may be papilloedema and retinal bleeds. This injury may kill the child; if it does not, if often leaves him mentally retarded, hemiplegic or blind.

The injury which can kill or leave the child with severe brain damage

All the baby's injuries must be noted in detail and photographed if possible.

A careful enquiry is essential. The parents often delay in bringing the child for medical attention. Their story does not accord with the injuries. Their explanation for the injuries may change if they are pressed. Their concern for the child may be inappropriate, they may show too much concern or anger or they may be off-hand and indifferent. Often they are relieved when hospital admission is advised. Sometimes they will talk at length about their own anxieties and problems and say how difficult and demanding the baby has been. It is very important to record precisely the history as it is given, with an evaluation of the parents' attitudes.

Child abuse occurs in families from all walks of life but it is more common in the under-privileged and in families where actions speak louder than words. As Professor Kempe has suggested, the setting in which child abuse might occur includes a number of elements:

1. The parents have usually had troubled childhoods themselves; they may be from broken homes or have suffered deprivation or abuse themselves when children.
2. There are problems with the marriage; for example the marriage may be between two young people from disturbed homes who married for the wrong reasons, perhaps because they wanted to leave home or were in need of affection. Some people mistakenly believe that a pregnancy will help to reverse a breaking relationship.
3. The child may be difficult to rear, he may have been premature or have a blemish or handicap. More often than not the child's problems are imaginary, the baby's first cry is seen as rejection, he fails to respond as his mother feels he should to her and this is felt to be his fault. An unloved child may be difficult, a difficult child may be unloved.
4. Against this background there may be added stresses, for example the father in trouble with the law or there may be financial or housing problems.
5. Finally, there are no life lines available, no close friends to whom the parents can turn for advice, support and relief.

Management. If a health visitor, social worker or casualty doctor suspects non-accidental injury the child must be admitted to a place of safety until a fuller enquiry has been made. This might be a police station, a social service institution or a hospital. If his parents are deliberately injuring him, society has a responsibility to protect him. If the parents are unwilling to release their child then he may have to be taken from them on the grounds laid down to obtain the necessary care order.

Whilst providing temporary protection, the primary medical responsibility is to identify and treat the injuries, attend to the child's general well being, and to exclude possible contributing factors and alternative diagnoses. It is equally important for others to evaluate the parents and the family situation and provide support and guidance if this is appropriate.

The distribution of the bruises is usually diagnostic. Babies when they begin to walk frequently fall and bruise their foreheads and shins, but do not bruise their upper arms and chests. Nevertheless bleeding diseases should be excluded. Brittle-bone disease is a rare condition where bruising as well as bone fractures occur with the slightest injury, but the fractures are in the shaft and not at the end of the long bones. Although some bony injuries are obvious, others are not, so a full skeletal survey by radiography is essential.

The social work team will usually take the lead in planning the strategy for management, but they depend on the full cooperation of medical and nursing personnel involved and the police. Initial policy is usually worked out at a case conference held as soon as possible after the diagnosis is firm. Subsequent management will depend on the background and on the attitudes of the parents. When investigations have been completed a full case conference with representatives from all agencies concerned in attendance is held to decide what legal action is required, what social work activity is to be attempted and what medical surveillance is desirable.

Many children may be allowed home, initially under supervision, and although they may not live happily ever after they do appear to thrive and to be content. Occasionally it is necessary to take the child away from his parents and put him into care of others. The decisions are very difficult and even those with most knowledge and experience can get it wrong. Unhappy experiences in this area can harden the hearts of the wisest and kindest of men and produce vicious reaction in others.

Child neglect

A child may also be harmed by omission. This might be due to unavoidable circumstances, or ignorance or ineptness on the part of his guardians as well as deliberate attempts to hurt or punish him. The children are generally under-nourished and undersized, the skin and hair are often in poor condition and they may be dirty and infested. Nasty rashes may be present in those places where the most dirt collects, the skin creases and nappy area.

Sexual misuse or abuse

Sexual abuse, that is a child being involved by an adult in sexual activities that he or she is not old enough to understand, or to give informed consent to, and which breaks the community taboos and expectations, appears to be on the increase. Although there is a notion that such activities happen at the hands of strangers, in fact it is three times more likely to occur within the family or within a circle of trusted friends. The first step is to recognize the problem for what it is, for both the adult and the child involved, need expert counselling.

Deprivation

A child in a repressive atmosphere may appear to be well nourished and clean, but still fail to thrive, his hands and feet may be cold and small, and his growth suppressed. These more subtle forms of negligence or abuse are more difficult to recognise and define. The management as with most of the problems in this chapter includes a thorough clinical evaluation, a detailed enquiry about him, his family life and his neighbourhood, and a programme of care which is realistic and accepted by all concerned.

Munchausen syndrome by proxy

This is a bizarre form of child abuse in which one of those who cares for a child, usually the mother, persistently fabricates symptoms and signs such that the child becomes ill or is in danger of, or is subject to, unnecessary investigations and treatment. The diagnosis should be considered in any child whose illness is unexplained and prolonged or extraordinary in some way; when the child's signs and symptoms seem particularly inappropriate or incongruous, or only occur when the parent is present. It should also be suspected when treatments are surprisingly ineffective or not well tolerated. As in other instances of child abuse the parent may be inappropriately concerned, or alternatively not concerned about the severity of the child's supposed problems, or they may in some way benefit from the child's illness by way of support, attention or money.

Making a firm diagnosis can be difficult. There is no alternative to taking a clear history, particularly noting the time and place of the events described, and then making enquiries from others for supporting evidence. This means seeking information from other members of the family and other health professionals concerned with the child's care. If the diagnosis is suspected, it is important that the child and the parent be observed carefully. Perhaps the easiest way of making the diagnosis is to see if the signs and symptoms disappear when the parents are excluded.

Management can be difficult and it is vital for the child's sake for it to be firm and determined. This will involve case conferences and may mean keeping the child in a place of safety at least in the short term until the situation has been clarified.

BIBLIOGRAPHY

Helfer R E, Kempe C H 1968 The battered child. The University of Chicago Press, Chicago
Pinkerton P 1968 Childhood disorders. Crosby Lockwood Staples, St Albans, U.K.
Rutter M 1972 Maternal deprivation reassessed. Penguin, London
Rutter M, Herson L 1977 Child psychiatry. Modern approaches. Blackwell, Oxford
Smith S M (ed) 1978 The maltreatment of children. M.T.P. Press, Lancaster

Essential Paediatric Formulary

The range of drugs regularly prescribed in general paediatric practice is considerably more limited than in adult medicine. This therapeutic caution is well founded. The pattern of many childhood disorders is short-lived and self-limiting, and does not justify drug therapy. Many common disorders are amenable to long established agents with a low incidence of side-effects. Simple measures, such as the use of glucose-electrolyte solution in gastroenteritis, make an enormous contribution to child health. On the other hand, casual use of anti-emetics and anti-diarrhoeal agents is indefensible. The prescribing habits of a doctor not only determine future demand for drug intervention, but also modify parental attitudes to their child's health.

The efficacy of a drug depends on the doctor selecting an appropriate preparation, calculating the correct dosage, and motivating the family to ensure regular administration. Infancy raises problems of immaturity of absorption, transport, enzymatic biotransformation and excretion. Drug dynamics may be profoundly altered in preterm infants reflecting not only immaturity but also altered body fluid compartments. The awareness of altered drug metabolism in young children has resulted in more restricted licensing of newly introduced drugs. The ethical and practical problems of drug trials add to this restraint. Paradoxically these same restraints may delay studies which bring to light side-effects in older established drugs. Fortunately carefully designed multi-centre studies have enabled certain paediatric subspecialities, such as oncology, to move rapidly ahead in the introduction of complex but effective drug regimens.

Selecting an acceptable oral preparation for a miserable child is usually dictated by finding a palatable liquid preparation. The formulary provides a useful range of these; the majority contain a convenient children's dose in a 5 ml spoonful. The British National Formulary (BNF) recommends that smaller doses be diluted so that they also match a 5 ml spoonful. Liquids containing sucrose promote dental caries and should be avoided for long-term use. Colouring agents are also coming under critical review.

Drug dosage in children is a potentially complex topic but, for most drugs, readily available guidance is based on either age or body weight. Age-related doses are appropriate when prescribing commonly used drugs with high therapeutic indices to average-sized children. Body weight calculations are also convenient but tend to underestimate dosage in infancy, and overestimate dosage in older or obese children. Body surface area measurements are less amenable but have a closer relationship to physiological functions which influence drug effects. Again caution is required in the immature infant with a disproportionately large surface area. The percentage method, derived from surface area, provides a simple scheme for calculating dose as a percentage of an adult dose.

Faced with these contrasting methods the wise doctor will not hesitate to reach for a reliable formulary rather than rely on a fallable memory. He must also be obsessionally careful about providing correct instructions for critically dose-dependent drugs such as digoxin.

This list has been selected from the British National Formulary to reflect drugs most commonly prescribed in our department. It does not encompass drugs used in specialised branches of paediatrics. It aims to provide an easily accessible guide to rational prescribing in childhood but is definitely not an alternative to more comprehensive formularies.

Abbreviations

I   indications
CI   contraindications
SE   side-effects
S/F sugar-free liquid
S/R slow release granules

GASTROINTESTINAL SYSTEM

ANTACIDS
Infant Gaviscon
Gaviscon®

I	Gastro-oesophageal reflux
CI	Prematurity, impaired renal function
SE	Gastric distension

Sachets — Infant
(aluminium hydroxide,
magnesium trisilicate,
sodium bicarbonate,
alginic acid
Na^+ 0.9 mmol/dose)

1–2 doses with feed

ANTISPASMODICS

Dicyclomine	I	Smooth muscle spasm e.g. of bowel
	CI	Infants under age 6 months
	SE	Respiratory irregularity, dry mouth, thirst, dizziness
Syrup 10 mg/5 ml Tabs 10 mg		6–24 months 5–10 mg before feeds (max 40 mg/day) 2–12 years 10–20 mg 3 times daily

ULCER-HEALING

Cimetidine	I	Peptic ulcer Gastrooesophageal reflux
	CI	—
	SE	Rare reversible liver damage
Syrup 200 mg/5 ml Tabs 200 mg		20–40 mg/kg/day in 3–4 doses

ANTIDIARRHOEAL

Loperamide	I		Prolonged non-specific diarrhoea
	CI		Infective gastroenteritis
	SE		Occasional rashes
Capsules 2 mg	4–8 years	1 mg 4 times daily
S/F syrup 1 mg/5 ml	9–12 years	2 mg 4 times daily

LAXATIVES

Stimulant

Senna	I	Chronic constipation
	CI	Undiagnosed abdominal pain
	SE	Mild discomfort

Tabs 7.5 mg
Syrup 7.5 mg/5 ml   5–20 ml once daily

Softener

Dioctyl/sodium sulphosuccinate

Paed syrup   12.5–25 mg 3 times daily
12.5 mg/5 ml

Osmotic

Lactulose

Elixir 3.35 mg/5 ml	Under 1 year	2.5 ml twice daily
	1–5 years	5 ml twice daily
	6–12 years	10 ml twice daily

PANCREATIN REPLACEMENT

Pancreatin	I	Pancreatic exocrine failure
	CI	—
	SE	Anal irritation

Creon®
capsules containing
enteric-coated
granules   5–15 capsules daily with meals
Pancrex V® powder   2–8 g daily with meals
Pancrex® tabs forte   8–20 tabs daily with meals

CARDIOVASCULAR SYSTEM

CARDIAC GLYCOSIDE

Digoxin	I	Heart failure, supraventricular arrhythmias
	CI	Hypokalaemia
	SE	Vomiting, bradycardia, arrhythmias

Elixir PG 50 mcg/ml		10 mcg/kg/day in 2 doses
Tabs PG 62.5 mcg		
Tabs 125, 250 mcg		

DIURETICS

Frusemide	I	Fluid overload, hypertension
	CI	Liver failure
	SE	Rashes, electrolyte imbalance

S/F liquid 1 mg/ml		1–3 mg/kg/day in 2 doses
Tabs 20, 40 mg		
Injection 20 mg/2 ml	IV	0.5–1.0 mg/kg/dose

Spironolactone	I	Fluid overload in liver failure
	CI	Hyperkalaemia
	SE	GIT upset, gynaecomastia

| Tabs 25 mg | | 1.5–3 mg/kg/day |

BETA-ADRENOCEPTOR BLOCKING DRUGS

Propranolol	I	Hypertension, supraventricular arrhythmias, thyrotoxicosis
	CI	Cardiac failure, asthma
	SE	Cardiac failure

| Tabs 10, 40 mg | | 1 mg/kg three times daily |

RESPIRATORY SYSTEM

BRONCHODILATORS

Beta$_2$ adrenoreceptor	I	Reversible asthma
stimulants	CI	—
	SE	Tremor, headaches, tachycardia

Salbutamol

S/F syrup 2 mg/5 ml	2–5 years	1–2 mg 3–4 times daily
Tabs 2, 4 mg	6–12 years	2 mg 3–4 times daily
Aerosol 100 mcg/puff		1–2 puffs 3–4 times daily max 4 hourly
Rotacaps 200 mcg, 400 mcg		200 mcg 3–4 times daily max 4 hourly
Nebulised solution 2.5 mg/2.5 ml		2.5–5 mg max 4 hourly

Terbutaline

S/F syrup 1.5 mg/5 ml	3–7 years	0.75–1.5 mg 3 times daily
Tabs 5 mg	7–15 years	1.5–3 mg 3 times daily
Aerosol 250 mcg/puff		1 puff 3–4 times daily
Nebulised solution 2.5 mg/1.0 ml		2.5–5.0 mg max 4 hourly

Xanthine bronchodilators

	I	Reversible asthma
	CI	Tachycardia
		Avoid i.v. infusion if established treatment
	SE	Tachycardia, vomiting, irritability, headache (measure plasma levels)

Theophylline

Capsules containing S/R granules		
60, 125, 250 mg	2–6 years	60–120 mg 12 hourly
	7–12 years	125–250 mg 12 hourly

Aminophylline

i.v. ampoule 250 mg/10 ml		Slow i.v. infusion
		Loading 5 mg/kg slow injection
		Maintenance 0.3–0.5 mg/kg/hour

ANTI-ALLERGY

Inhaled corticosteroids

	I	Asthma
	CI	—
	SE	Oral candidiasis

Beclomethasone

Inhaler 50 mcg/puff	50–100 mcg 2–4 times daily
Rotacaps 100 mcg,	100 mcg 2–4 times daily
Nebuliser 50 mcg/ml	50–100 mcg 2–4 times daily

Prophylactic drugs

	I	Asthma
	CI	—
	SE	Upper airway irritation

Sodium cromoglycate

Inhaler 1 mg/puff	2 mg 4–6 times daily
Spincaps 20 mg	20 mg 4–6 times daily
Nebulizer 20 mg/2 ml	20 mg 4–6 times daily

Antihistamines

	I	Hayfever, urticaria, emergency treatment of anaphylaxis
	CI	Caution in epilepsy
	SE	Sedation, dry mouth

Chlorpheniramine

Tablets 4 mg	1–5 years	1–2 mg 3 times daily
Syrup 2 mg/5 ml	6–12 years	2–4 mg 3 times daily
Injection 10 mg/ml	IV	200 mcg/kg slowly

Promethazine HCl

Tabs 10, 25 mg	6–12 months	5–10 mg at night
Syrup 5 mg/5 ml	1–5 years	5–15 mg at night
	6–12 years	10–25 mg at night

Terfanidine

Tabs 60 mg	6–12 years	30 mg twice daily
Suspension 30 mg/5 ml		

CENTRAL NERVOUS SYSTEM

HYPNOTICS, SEDATIVES

Chloral	I	Sedation
	CI	Airways obstruction
	SE	GIT upsets, rashes
Elixir paediatric		
200 mg/5 ml		30–50 mg/kg at night
Mixture 1 g/5 ml		(max 1 g)

Trimeprazine	I	Sleep disturbance with pruritus
	CI	Epilepsy, infants under 6 months
	SE	Paradoxical stimulation
Syrup 7.5 mg/5 ml		
Syrup forte		
30 mg/5 ml		3 mg/kg at night

Temazepam	I	Sedation in burns, painful trauma
	CI	—
	SE	—
Caps 10 mg		0.75–1.0 mg/kg
S/F elixir 10 mg/5 ml		premedication

NAUSEA, VERTIGO

Metoclopramide	I	Nausea particularly with migraine and cytotoxic therapy
	CI	Young children — acute GI disorders
	SE	Severe extrapyramidal reactions
S/F elixir 5 mg/5 ml	1–3 years	1 mg 2–3 times daily
Injection 5 mg/ml	3–5 years	2 mg 2–3 times daily
	5–14 years	2.5–5 mg 2–3 times daily

ANALGESICS/ANTIPYRETICS

Paracetamol	I	Mild to moderate pain, pyrexia
	CI	Liver impairment
	SE	Liver damage in overdosage
Tabs 500 mg	0–1 years	60–120 mg 4–6 hourly
S/F elixir 120 mg/5 ml	1–5 years	120–250 mg 4–6 hourly
	6–12 years	250–500 mg 4–6 hourly

ANTIEPILEPTICS

Sodium valproate	I	Generalised epilepsies, prophylaxis of febrile convulsions
	CI	Hepatic impairment
	SE	GIT symptoms, lethargy, weight gain, thrombocytopenia, liver toxicity, pancreatitis
Tab 100, 200, 500 mg S/F elixir 200 mg/5 ml		20–40 mg/kg/day divided doses
Carbamazepine	I	Partial epilepsies
	CI	Hepatic impairment
	SE	Lethargy, dizziness, transient rash, rare marrow, liver toxicity
Tab 100, 200 mg S/F syrup 100 mg/5 ml		10–20 mg/kg/day
Phenobarbitone	I	Short-term seizure control e.g. encephalopathy
	CI	Acute intermittent porphyria
	SE	Lethargy, behaviour disturbance, rashes
Tabs 15, 30, 60, 100 mg S/F elixir 15 mg/5 ml		loading dose i.v. 15–20 mg/kg once Maintenance i.v./oral 5–10 mg/kg/day
Injection 15, 30, 60, 200 mg all in 1 ml		

Phenytoin	I	Generalised and partial epilepsies
	CI	Hepatic impairment
	SE	Nausea, ataxia, gum hypertrophy, rashes, facial coarsening, haematological effects, rickets
Phenytoin sodium S/F tab 50, 100 mg Phenytoin base susp 30 mg/5 ml		4–8 mg/kg day
Ethosuximide	I	Petit mal (absence seizures)
	CI	—
	SE	Nausea, headaches, rashes, bone marrow depression
Caps 250 mg Syrup 250 mg/5 ml		20–40 mg/kg/day
Clonazepam	I	Myoclonic seizures
	CI	—
	SE	Drowsiness, salivation
Tabs 500 mcg, 2 mg		50–200 mcg/kg/day Gradual introduction recommended

DRUGS USED IN STATUS EPILEPTICUS

Diazepam	I	Status epilepticus
	CI	—
	SE	Respiratory depression, venous thrombophlebitis at injection site (minimised by using an emulsion)
Injection 5 mg/ml Rectal tube 5, 10 mg	Slow i.v. 1–3 years Over 3 years	200–300 mcg/kg 5 mg 10 mg

Paraldehyde	I	Status epilepticus
	CI	Hepatic impairment
	SE	Sterile abscesses, rashes
Injection 5, 10 ml ampoule	Deep i.m.	0.1 ml/kg to max 5 ml

JOINT DISEASE

ANTI-INFLAMMATORY

Aspirin	I	Juvenile chronic polyarthritis, rheumatic fever
	CI	GIT bleeding, liver impairment, salicylate hypersensitivity
	SE	GIT symptoms, tinitus, hyperventilation, hypersensitivity
Tabs 75 mg, 300 mg	Child	Up to 100 mg/kg/day Titrate with blood levels

Ibuprofen	I	Juvenile chronic polyarthritis
	CI	GIT bleeding
	SE	Mild GIT symptoms, rashes
Syrup 100 mg/5 ml	Child	10 mg/kg 3 times daily
Tabs 200 mg	Max.	500 mg/day in child under 30 kg

Indomethacin	I	Juvenile chronic polyarthritis, ankylosing spondylitis
	CI	GIT bleeding, salicylate hypersensitivity
	SE	Headaches, GIT symptoms, blood dyscrasias
Suspension 25 mg/5 ml Caps 25 mg, 50 mg		2.5 mg/kg/day

Naproxen	I	Juvenile chronic polyarthritis
	CI	GIT bleeding
	SE	GIT symptoms
Suspension 125 mg/5 ml Tabs 250 mg		5 mg/kg twice daily

ENDOCRINE

Insulin	see p. 231
Thyroxine	see p. 226

ANTITHYROID

Carbimazole	I	Thyrotoxicosis
	CI	—
	SE	Nausea, headache, rashes, rare bone marrow depression
Tabs 5 mg	Infants	0.5–0.75 mg/kg/day
	Children	5–15 mg/day

Propranolol	I	Thyrotoxicosis
	CI	—
	SE	—
dose		See p. 314

CORTICOSTEROIDS

Hydrocortisone	I	Cortisol replacement, pituitary and adrenal failure
	CI	—
	SE	Excess dosage causes growth failure
Tabs 2.5, 10, 20 mg		10–20 mg/m²/day surface area
Injection 100 mg		Dose increased during illness or other stress

Fludrocortisone	I	Mineralocorticord replacement in adrenal failure
	CI	Salt retention, hypertension
	SE	Hypertension, cardiac failure
Tabs 100 mcg		50–200 mcg/day

ANTIBACTERIAL DRUGS

Selection is based on
- clinical features e.g. otitis media
- microbiological data
- patient age, health e.g. renal impairment and drug hypersensitivity
- hospital antibacterial policy

VITAMINS

VITAMIN D

Calciferol

	I	Prematurity Nutritional deficiency
Low dose therapy	CI	—
1 mcg=40 i.u.	SE	—
Oily sol. 75 mcg/ml	Neonate	12.5–25 mcg daily
Tabs 75 mcg	Children	12.5–25 mcg daily

Calciferol

High dose therapy	I	Malabsorption, liver disease, renal disease, hypoparathyroidism
	CI	—
	SE	Hypercalcaemia, renal damage
Tabs 250 mcg		Dose individual titration 250–1250 mcg daily

Alfacalcidol

	I	As above Advantage of short-half life allowing reversal of hypercalcaemia
	CI	—
	SE	—
Drops 250 ng/dp		Dose individual titration 50 ng/kg/day
Caps 250 ng, 1 mcg		

VITAMIN E

Alpha tocopheryl acetate	I	Prematurity: possible role in preventing retinopathy and anaemia, chronic cholestatic jaundice to prevent neuropathy
	CI	—
	SE	—
Liquid 500 mg/5 ml Tabs 10, 50, 200 mg	Preterm Children	10 mg daily 5–100 mg daily

VITAMIN K

Phytomenadione	I	Routine administration to newborn, malabsorption, liver disease
	CI	Avoid synthetic analogues in neonate
	SE	Hypotension after rapid i.v. injection
Injection 1 mg/0.5 ml active orally Tab 10 mg	Neonate Children	1 mg orally/i.m. single dose 5–10 mg weekly

FOLIC ACID

Folic acid	I	Anaemia of prematurity, haemolytic anaemia in newborn, folate deficiency in chronic haemolysis e.g. HbSS
	CI	—
	SE	—
Syrup 2.5 mg/5 ml Tabs 100 mcg, 5 mg	Neonates Children	200 mcg daily 5–10 mg daily

ORAL IRON see p. 189

EYE

Chloramphenicol	I	Local infections
	CI	Ineffective against chlamydia
	SE	—
Drops 0.5%		Apply ×4–6 per day
Ointment 1.0%		
		Note. Systemic penicillin therapy is recommended in addition to topical therapy for gonococcal conjunctivitis
Sodium cromoglycate	I	Allergic conjunctivitis
	CI	—
	SE	—
Drops 2%		Apply × 4 per day
Tetracycline	I	Chlamydial conjunctivitis
	CI	—
	SE	—
Drops 1.0%		Note. Oral erythromycin therapy is combined with topical treatment

NOSE

NASAL DECONGESTANTS	I	Nasal congestion
	CI	Caution in infants under 3 months
	SE	Rebound congestion
Ephedrine HCl Drops 0.5%		1–2 drops per nostril 4 times daily
Oxymetazoline HCl Drops 0.025%		1–2 drops per nostril 2 times daily
Xylometazoline HCl Drops 0.05%		1–2 drops per nostril 2 times daily

MOUTH

MOUTH ANTIFUNGAL AGENTS	I	Oral candidiasis
	CI	—
	SE	—

Nystatin
Suspension
100 000 units/ml   1 ml 4 times daily

Miconazole
Oral gel 2%

0–2 years	2.5 ml 2 times daily
2–6 years	5 ml 2 times daily
over 6 years	5 ml 4 times daily

SKIN

BARRIER PREPARATIONS

Zinc and caster oil   I   Napkin dermatitis

Ointment   Apply at frequent napkin changes

ANTI-CANDIDA PREPARATIONS

Hydrocortisone 0.5%   I   Skin candidiasis
Nystatin
Barrier agent
ointment/cream

Nystaform HC®   Apply 3–4 times daily at napkin
Timodine®   changes

CORD INFECTION

Alcohol/chlorhexidine
Swabs   Apply as required

Index